Fire Your Doctor!

How to Be Independently Healthy

By
Andrew Saul, Ph.D.
Foreword by Abram Hoffer, M.D.

EasyRead Large

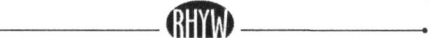

Copyright Page from the Original Book

The information contained in this book is based upon the research and personal and professional experiences of the author. It is not intended as a substitute for consulting with your physician or other healthcare provider. Any attempt to diagnose and treat an illness should be done under the direction of a healthcare professional.

The publisher does not advocate the use of any particular healthcare protocol but believes the information in this book should be available to the public. The publisher and author are not responsible for any adverse effects or consequences resulting from the use of the suggestions, preparations, or procedures discussed in this book. Should the reader have any questions concerning the appropriateness of any procedures or preparation mentioned, the author and the publisher strongly suggest consulting a professional healthcare advisor.

Basic Health Publications, Inc.
28812 Top of the World Drive
Laguna Beach, CA 92651
949-715-7327

Library of Congress Cataloging-in-Publication Data

Saul, Andrew W.
    Fire your doctor! : how to be independently healthy / by Andrew W. Saul;
foreword by Abram Hoffer.
      p. cm.
    Includes bibliographical references and index.
    ISBN-13: 978-1-59120-138-0
    ISBN-10: 0-59120-138-1
    1. Self-care, Health. 2. Health. 3. Medicine, Popular. I. Title.

    RA776.95.S28   2005
    613—dc22
                                              2005022059

Editor: John Anderson
Copyeditor: Susan Andrews
Typesetter: Gary A. Rosenberg
Cover design: Mike Stromberg

Printed in the United States of America

10   9   8   7   6   5   4   3   2   1

ReadHowYouWant partners with publishers to provide books for ALL Kinds of Readers. For more information about Becoming A (RHYW) Registered Reader and to find more titles in your preferred format, visit:
www.readhowyouwant.com

ReadHowYouWant partners with publishers to provide books for ALL Kinds of Readers. For more information about Becoming A **RHYW** Registered Reader and to find more titles in your preferred format, visit:
www.readhowyouwant.com

TABLE OF CONTENTS

To my best teachers,
the ones who took me seriously.

And to my beloved parents,
who really had no choice.

Foreword

Why do we need a book educating patients on how to stay healthy? Is it not the responsibility of the medical profession and other allied health professions to look after all our needs? Are we not all supposed to be medically pious, meaning that we look upon medical advice as the word from all high, as writ in stone? To answer these questions we need only to read the headlines in the daily press, where constant and recurrent cries are heard about the costs of treating the sick, the number of sick, the death rates, the increase in cancer, the resurgence of tuberculosis, the great calamity of HIV/AIDS, the number of Alzheimer's patients. If the healthcare professions were able to maintain our health, then why are we in such poor shape?

The main problem is that often the best information gathered so painfully by the professions remains hidden within the obscure journals that were rash enough to publish them, and most people have not heard of, nor know how to use, the findings. This is still the hangover from the centuries-old tradition of guilds who maintained their secrets at all costs.

Modern medicine has failed, not in discovery, but in effectively bringing the attention of the people to the discoveries that have been made. The one field that has not failed in its educational effort is the drug industry, which has an enormously successful history of informing the public about the advantages of the drugs that they sell. The other discoveries, those dealing with nutrition, with herbs, with innovative treatment, remain buried in the tons of literature published every year. We need books such as this one by Andrew Saul to fill in the gap, to bring to the public what they need to know to get well and stay well, and to learn this in spite of lack of medical interest.

Even worse are the attempts of the medical profession to suppress valuable information if it does not conform to the conventional viewpoint. It takes at least forty years for major paradigm shifts in medicine, and while the battle of the paradigms rages, patients are deprived of the information that may save their lives. Excessive conservatism is very costly. When my colleagues and I first published our paper on the use of vitamin B3 for treating schizophrenia in 1957 (Hoffer, A., H. Osmond, M.J. Callbeck, and I. Kahan. "Treatment of Schizophrenia with Nicotinic Acid and Nicotinamide." *Journal of Clinical and Experimental Psychopathology* 18(1957):131–158), it was mostly ignored because the popular paradigm did not consider schizophrenia to be a biochemically based disease. Rather, it was a way of life and therefore could not have any connection with the use of simple vitamins in above-average doses. But as we continued to publish our findings, based upon double-blind studies, orthodox medical resistance actually began to mount. By the 1970s, the bias of the American Psychiatric Association had denounced orthomolecular (nutritional) psychiatry. Their position has been used as a shield to protect psychiatry from the vitamin heretics like myself, who found that patients truly recovered with nutritional treatment.

Orthomolecular medicine involves active participation between people and the professions, for it involves dietary and lifestyle changes, which cannot be done by the doctor alone. There is a keen need to educate the public, and motivate people to read and learn for themselves. *Fire Your Doctor!* is precisely about this (and certainly not about performing one's own thoracic surgery, as a hostile critic might choose to mistakenly presuppose). The great orthomolecular educators, like Linus Pauling, have long aimed their work directly at the general reader. They did so because life-saving knowledge is too important to be passed over, and the academics, physicians, and physician associations were not listening. In this tradition, *Fire Your Doctor!* takes it straight to the people.

In 1945, we were taught to write prescriptions in Latin. Over the past sixty years, things have changed enormously. Now patients have access to whole libraries of material via the Internet. There are so many different information sources that many people get confused. We are flooded with new books for every known disease. Treatments are described in detail and for every known condition. The whole diversity of modern medicine, including the alternatives, is so diverse that it is impossible for lay people to properly assess the value of the treatment described.

The information world has changed from one with hardly any useful information written for the public to one where there is too much, and it is accumulating ever more quickly. We are compelled to turn to people who are knowledgeable and trustworthy, and who are more interested in healing the sick than they are in prestige or money. Such people sift the amazing amount of information, blow away the chaff, and harvest the kernels of truth.

Health-promoting information must include the correcting of misinformation that is so prevalent in the current medical literature. A professor of medicine once started his lectures by advising his students that only half the information he would give them was correct and he was not sure which half it was. I once opened a lecture at Columbia University by telling the students that most of the stuff they were being taught in psychiatry was wrong. The third-year medical students got up and gave me a standing ovation.

Misinformation is used to support, or to attack, a popular belief system. When it came to nutrition, the dietary evils of sugar and chemical food additives were supported by misinformation to counter the facts. When vitamins were found to be very helpful, the establishment quickly mobilized and released tons of misinformation about nonexistent evils of vitamins. Vitamin C was alleged to cause kidney stones; it does not happen. Niacin was supposed to cause liver damage; it does not. The construction of dangerous toxicity is limited only by the imaginations of the doctors. Factoids are created with wild abandon. The truth is that vitamins do not cause kidney damage, do not cause pernicious anemia, do not decrease fertility, do not cause liver damage, do not cause iron overload, do not interfere with glucose blood tests, do not decrease the effectiveness of chemotherapy or radiation therapy.

Authors of health books should also be healers, should know what to emphasize, should know what are the values and defects of any therapeutic program, and above all, should write for the public. Good health books are now indispensable to help readers efficiently sort through the enormous amount of material so that it becomes meaningful for them. Each person must develop the diet that works best for him or her. But in order for them to do so, they have to understand the treatment options that are available. *Fire Your Doctor!* helps the reader do precisely this.

So, from an era fifty years ago, when no information was provided, we come to the present, where so much conflicting information is available that we depend on books such as this one to glean from the vast literature some of the main tenets of modern nutritional treatment. New information raises new questions, and this in turn creates new ways of dealing with the problems. Experience has taught us that we cannot depend upon the professions to make alternative health information available. Much of it is still controversial, but that is the nature of medicine. *Fire Your Doctor!* is about the medicine of nature, orthomolecular medicine.

—Abram Hoffer, M.D.

Preface

Another health book? Why?

Either the good ones are not being read, or the ones being read aren't that good. Look around you at your family and friends: The need is there; a lot of people are just not healthy.

Can a book offer anything that well over one trillion (that's a million million!) dollars per year spent on American "health care" hasn't? Quite possibly. I can tell you that what is in this book has worked for me, for my family, and for people I have known over of the past thirty years. It may help you, too.

The biggest deception ever perpetrated upon the American people is the myth that improving your health with vitamins and natural living is somehow difficult or dangerous. Better health is not difficult; it is only perceived as difficult. And dangerous? It is conventional drug treatments for disease that are dangerous. But in newspapers, magazines, and on television, the public has been warned off the very vitamins and other supplements that have been repeatedly proven to reduce illness in practically every instance. The effective use of food supplements and natural diet saves money, pain, and lives ... and you have been told not to do it.

If you want something done right, you have to do it yourself. This especially includes your health care.

One of the most common questions about vitamin therapy is, "Are huge doses safe?" This book will help answer that question once and for all. And while we're at it, here's the answer in advance: Yes, megadoses of vitamins are very safe. Vitamins do not cause even one death per year. Pharmaceutical drugs, taken as directed, cause over 100,000 deaths annually.

Still, it is granted that we need access to all the tools that medicine and technology can provide, when used with caution. We must also fully use our "natural resources" of therapeutic nutrition and vitamins. To limit ourselves to pharmaceutical medicine is like going into the ring to fight the champ with one hand tied behind our backs.

For these reasons, there is a need for at least one more health book. And here it is. Brace yourself.

VITAMIN THERAPY WORKS

She sat in the corner, silently. The fifty-five-year-old woman's face was in shadow, invariably turned down and toward the wall. And that's where she stayed, day after day. She had no appetite and she never spoke to anyone. Her family had tried seemingly everything. Yes, she was under the care of a psychiatrist and, yes, she was on medication.

"Actually, she's been on a whole lot of different medications," her daughter told me. "None of them has helped her and several made her worse. She tried to kill herself several times. Now she seldom moves from her corner, and she never says a word. Is there anything you can do?"

At times like this, what you want is a wand to wave, but life so rarely resembles a Harry Potter story. This was all too real. Maybe the patient was past caring, but her family sure did. As I talked to one of her sons, the living room started to fill with relatives. I don't know where they all came from; this working-class neighborhood house must have had a really big kitchen. Presently, all the relatives had created a semicircle around me waiting to hear something profound, something encouraging.

I felt uneasy (and who wouldn't?) face to face with the entire family in an unresponsive, if not downright despairing, situation. But I had been asked to offer an opinion, and the time had come. I suggested the best orthomolecular (nutritional) therapy I knew of: megadoses of niacin, in multigram doses. Then, I mentally braced myself for their reaction.

There was no reaction. But they didn't run off, either.

So I continued. "Because she is so sick, your mother might need an exceptionally large amount of some vitamins, especially C and B complex. But her foremost need is for niacin, really large quantities of niacin."

"How large?" asked a male relative on my left. That question you can count on.

"Thousands of milligrams a day, in divided doses," I answered. "Possibly even 10,000 milligrams or more, every day."

They all listened. I got the distinct impression that they were weighing the gravity of what must certainly have felt like a hopeless situation against what must have sounded like a pretty simplistic solution. But still they did not run off. Some of the family now sat down, on chairs, the old sofa, and on the well-worn gray carpet.

The inquisition shall now begin in earnest, I thought.

Not at all. I was asked a series of intelligent, commonsense questions about the safety and administration of high doses of niacin. I explained niacin's low toxicity and the need for large and divided doses. I told them to expect, at least initially, some pretty strong but harmless "niacin flush" side effects. And, I presented the need to educate their attending doctors as to what the family was doing. Finally, I outlined a therapeutic trial starting with 1,000 milligrams per day of niacin, and gradually but steadily increasing the dose by an additional 1,000 milligrams every day.

"How will we know when to stop increasing the dose?" asked a son-in-law.

"When she responds," answered his wife. "Right?"

"Yes," I said. "The goal is to give enough niacin to see good results. You all will be the judges of that."

"Will she have to keep taking niacin forever?" asked another daughter.

"Yes, but not necessarily as much as she'll need initially. We first need to see if she responds at all. But if it works, why stop it?"

Everyone nodded. Nobody smiled. Tough crowd. I left with a distinct feeling that I had contributed precious little to that family's hopes.

Was I ever wrong. I got a call about two weeks later from a profoundly relieved, and positively delighted, daughter.

"Mom is just fine," she said happily. "She sits at the dinner table now. She talks to us, talks like nothing happened. It's incredible. She's off all medications. It's the niacin: it made all the difference in the world."

"That is wonderful news," I said. "How much niacin is your mother taking now?"

"11,000 to 12,000 milligrams every day."

"Do you happen to remember at what level she experienced a niacin flush?" I asked.

"That's easy to answer," replied the daughter. "She never flushed at all."

Wow—11 or 12 grams of niacin a day and no flush. This meant she had been severely deficient. But results are what matters in any therapeutic trial. A huge amount of niacin, along with the other B vitamins and vitamin C, had done the job. A very big job.

"This is great!" said the daughter. "We have our Mom back!"

That was a beautiful moment.

Later that month, the family took the fully mobile and positively talkative mother to see her psychiatrist. She didn't need to go, but they all wanted the doctor to see the recovery with his own eyes. I was not there, but I heard about it afterward.

"The doctor told all of us that there could be some side effects with that much niacin," said the daughter. "Especially changes in liver function. Also, he said that Mom's skin looked slightly darker to him. The doctor said she should not take niacin because of it."[1]

"None? At all?" I said.

"Right: none. He told her, and the rest of the family, that she should be on medication, not on some vitamin."

"It is usually the medication that has harmful side effects, not the niacin," I said. "Dr. Abram Hoffer and other physicians with extensive experience administering niacin have found that niacin is not liver toxic. They report that niacin therapy can increase liver function tests, but they also point out that this elevation means that the liver is active. It does not indicate an underlying liver pathology.[2] If your doctor wanted to do monitoring tests, that is one thing. But to take a successful, already working therapy away from a seriously ill patient is quite another."

It really mystified me then, and it still does today: Just why are so many physicians prejudiced against vitamin therapy? Decades ago, Frederick Klenner, M.D., was so frustrated by his colleagues' flat rejection of megavitamin therapy that he wrote that some doctors would rather see their patients die than use vitamins.

I asked her what the family had decided to do now.

"We've already done what the psychiatrist said, and Mom no longer gets niacin. She is back on drugs, three of them."

The daughter then paused. I knew the worst was yet to come.

"And," said the daughter, with a choke in her voice, "Now my mom is back in the corner."

Indeed, this was no Harry Potter story. It was, I am sorry to say, much more like the medical tyranny illustrated in *One Flew Over the Cuckoo's Nest.* When doctors prefer patients to people, we have a problem.

We also have a solution: just say no. Fire your doctor. And take your vitamins.

Part One

Tools for Healthy Living

A Pep Talk to Get Started

"Fire your doctor? Just what kind of a nut would say that?"

A health nut, that's who. Here's my question to you: If you are not a health nut, just what kind of a nut would you rather be? Still, merely saying, "Nuts!" to your physician is not enough. There must also be a set of positive, proactive, and practical alternatives ready for you to use. *Fire Your Doctor!* provides a pack of them.

Health is a big subject and so is natural healing. There seem to be more areas of study, more *-ologies* and *-opathies,* than you can possibly shake a stethoscope at. It takes some distillation to concentrate it down to good stuff, but that is likely why you picked up this book.

You do not need to know every aspect of mechanics to be able to drive your car. You do not need to master every detail of electronics to use your computer. And, by golly, you do not need to have an exhaustive knowledge of physiology or pharmacology to use your body. Rather, you need to know what works best to get you well and keep you well. That is the focus of this book: how we can get better using practical, effective, and safe natural therapies. Starting today; right now, in fact.

Fire Your Doctor! is also about an attitude. It is about empowering yourself. First off, you have got to want it. Are you sick of sickness? Then, say the Chinese, you are no longer sick.

Secondly, *Fire Your Doctor!* is about knowledge. You need to know what to do and how to do it. This we gain through reading others' work and by our experience confirming their experiences. It just so happens that these "others" are physicians. I am not a physician and I am certainly not smart enough to make up this stuff. I am, however, able to find out which researchers and physicians are getting successful results and share their knowledge with you.

Mostly, *Fire Your Doctor!* is about asserting yourself. For nearly thirty years, I have worked with lots of folks who have made the transformation from being somebody else's fear-filled patient to being their own self-reliant, naturally healthy Self. It can be done, and you can do it.

WHY PEOPLE NEEDLESSLY SUFFER

Reason One: Fear

As a scrawny teen, high-school wrestling scared me green. I was quite terrified. Awaiting my turn to get creamed on the wrestling mat, I knew I'd had it. Our gym teacher, a paragon of gladiatorial efficiency, always paired us off by height. The problem was that I was tall but very skinny. My equally tall adversary invariably turned out to be a varsity football lineman, easily three times my weight. That's why I knew my number was up.

Faced with the certainty of imminent pain, I had to gain the essentials not of wrestling, but of survival, and very quickly. I therefore developed the world's fastest sit-out, followed by my immediately turning over and lying spread-eagled on the mat. Yes, I made a big human "X," face down into the canvas. It worked, and I am here to tell the tale. I never won a match, but no one could pin me either.

Fear had very nearly crippled me, but my circumstances forced the learning curve far beyond what I thought I was capable of. Maybe you find yourself in an analogous position. If you are afraid of illness (and who isn't?), you know what I mean: you may be ready to take matters into your own hands. With this book, you will have a stack of therapeutic alternatives and preventive strategies to protect your health. And all are drug-free.

Okay, never getting pinned in wrestling is one thing; raising healthy kids is quite another. I raised my kids to college age and they never had a single dose of any antibiotic. This book is about how you can learn to use natural therapies as we did.

While talking with General George "Blood and Guts" Patton, a soldier confessed that he was afraid of battle. Patton replied, "So am I, son." The soldier, truly surprised, said, "You, General? You're not afraid of anything!"

Patton answered, "Anyone who tells you that they are not afraid of battle is either a liar or a fool." General Patton's advice to this soldier, and to the rest of us, still rings true today: "Never take counsel of your fears." Note that he did not say, "Don't have them." He said, "Don't listen to them."

We are all afraid of something. Just try to tell a four-year-old not to be afraid of a hypodermic needle. Or try to tell a teenage boy not to be afraid of calling up a girl and asking her for a date. Just try to tell a student pilot not to be afraid of flying an airplane solo for the first time. Or tell someone not to be afraid of major surgery. Just telling someone not to be afraid doesn't work. The way to eliminate fear is to expose it for the fraud it is. Truth banishes fear. As there is no fear greater than the fear of getting a disease, we need the knowledge and tools to set ourselves free by taking control of our own health.

Years ago, while waiting for a train at London's Euston Station, I was unavoidably involved in a conversation with a drunken derelict in search of a handout. As he coughed in my face, he told me he had recently gotten out of prison. He sought to prove his honesty by producing tattered but nonetheless recognizably official discharge papers. I happened to note, as he continued coughing, that he also had been diagnosed with tuberculosis (TB). I gave him a 50P coin to send him on his way so that I could breathe clean air again.

For a long time afterward, I worried about getting tuberculosis. I mean, what an exposure! Then, to compound my anxiety, when I first started out as a college instructor, the only teaching job I could get was in state prisons. My "captive audience" also coughed a great deal. One in eight prisoners tested positive for TB. I spent many hours in mostly unventilated rooms with a lot of very unhealthy men and women. As a condition of employment, prison faculty had TB tests, and fortunately mine remained negative.

The conclusion I drew from this? The body's immune system is more important than is pathogen exposure. Or, as the great bacteriologist Louis Pasteur put it, "The germ is nothing; the terrain is everything." Our terrain is our body—the territory that you have responsibility for and authority over. We live in a world full of germs. What you can do is strengthen your body's defense systems to combat them.

Reason Two: Erroneous Belief Systems

But sometimes we remain timid. Most people's fear of self-care centers on three common fallacies:

1. "You are not educated enough to treat yourself. That's what doctors are for."
2. "Natural therapies aren't powerful enough to cure real diseases."
3. "Megavitamin therapy is dangerous."

These are not facts; these are beliefs. And, as this book will demonstrate, they are all unfounded. Jazz musician Eubie Blake said it best: "It's not what we don't know that harms us, but what we do know that ain't so."

If your doctor "does not believe in using vitamins," not only is that doctor behind the times, that doctor is not being scientific. Therapeutic nutrition is not a matter of belief; it is a matter of confirmed clinical experience.

Belief systems can be wrong. It is not a matter of belief that vitamin C powder applied directly to herpes sores heals them overnight.

It is not a matter of belief that high doses of oral vitamin C is the best systemic antiviral on Earth. Nor is it a matter of belief that vitamin E stops heart disease.

Try these and see for yourself. Seeing is better than believing anyway.

Reason Three: Never Tried It

One of my favorite sayings is, "If you do what you've always done, you'll get what you've always gotten." If you know something does not work, why belabor the issue? Try something else. Do not let fears or belief systems keep you from the most powerful, commonsense conclusion: There may be something you do not know about that may help you. There is no guarantee that the new is better than the old, but if you decline to investigate the new, there is an absolute guarantee that all you'll have to choose from is the old. Explore your options and look for yourself.

WATCH ONE, DO ONE, TEACH ONE

"Watch one, do one, teach one—that's how we learn," a surgical resident told me over three decades ago, when I first gowned up as a student observer in the operating room. "Watch a procedure, then do it, and then teach it. Here," he added, "Hold that clamp like this. Yes, that's it." He had no business letting me assist with surgery, but I began to learn how to learn: watch and copy.

Interestingly enough, that's also how I learned to fly an airplane. "Pay attention," my 275-pound, red-faced flight instructor said. "If you get it right on the first attempt, the flight examiner won't ask you for more." As much as I dreaded the flight test, I actually paid attention for a much stronger reason: I considered my overweight and hypertensive instructor to be a prime candidate for a mile-high heart attack. If he was going to die in the air, I was not about to let him take me with him. I wanted to be able to control and land that plane in the worst way. I wanted to live.

Motivation is a wonderful thing. Survival is probably the most powerful motivator: the breath of life is everyone's number-one concern. No one wants to sicken and die, and sick people very much want to get well. That is why the most common Internet searches are for information on health and disease.

The title of this book is meant to confirm the notion that you can learn to manage your own health care. But how, when physicians are generally unwilling to teach us? There is only one path left to us: we'll teach ourselves. Face it—most doctors do not explain their trade secrets any more than medieval guild members would show peasants how to make their own swords, purify their own silver, or read Latin. If you made your own sword, why have craftsmen? If serfs had access to their own silver, they would buy their freedom. If everyone could read, well, history would change.

Changing your present, and thereby your future, sounds even better, doesn't it? When I am asked my goal in all of this, I answer, "Each their own physician, today." I think one way to do this is to demystify medicine of its needlessly confusing terminology. Another way is to simultaneously present both the validity and the simplicity of natural health care.

"EASY" VERSUS "SIMPLE"

Asking me what to do, or seeking a physician to do it for you, is easy. Neither will work. If you want to be a pilot, you have to hoist yourself into the left seat of an aircraft and take the time to learn to fly. If you are content to be a passenger in the medical system, you are reading the wrong book. If you want something done right, you have to do it yourself, and this especially includes your health care. You can learn it, you can do it, and you can share the way with others.

Change your lifestyle and you can dramatically improve your health. "That's so simplistic!"

rails our inner critic. We doubt natural therapy because it seems too simple to work and we doubt self-care because we doubt ourselves. We've been educated to be good consumers, and that includes becoming consumers of healthcare services. We have not been educated to be self-reliant.

The good news is that therapeutic nutrition is cheap, simple, effective, and safe. Of course, we have been taught that anything cheap, simple, and safe cannot possibly be effective against real diseases. And when, by our own verified experiences, we find that megavitamin therapy is cheap and effective, there are plenty of "pharmaphilic" (drug-loving) fear-mongerers trying to tell us that it can't be safe. But vitamin therapy is safe. There is not even one death from taking vitamins per year.[1]

PHARMACEUTICAL MEDICINE: DANGEROUS AND DEADLY

In fact, the evidence proves that it is drugs and doctors that are dangerous. Over 770,000 hospital patients suffer adverse drug reactions from taking properly prescribed drugs in the prescribed doses. And this figure is for just one year in the United States. Furthermore, there are 140,000 deaths attributable to properly prescribed prescription drugs every year, according to recent studies.[2] If overdoses, incorrect prescriptions, and drug interactions are figured in, total drug fatalities number over a quarter of a million.[3]

Hospitals are dangerous places. A hospital is, by definition, a collection of sick people. Aside from exposure to other people's illnesses and infections, hospital drug treatment virtually guarantees side effects, many of which are dangerous and all of which are expensive. In one study of hospitalized patients, "there were 247 adverse drug events among 207 admissions ... of which 60 were preventable." Preventable adverse drug events added 4.6 days to the average hospital stay, at an extra cost of nearly $5,000. "Moreover, these estimates are conservative because they do not include the costs of injuries to patients or malpractice costs."[4]

Ultimately, we have to decide who we are going to listen to, particularly when it comes to our health. Read the research and see for yourself. Everything changes the day you decide to no longer let your healthcare providers treat you like a child. At first, it may not be easy to face down a domineering doctor or even to negotiate with family members. But you can indeed do both, especially when you know your available alternatives. It is a challenge, but it is also absolutely vital.

SOME PROPHETIC RANTING AND RAVING

I find medicine is the best of all trades because whether you do any good or not you still get your money.
—JEAN-BAPTISTE POQUELIN DE MOLIÈRE, THE PHYSICIAN IN SPITE OF HIMSELF (1664)

If we doctors threw all our medicines into the sea, it would be that much better for our patients and that much worse for the fishes.
—OLIVER WENDELL HOLMES, M.D.

I have seen the foolishness of conventional disease care. I have seen hospitals feed white bread to patients with bowel cancer and Jell-O to leukemia patients. I have seen schools feed bright red "Slush Puppies" to seven-year-olds for lunch and then children vomit up red crud afterward. And, I have seen those same children later line up at the school nurse for hyperactivity drugs.

I have seen hospital patients allowed to go two weeks without a bowel movement. I have seen patients told that they have six months to live, when they might live sixty months. I have seen people recover from serious illness, only to have their physician berate them for having used natural healing methods to do so.

I have seen infants spit up formula while their mothers were advised not to breast-feed. I've seen better ingredients in dog food than in the average school or hospital lunch.

And I have seen enough.

Don't bother looking in the history books for what has slaughtered the most Americans. Look instead at your dinner table. There's an old saying: "One-fourth of what you eat keeps you alive; the other three-fourths keep your doctor alive." We eat too much of the wrong things and not enough of the right things. Scientific research continually indicates nationwide vitamin and mineral deficiencies in our country, and then we spend over $1 trillion each year on disease care in America.

Nearly two-thirds of a million men died in the Civil War. All other U.S. wars put together add about another two-thirds of a million soldiers killed. That means that about 1,300,000 Americans have died in total in all the wars in U.S. history. That is a lot of deaths. Today, we lose more than that number of Americans each *year* because of cancer and heart disease.

So always remember that disease is the real enemy.

Nearly 10 million soldiers were killed in World War I, charging machine guns and getting mowed down month after month. A terrible slaughter went on for four years. Yet, in just the two years following the war, over 20 million people died from influenza. During the American Civil War, three times as many soldiers died from disease as from battle. Today, alcohol and tobacco kill nearly as many Americans in one year as the entire Civil War did in four.

Results are all that matter to me. Alternative medicine works. The natural treatment and prevention of illness can be accomplished safely, inexpensively, and effectively. It is time to see for yourself what really works.

My work is not prescription, but rather description. As a people, we should be free to utilize any reasonable healthcare approach. To make such a decision, we need education far more than we need medication. The proposed treatment regimens included in *Fire Your Doctor!* are not mine. I do not stay up late at night making all this up. I have collected the safest and most effective healing approaches from physicians worldwide.

Natural healing is not about avoiding doctors; it is about not needing to go to doctors. A dentist is not upset if you are cavity free; a doctor should not be upset if you are healthy. The idea is to be well. The first step is wanting to be healthy. The second step is to do something now to improve your health. Each of us is ultimately responsible for our own wellness and we should consider all options in our search for better health. You get out of the body what you put into it: your body *will* respond to efforts to improve your health.

The time to start is right now. Another old saying: "If not now, when? If not here, where? If not you, then who?"

It's supposed to be a secret, but I'll tell you anyway. We doctors do nothing. We only help and encourage the doctor within.
—NOBEL LAUREATE ALBERT SCHWEITZER, M.D.

HOW I GOT STARTED

It was either the shots or the blood.

Since the earliest I can remember, going to the doctor meant getting a needle in the rear end. When I was a preschooler, our family doctor seemed genuinely old. He had been a general practitioner for thirty years before I went to him. I noticed that his ancient medical degree dated from the 1920s. His methods were not refined: he gave me what he thought was a smile, had my parents forcibly flip me upside down onto his paper-covered black leather examination table, and jabbed me in the keister. I couldn't have been thinking too deeply at that age, but evidently the impression those hypodermic needles made on me were deep in more ways than one. Somewhere in the back of my mind, it seemed that there must be more to medicine than silver-colored instruments and pain.

While in high school, I looked, and occasionally acted, like the type of kid who would someday be a doctor. I was the kid who could cut up anything in biology class and I dissected toads, bullheads, and fetal pigs at home on Saturdays. I turned my bedroom into a chemistry lab. I started a science club at school and attended future physicians' seminars.

Once, at a meeting of the local medical society, we watched a movie showing surgical operations. From the first foot-long incision, I knew I had a problem. During the discussion afterward, I asked if anyone had ever become a doctor who could not stand the sight of human blood. The responding doctor said, politely smiling, that rather few had done so.

During my second and third years in college, I arranged to observe surgery at various hospitals. This seemed like a good way to overcome my aversion to slicing into a live person. It took over two hours by bus to get to see my first operation at a small hospital in Dansville, New York. I was the first gowned-up non-nurse in the operating room when they wheeled in the patient. She was old enough to be my great-grandmother and was in for a breast biopsy. As she turned toward me, she could not have missed seeing that I was as white as my mask. Perhaps she noticed the cold sweat on my forehead.

She quietly said, "You're not the doctor, are you?"

"No, ma'am," I answered.

"Oh, good!" she said, smiling, and closed her eyes.

I had brought comfort on my very first day.

I managed to remain vertical through the opening incision, saw that fat was bright orange, and the lump proved benign. I knew now that I could handle an inch-long incision without passing out.

From that time on, I watched more extensive operations at larger hospitals. One procedure is particularly memorable. Another elderly woman was in for an adrenalectomy (excision of the adrenal glands). I was told that this was to help relieve her severe arthritis pain. Having by now seen enough abdomens opened up, I watched with surprise as the operating team turned her over and made generous cuts at the level of the lowest rib. It then occurred to me that, of course, this was the shortest route to the kidneys (on which the adrenal glands are perched). The kidneys are each protected by ribs. I waited for the rib-spreaders next. In a stainless-steel flash, the chief surgeon instead produced a large pair of tin snips, massive metal-cutting scissors that would probably cut through a Buick.

Oh, no, he's not really going to...

"...Crunch!"

Yes, as a matter of fact, he was.

"Crunch!" Those were the genuinely loud sounds of human ribs being cut. Oh well, I thought, they'll put them back when they're done. They didn't. The ribs were removed, casually placed in a pan, and that was the last of them. The adrenals were easily removed after that. You might think that I'd immediately begin a passionate search for a painless, natural cure for arthritis. No, for I could now better withstand the incisions and the blood, and I wanted to be a doctor.

It was one of my professors, John I. Mosher, at the State University of New York College at Brockport, who first asked me to reconsider what "being a doctor" actually meant. Was it about being the M.D. in the white coat or was it about really helping people get well? It was a good point, and I largely ignored it. After all, I already assumed that it was essential to be a medical doctor in order to do healing. I wanted to be one of the guys at the top of the health heap!

Dr. Mosher told me to read a book called *The Pattern of Health* (now out of print) by English physician Aubrey T. Westlake. It changed everything. Dr. Westlake wrote that during his long experience as a practitioner, he had mostly been engaged in "bailing out leaking boats." I followed his narrative with increasing fascination as he described his search for real healing. He ended up way outside of conventional medicine: herbology, homeopathy, naturopathy, approaches that were utterly new to me. Yet Dr. Westlake, a fully qualified doctor, saw value in these unorthodox treatments. I could not simply disregard them anymore—there appeared to be something to these natural healing methods after all.

That was only the beginning. The really subversive thing about reading books is that each good one leads to many others. If there wasn't a blacklist of health heresy in print, I came reasonably close to creating one during college and graduate school. I read *Limits to Medicine: Medical Nemesis, the Expropriation of Health,* by Dr. Ivan Illich, *Who is Your Doctor and Why,* by Alonzo Shadman, M.D., and dozens of papers on nutritional research. Works by a number of respected authors, including Linus Pauling, Abram Hoffer, Wilfred and Evan Shute, Paavo Airola, Ewan Cameron, Richard Pass-water, Robert Mendelsohn, Roger J. Williams, Edward Bach, and William J. Mc-Cormick, eventually persuaded me that natural healing was not only valid but was generally superior to conventional drug-and-surgery medicine.

As an undergraduate, I spent a year studying at the Australian National University. While there, a friend and I calculated that a person would have to eat approximately 700 oranges a day to get the amount of vitamin C recommended by Linus Pauling. That seemed like a lot to me, but I soon began to take a daily vitamin C supplement. While doing graduate work, I began practicing vegetarianism. To tell you the truth, I did this mostly to have fewer dishes to wash. I also found that vegetarian meals were cheaper and took less time to prepare. I avoided a lot of greasy pots and pans and, as a side benefit, began to feel better as well.

Around this time I tried fasting—something I learned from my dog. It happened that the dog developed a high fever and curled up in a corner of the dining room all day and night. I checked with the veterinarian, and he said that it was not dangerous to leave the dog to itself, so I did. That dog stayed in the corner for three days. It moved only for water and to go outside for the usual purposes. The dog ate nothing at all during those three days. It slept, and I watched. On the fourth day, the dog got up and was its own doggy self again; the fever was gone.

This got me thinking.

Not long afterward, I got sick. Sick enough that neighbors stopped by to check on me. I began to fast, basically duplicating what my dog had done, with the exception that I did not sleep in the corner. (I also did not use the outdoors for excretory purposes.) To my surprise, I was comfortable eating nothing. Like the dog, all I wanted were liquids and sleep. The illness was over quickly, without any medicines. The result was good, but it was the process by which I'd gotten better that really intrigued me. This sounds odd, but while fasting I'd felt the best I had ever felt while feeling bad. Certainly I had been very ill, yet this simple cure was completely satisfactory.

I continued with my informal study of naturopathy. This kept me reading more books on natural healing written by experienced doctors. These physicians treated serious diseases with fasting, diet, herbs, homeopathy, minerals, and vitamins. I finally began taking a multiple vitamin every day.

From reading we can soak up many facts, but it is having children that really tests our knowledge. Raising a family provides plenty of opportunities to see whether or not an idea is any good. What it repeatedly demonstrated is that nature-cure works.

Yes, it turns out that natural therapeutics are as good, or better than, allopathic (drug-based) medicine. During my bouts with pneumonia, experience showed me that drugs would not cure it as fast as high-dose vitamin C therapy. My father got rid of his angina by taking high doses of vitamin E each day. He found that the vitamin works better than the prescriptions he'd been taking and doesn't have the side effects, either.

Outside my family, I have seen "hopeless" cases turn around with natural therapy: impending blindness reversed, multiple sclerosis improved, mental illness ended, hips rebuilt without surgery, malignancies shrunk, immune systems restored, severe arthritis eliminated—all these and many more, all cured without drugs. After you see this happen again and again, it begins to reach you: these truly are simple, safe, economical, and effective treatments. And, they work on real diseases.

Does health care have to hurt and cost a fortune? Are blood and drugs prerequisites for healing? Is a hospital really the best place for getting better? Have medical doctors cornered the market on healing knowledge? Is nature-cure a lot of hooey? Don't believe it. Instead, see for yourself. Read a few of those books at the health food store. Change your diet. Next time you are sick, try a natural alternative instead. Find out for yourself. That's what I did, and it has worked.

Do not fear to be eccentric in opinion, for every opinion now accepted was once eccentric.
—BERTRAND RUSSELL

TEACHING THE DOCTORS

It's still hard to believe that it was thirty years ago that I was dropped into the deep end at the intensive care unit (ICU) of Boston's Brigham Hospital. I was then a clinical counseling student. A never-ending stream of the critically ill was wheeled through the Levine Cardiac Unit, where I'd hung my hat for a semester. What a place: It was as full of electronics, dials, and overhead monitors, as is the control room of a submarine. And just as crowded. In the few corners not taken up with life-saving equipment, space had somehow been found for patients' beds. If you ducked under some wires and walked over others, you could usually locate your patient. And there I found Sammy.

Samuel, a seventy-four-year-old retired firefighter, had just experienced a heart attack. I had an instant rapport with this delightful grandfatherly man, who was quick with Yiddish humor and had a disarming smile. His kindliness toward me went a long way toward hiding my nervousness, inexperience, and youth. As counseling students, we were supposed to get seriously ill patients to talk, open up, and feel better. But although he told me about himself, usually it was he who got me to talk. It was as if he was the real counselor and, looking back, I think he was. I looked forward to our visits, but one day his bed was empty—Sammy had died the night before. The bed was not vacant for long.

For most ICU patients, the survival odds were about 50-50. One day, I was asked to visit a forty-year-old football coach who'd had a massive heart attack. He was well aware of his chances and told me so without batting an eyelash. "I've played games with worse odds than those," he added with a grin. His bed was vacant a week later—that's because he'd gone home, alive.

Downstairs a few floors, I was assigned to a thirty-four-year-old woman with cancer. She was dying and the most advanced medical technology had nothing to offer her. Unlike the intensive care patients, who usually came or went within a week, I visited her for an extended period of time. I got to know her husband, too. They were not happy people. Sure, I could sympathize, but I felt useless. There was so little I could do, aside from visiting and listening. She died shortly before the semester was over. The last thing I remember is her husband, sitting alone on a wooden bench in the old whitewashed hospital corridor, with his head bent over a medical textbook. He was still trying to figure out what had happened.

Those images are part of the reason why I am in my line of work today. Do I now have the "magic bullet" cure for these diseases? No. But I can offer you a piece of the answer and that's worth doing. Modern drug-based medicine is as incomplete as a novel written with three vowels, as discordant as a symphony constructed with only some of the notes. High-dose nutritional therapy is the much-needed missing part of our vocabulary of health care. The fight against disease needs all the help it can get.

"Health is the fastest growing failing business in western civilization," writes Emanuel Cheraskin, M.D., D.M.D[5] Far more scathing attacks on modern medicine's dangers will be found in *Confessions of a Medical Heretic* by Robert Mendelsohn, M.D.; *The Truth About Drug Companies* by Marcia Angell, M.D.[6], and *Death by Modern Medicine* by Carolyn Dean, M.D.[7] Some people will never read these books, as they are too disturbing. I have an entire family full of doctor-worshippers; perhaps you do, too. Do doctors command more respect than they've earned? It amounts almost to a religion, when we put so much faith in mortals. Consider that you may well be born without being baptized and die without seeing a rabbi or priest, but you will not even officially exist until a doctor signs your birth certificate, and you are not free from the Internal Revenue Service (IRS) until a doctor signs your death certificate.

Between these events, doctors enjoy high incomes, high social status, and immense authority. Napoleon is said to have declared that in the next world, doctors would have more deaths to account for than generals. Author and Ayurvedic physician Deepak Chopra, M.D., has said that more people live off cancer than die from it.

Abram Hoffer, M.D., offers this comment: "Modern medicine is not scientific; it is full of prejudice, illogic, and susceptible to advertising. Doctors are not taught to reason. They are programmed to believe in whatever their medical schools teach them and the leading doctors tell them. And over the past 20 years, the drug companies with their enormous wealth have taken medicine over and now control its research, what is taught, and the information released to the public."[8]

The good news is that the people know better. When it comes to natural healing and vitamin therapy, patients are now teaching the doctors.

SEE FOR YOURSELF

It was a society luncheon and I was speaking to a large roomful of elderly folks on the benefits of therapeutic nutrition, natural healing, and wellness self-reliance. Apparently they really loved my talk: lots of bifocaled eye contact and positive nods from many a gray-haired head. After the presentation, I invited people to come up if they had a question. The response to this offer was overwhelming: they crowded onto the stage and someone actually stole my lecture notes right off the podium.

A natural lifestyle really works and people can instinctively sense it. Then they try it, they feel better, and they tell others. I recently received a couple of delightful phone calls. One was from a lady, now eighty-eight, who said that she's been following the natural foods and supplements way for nearly thirty years. She'd previously had an assortment of health problems, until she totally reformed her diet and started taking vitamins. Now, she said, "I take no medicines at all and I feel wonderful." Another lady, now ninety-three, phoned and said that, back in 1970, her husband had a severe heart attack and his prospects were not great. Dr. Evan Shute placed him on 1,600IU of vitamin E daily. Did it work? Looks like it might have: her husband is now ninety-two and still takes 1,200IU of vitamin E every day. A third of a century on megadoses of vitamin E and no side effects, but great success!

Shh! Don't let word of this get out! Do not learn about megadose vitamin therapy. Warning: Doing so may be helpful to your health. If you are healthy, and if your family and friends get wind of what you are doing, it could undermine our medical and pharmaceutical industries. We don't want that now, do we?

Of course, if you are bound and determined to get well and stay well, then I expect you'll want to go ahead and read some more of this book.

Educating Yourself

The inventor of the microwave oven, Percy Spencer, had just a third-grade education.

Bill "Learjet" Lear had only an eighth-grade education, but had over 150 patents to his name. He also invented the 8-track tape player, but you can't win them all.

The great silent film comedian Buster Keaton spent a total of one day in school. His film work is regarded worldwide as among the best ever.

In 1939, Richard Dillworth designed and built the General Motors Electromotive FT Diesel Locomotive, the streamlined locomotive that revolutionized modern rail transit. He had one-half day of schooling in his entire life.

And Irving Berlin, arguably the most successful songwriter in history, never learned to read music.

What does this mean? You (yes, you) can learn far more about being your own doctor than you may have thought. It's not about schooling; it's about knowledge.

Of course, if you go to medical school, you will learn drug-based medicine. But in medical school, you will probably not also learn how to avoid the use of medicine. You will most certainly not learn how to substitute high-dose nutritional therapies (also known as "ortho-molecular" treatments) for drug treatments.

So, we need to go to "nonmedical school" to learn alternatives. *Fire Your Doctor!* is your freshman textbook. For lesson one, I'd define "modern medicine" as "the experimental study of what happens when poisonous chemicals are placed into malnourished human bodies." Politically powerful medical quackery is nothing new. Drug-and-cut doctors have been ignoring nature's cures for a long time, with disastrous results.

WHY GEORGE WASHINGTON SHOULD HAVE FIRED HIS DOCTOR

"General Washington was taken in the night (in December 1799) with a sore throat. The 'bleeder' being sent for; he took from him 14 ounces of blood. The following morning, the family physician arrived, and proceeded to bleed him copiously, twice within a few hours, and again the same evening, giving him thereafter a dose of calomel (mercury). Next morning he was given another dose. The next day another physician was called in consultation, and the result was that they took an additional 32 ounces of blood from General Washington.

There was no alleviation of the disease. Ten grains more of calomel were given, followed by a tartar emetic in large doses. To his extremities blisters were applied, and to his throat poultices. General Washington died."[1]

President George Washington, the father of our country, died from a sore throat? No, he died from the treatment. Washington had the best scientific medical attention of his day. They bled him no fewer than five times in three days. Let's do the grisly arithmetic. The first bleeding removed 14 ounces; there were then three bleedings of unspecified quantity, collectively described as "copious"; and then a final full quart was removed. Assuming that the three "copious" bleedings were also 14 ounces each, that is another 42 ounces lost. Adding up, we have some 88 ounces of blood taken from Washington. The human body contains about 10 pints (5 quarts) of blood. That 88 ounces is close to 3 quarts, well over half the blood in a person.

It doesn't take a conspiracy, nor an assassin, to kill a great man. Stupidity will do it just as well.

IF NOT YOU, WHO? IF NOT NOW, WHEN?

The world cares very little about what a person knows; it is what the person is able to do that counts.
—BOOKER T. WASHINGTON

If you want the government to save you money on health care, you are in for a long wait indeed. If you want to avoid doctors and drugs, you need to know how to use vitamins and other natural methods to get well and stay well. This means you must become a "health homesteader," take matters into your own hands, and find out what your options are. You, not your doctor.

You might think that you could expect your physician to do the learning for you. I think that is like expecting to be served chow mein in a French restaurant. When is the last time a medical doctor told you to not pick up a prescription? And when is the last time your doctor told you exactly what to do instead?

An old proverb says, "Give someone a fish to eat today and you must give him a fish tomorrow. Teach someone to fish, and he can always have food." Dare to apply this to health care. Physicians should teach more than prescribe; clearly they do the opposite. For drug therapy, we will always be dependent on pharmacies and doctors. For health, we will ultimately be dependent upon ourselves. We must learn how to live, and the sooner, the better.

Perhaps you think you can ask me your questions, but I do not provide such a service. The service I provide is in your hands, and it must be read. Hitting the books and reading the papers is our privilege and our job. When you do so directly, the medical professions are bypassed. And since the medical professions do not prosper when you do not use them, they will not support you when you go off on your own, to your local health food store or to your own library or Internet research. In fact, many doctors can be counted on to belittle the health homesteader.

If you've ever met a plumber or electrician or auto mechanic who said, "Here, let me show you how to do this," then you have been singularly fortunate. It is infinitely more rare for a health professional to teach you exactly how to dispense with their services. An underlying assumption implicit in fee-for-service medical care is that you cannot do what the doctor does and you are a fool for thinking you can. I disagree.

Once I was stranded out of state with my car's radiator fluid bleeding out around me, staining the parking lot nicely green. It was

Sunday and I could not find a mechanic who would come to fix the car, and I had no money for a tow or for an overnight stay to wait for the job to be attended to. So I pleaded with, and ultimately convinced, a gas station attendant to loan me a few tools and drop a hint about how to replace coolant hoses. That might sound like small potatoes to you, but I was a nineteen-year-old egghead, and up until then, had never worked on a car in my life. The prospect actually frightened me. But I learned that desperation and elbow grease will loosen even the frayed plumbing of an old Ford. I replaced the hose, filled the radiator, returned the tools, and drove away.

Car self-repair and health self-repair require a common attitude: "This is learnable, this is doable, and I can learn to do it."

Consider the financial aspects of this: What if we were determined to do without doctors? The medical-pharmaceutical assumption: certainly we can't. The health homesteaders' assumption: maybe we can. No longer a patient, the health homesteader takes back control and gains knowledge, experience, and self-reliance, in that order.

Now don't go off saying that this is silly, breathlessly citing crisis care as requiring physicians. Grant you there are times when we absolutely need professional help. But we can act to greatly reduce the frequency of those times, and far beyond what we've been told. The word *doctor* is derived from the Latin word for "teacher." If your physician is a good health coach, great. If not, then you absolutely need to doctor (teach) yourself.

Here is a quick way to evaluate your doctor's alternative health potential. Ask her if she agrees with this statement: "There is a natural substitute for nearly every drug. I do not want to use nutrition and vitamin supplements along with drugs. I want to use them instead of drugs."

If your doctor is intolerant of such a position, or simply not up to speed, you can help fill the void with the references provided in this book. The biggest health care mistake made by both physicians and patients is to assume that there is a prescription drug solution to nearly every bodily problem. I call such an assumption "pharmaphilia," or the "love of drugs." It is high time for all of us to grow out of it.

POWER TO THE PATIENT!

Do not let either the medical authorities or the politicians mislead you. Find out what the facts are, and make your own decisions about how to live a happy life and how to work for a better world.
—LINUS PAULING

Why do people wait for hours to see a doctor? Is the doctor's time more important than yours? The answer is: yes, it is. Do you make hundreds of dollars an hour? Is your income far into six-figures? That's why you are sitting there waiting.

Now, let's say the tables are turned and the doctor is home with a flooded bathroom, waiting for the plumber. Let's say the wait is two hours. Whose time is more valuable now? Nice poetic justice though that may be, in each case the real problem is helplessness. I have learned (by necessity) to use a plunger, a plumber's snake, and have become adept with a closet auger. I can also fix and install toilets, fixtures, drains, and faucets. All of this means I don't call plumbers, for I have become one. Of course, I know my limits—I won't be bidding to install industrial, high-pressure, hot-water systems any time soon.

There are certainly practical limits to being your own doctor, but that should not be construed to mean your medical self-care potential is small. You can do far more than you think. For those who say they don't have time to learn self-reliance, remember this: there's always time available to you. Just use the time you spend in waiting rooms to bone up on your options. What's more, the average person spends several hours a day watching

TV; turn off the tube and do your research then.

LEARNING MADE EASIER

Be careful in reading health books. You may die of a misprint.
—MARK TWAIN

Language remains a big barrier for health homesteaders. Complex medical terms and fancy technical words are stumbling blocks for many people who seek to become their own doctor. You can sidestep this problem with a medical dictionary and an Internet search. I recommend, and regularly use, the *Merck Manual* when I have to look up a disease. (Your library has one or you can purchase it.) And when you use it, don't be bashful; remember what Einstein supposedly said when asked how many feet are in a mile: "I don't know." The questioner was flabbergasted at such an answer from such a man, but Einstein merely added, "Why should I clutter my head with things I can look up?"

A *Merck Manual* plus a medical dictionary (such as *Dorland's* or *Taber's,* or any of the numerous, online Internet dictionaries) will help take most of the mystery, and all of the puffery, out of medicine.

I get a lot of mail from people who are reluctant (if not downright unwilling) to search and find and read for themselves. Folks often send me, unrequested, their detailed medical histories. They fully expect me to review the matter and advise them on precisely what to do. That's not going to happen with me. Remember, I am not a physician. If you need that kind of service, see a doctor. To be free of such a need, see your librarian.

Fanatically interested persons who just cannot get enough health knowledge (you know who you are) will have a good time with all of this. There is so much good, useful information out there, just waiting for you to hit the trail and learn to fend for your health needs yourself. Many people commence their search via the Internet. It is far more than a convenience; public and university libraries the world over are accessible to you online.

We do not need to fear illness; we need to learn what to do to avoid it and to safely treat it when it is suddenly upon us. Sure, asking another to do it for you is almost irresistibly easy. Learning to do it yourself isn't.

BEST BOOKS ON NATURAL HEALING

"There are so many health books out there!" people say to me. "Where should I start reading?" Here is a list of what are in my opinion some of the best books on natural healing. Look for them at your favorite bookseller or your public library. Remember: even if a book is "out of print," it is still at a library. Ask your public librarian for help obtaining the books your body needs to read. Additional titles are listed in the bibliography at the back of this book.

Therapeutic Nutrition

- Balch, James F., and Phyllis A. Balch. *Prescription for Nutritional Healing,* 3rd ed. Garden City Park, NY: Avery, 2000. A fine presentation of specific therapeutic, natural, nutritional procedures (protocols) for a great many illnesses. Concise, easy to use, and especially for the skeptic, it is authored by a nutritionist-physician team.
- Pauling, Linus. *How to Live Longer and Feel Better.* New York: Freeman, 1986. Nobel Prize–winner Dr. Pauling presents an exceptionally thorough case for mega-

doses of the various vitamins. He also answers critics with facts from peer-reviewed scientific journals. Dr. Pauling has a rare gift for making the complex understandable. He covers vitamins and cancer, heart disease, aging, infectious diseases, vitamin safety, toxicity and side effects, medicines, doctors attitudes, nutrition history, vitamin biochemistry, and more. If you were to read only one health book, this would be the one.

Homeopathic Medicine

- Clarke, John H. *The Prescriber,* 9th ed. Essex, England: C.W. Daniel, 1972. This book is the next best thing to having a personal homeopathic doctor, because it is written by one. You will first find the best introduction ever written on how to use homeopathic remedies, and then over three hundred pages of foolproof repertory. Though out of print, an interlibrary loan or Internet used-book search is well worth your trouble for this essential reference for a healthy home.

Cancer

- Gerson, Charlotte, and Morton Walker. *The Gerson Therapy.* New York: Kensington Publishing, 2001. Max Gerson, M.D., cured cancer. He did so with a strict fat-free, salt-free, low-protein, essentially vegetarian dietary regimen, based on great quantities of fresh vegetable juice, supplements, and systemic detoxification. This book, written by the doctor's daughter, explains it all with treatment specifics, instruction, hints, cautions, recipes, case histories, and references, all held together with an authority that only experience can bring. The Gerson approach has been shown, for over six decades, to significantly improve both quality of life and length of life in the sickest, the most hopeless, of cancer patients.

- Hoffer, Abram. *Alternative and Natural Therapies for Cancer Prevention and Control.* East Rutherford, NJ: Basic Health Publications, 2004. This is an expansion of Dr. Hoffer's previous, and excellent, *Vitamin C and Cancer: Discovery, Recovery, Controversy* (Kingston, ON: Quarry Press, 1999). There are many controlled studies that demonstrate that vitamin C is indeed effective against cancer. Plus, vitamin C reduces the side effects of chemotherapy, surgery, and radiation therapy. The number of conventionally educated, hospital-trained doctors that support vitamin C therapy is growing. Dr. Hoffer was among the first. Your oncologist could be next.

Vitamin C Safety and Effectiveness

- Hickey, Steve, and Hilary Roberts. *Ascorbate: The Science of Vitamin C.* Morrisville, NC: Lulu, Inc., 2004; ISBN 1-4116-0724-4. Thorough, up-to-date summary of important medical research supporting very high doses of vitamin C. The authors present ascorbate C therapy with a clear and easily understandable style. Debunks vitamin C myths like no other book. It is nontechnical and yet contains 575 supporting references. Well written and most highly recommended.

- Levy, T.E. *Vitamin C, Infectious Diseases, and Toxins: Curing the Incurable.* Philadelphia: Xlibris Corp., 2002. Vitamin C is the best broad-spectrum antibiotic, antihistamine, antitoxic, and antiviral substance there is. Dr. Levy, a board-certified cardiologist, writes: "The three most important considerations in effective vitamin C therapy are 'dose, dose, and dose.' If you don't take enough, you won't get the desired effects Period!" Dr. Levy's book presents clear evidence that vitamin C cures disease, using over 1,200 supporting scientific references.

It does not mince words. It is disease specific, dose specific, practical, and readable. Astounding detail; hand this book to your doctor.

- Smith, Lendon H. *Clinical Guide to the Use of Vitamin C:* The Clinical Experiences of Frederick *Klenner, M.D.* Tacoma, WA: Life Sciences Press, 1991. Orthomolecular medicine pioneer Frederick Robert Klenner, M.D., spent nearly forty years successfully treating patients by administering enormous doses of vitamin C. "Vitamin C should be given to the patient while the doctors ponder the diagnosis," wrote Dr. Klenner. "I have never seen a patient that vitamin C would not benefit." Only sixty-eight pages, yet amazingly valuable.
- Stone, Irwin. *The Healing Factor: "Vitamin C" Against Disease.* New York: Grosset & Dunlap, 1972. Humans have inherited a genetic trait to need but not manufacture vitamin C. This book contains over fifty pages of scientific references, making it required reading for you, and especially for your doctor. Topics covered include infections (bacterial and viral), allergies, asthma, eye diseases, ulcers, cancer, heart disease, diabetes, fractures, wounds, pregnancy complications, and glaucoma. The full text of this

book has been posted on the Internet: ww w.vitamincfoundation.org.

Orthomolecular (Megavitamin) Psychiatry

- Hoffer, Abram. *Healing Schizophrenia.* Toronto, Canada: CCNM Press, 2004. Here is a new and up-to-date work encompassing several of Dr. Hoffer's classic books on megadose niacin treatment for schizophrenia, psychosis, and related mental illnesses. You can learn exactly how Dr. Hoffer, regarded as the pioneering "Father of Orthomolecular Medicine," has achieved spectacular psychiatric cures for over fifty years using vitamin B3.
- Hoffer, Abram. *Healing Children's Attention and Behavior Disorders.* Toronto, Canada: CCNM Press, 2004. There are genuine nutritional alternatives to drug therapy for ADHD children. "Battered parents" (Dr. Hoffer's term) need to know what to do, and now. Saying "no to drugs" also requires saying "yes" to something else—that something else is nutrition, properly employed. This book presents the most comprehensive review of vitamin therapy for ADHD that I have yet seen. Invaluable

guidance from the foremost authority on the subject.

Cardiovascular Health

- Shute, Wilfrid E. *Vitamin E for Ailing and Healthy Hearts.* New York: Pyramid Books, 1969. Dr. Shute and his brother, Evan, were arguably the world's most experienced cardiologists, having treated tens of thousands of patients with vitamin E. Do not be dissuaded by the publishing date: vitamin E works as well today as it did when the Drs. Shute so successfully used it. As the risk of heart disease in America is double that of cancer, everyone would benefit greatly from this easy-to-understand and valuable book.

THE FIRE YOUR DOCTOR! GUIDE TO SURFING THE INTERNET

When looking for health information on the Internet (see "Quick Reference Guide to Additional Health Conditions"), a few precautions are in order:
- Beware of websites that have a product for sale. Such sites have an inescapable vested interest in selling that particular

product, and therefore their objectivity may be questionable. How can you expect otherwise? You may have to look very carefully to find the product affiliation within a website, but it is worth looking nonetheless.

- Beware of so-called consumer protection sites that draw conclusions such as, "You can get all the nutrients you need from your balanced daily diet" or "Natural healing is unscientific." Such misinformation is fifty years out of date and will not stand up to experience. If a site tells you to *not* read something, you should make a point to read it immediately.

- Be cautious of sites run by private physicians or other individuals who make their money through consultation services. Such professionals have an interest in offering you some promising free information and then charging you for the real service. If a physician puts up a large quantity of freely available information for you to read, such as the complete text of their book or a lot of articles, the site may still be considered useful.

- For that matter, be cautious of any site run by anyone. This includes my own website, www.doctoryourself.com. Use my CELERY system: Check Every Literature reference and personal Experience and Read for Yourself.

- When in doubt, follow the money. I think it is a good idea to examine the website to see where its funding comes from. While a complete financial disclosure cannot be expected of everyone, it certainly can be a powerful recommendation. (Incidentally, the only source of funding for my website, doctoryourself.com, is the sale of my books. I have no financial connection with any supplement company or any part of the health products industry.)

If this all sounds like work, of course it is. Life is work. You have to eat anyway; you might as well eat right. You have to spend time on your health; it might as well be at the library as in a doctor's waiting room. Time in front of the computer screen can teach us a lot more than time in front of a movie screen.

But hasn't health information on the Internet been described as the mother lode of all quackery? Of course it has. But as you learned in kindergarten, calling names does not make it so. There is a practical alternative to "blind trust": use your noodle and see for yourself. Be your own doctor, manage your own case, and change your life and live healthier, today.

SHARE THE HEALTH

For decades, I have been advocating that people form their own neighborhood health self-reliance cooperatives. These could be organized along the lines of a club, day-care pool, or neighborhood watch team. The benefits might be considerable. Imagine if all your neighbors pooled their knowledge of what they'd found to be effective for, say, baby's colic. What a great, free, three-in-the-morning resource for the new parent! How about sharing the best cough or fever remedies? How did your friends get their kids into the local public schools without having them vaccinated? Which doctors near you are any good? Who in town will let you borrow their copy of that hard-to-find health book you want to read? The possibilities are virtually limitless.

Such a group assumes that people want to take the time to learn and then take the time to unselfishly share. That's a lot of assumption, but it is vital. In a group, it takes everyone to make it work and only one to ruin the experience for all.

There may also be legal considerations. You may treat yourself and your immediate family with little threat from the powers that be, but your physical assistance to a neighbor might cross legal lines. Good Samaritan laws notwithstanding, nonemergency aid to another family would have to be provided only as education. As long as input is free of charge, and strictly educational in nature, I do not think there is a jury that would convict.

These turn out to be among the reasons why we have doctors, why they charge fees, and why we are generally content to go to them. And this is why you might at first feel like you are on your own when it comes to learning about what ails you. But that is not true. I think you and your family can be an effective co-op of your own. If your friends or work colleagues join in, so much the better.

You can also take advantage of online discussion groups on health-related topics. This is a way to share knowledge with people all over the world who may have similar health concerns and experiences.

IS NATURE-CURE TOO SIMPLE TO WORK?

Every problem is simple when it is explained.
—SHERLOCK HOLMES TO DR. WATSON

A rule in the teaching profession is, "You can't make it too simple." I have also heard this expressed as the "KISS" rule: "Keep it simple, stupid." The human body is certainly complex, but what it asks of us is very simple. An automobile is made up of about 15,000 parts and is also complex. Remarkably, all you do is turn the key and it starts. With your body, the ignition key is eating right. Good nutrition provides preventive maintenance, but it also provides so much more.

Unlike a car, your body is self-repairing. Even the medical profession candidly admits that most illnesses go away when doctors do nothing at all. I have grown to respect physicians who are reluctant to interfere with the normal healing process. Believe it or not, during the nineteenth century, there was a movement among some American doctors to see patients and give them pills containing no medicine. These doctors were very popular because fewer of their patients died! If a good bedside manner and a placebo (a drugless sugar tablet) leads to a cure, that's good. To do something harmless and be helpful is good medicine. Eating right is better still.

Good nutrition and vitamins do not directly cure disease; the body does. You provide the raw materials and the inborn wisdom of your body makes the repairs. You provide the bricks and mortar and the mason builds the wall. Without supplies, the most skilled workman on earth can build nothing. Without plenty of nutrients, the body can't either. Our role is so simple because the body is so capable.

It comes down to this: Living healthfully is prevention and cure for most chronic killer diseases of humanity. That is indeed simple. It is also true and it works.

ELIMINATE SYMPTOMS FROM THE INSIDE OUT

The body has ways of letting us know when something is not right. A symptom such as pain is one such way of telling us that whatever we're doing, we should stop doing what caused it. To have pain and then to take a pain reliever so it will go away is like driving a car with the low oil-pressure light on and putting black tape over it so that you won't notice the warning anymore. If you keep driving that way, you can easily ruin your engine, whereas if you'd stop and look under the hood, you could well prevent any further trouble.

Every day, millions of people drive their bodies without paying attention to the warning lights of pain or discomfort. Pain relievers do nothing to relieve the source or the reason for the pain—they are just bottles of black tape to hide the body's warnings. When people find themselves flat on their backs in a hospital, they wonder what happened. The body was not attended to: no one looked under the hood and the body was driven into the ground, as if it were a junker car.

We need to respect symptoms and see them for what they are—errant lifestyle indicators. The best way to eliminate recurrent symptoms is to end their fundamental, underlying cause and change what's wrong in your life. Drop your bad habits and your excuses for keeping them. Instead, eat right, exercise, juice vegetables, and take your vitamins. Even the most conservative medical and dietetic professionals will admit that at least two-thirds of illness is caused by poor health behaviors. I think the percentage is far higher.

Aimlessly chasing symptoms with drugs is a waste of time and money. During instrument pilot training, I was taught "don't chase the needle"—if you do, you fly the airplane all over the place. The same holds true for an obsession over symptoms. If you wander about after every symptom, you will likely spend your life adrift in the pharmaceutical aisles.

It is a cornerstone of allopathic (drug-oriented) medicine that symptoms are to be eliminated. Just look at all the over-the-counter and prescription medicines on the market. Runny noses are to be stopped up and stuffy noses are made runny again; coughs suppressed, sneezes stifled, constipation loosened, fevers lowered, rashes salved over, and upset stomachs neutralized, all by various pharmaceutical products.

It is a huge business. In 2003, worldwide pharmaceutical sales reached nearly $492 billion. In North America alone, pharmaceutical sales totaled over $229 billion and grew at an inflation-clobbering 11 percent. Drug profits are solidly based on a drug philosophy that holds that each symptom is in itself an illness to be treated. Such treatment is accomplished by chemicals introduced into a body that has no idea what to do with them.

Surgery is a logical business partner to drug therapy: when drugs fail, then cut out what's not working. And, if possible, plug in a new one. Body parts are removable if broken and replaceable if a donor can be found. It's like the real estate business: Money is made on transactions in either direction—remove or transplant, there's a fee either way.

Nothing could be more threatening to this system than healthy people who do not need either drugs or surgery. I propose that you become one such person.

As drugs and surgery are the twin prongs of modern medicine, there are also two powerful natural options: nutrition and detoxification. Nutritional ("orthomolecular") medicine provides the body with substances (vitamins and minerals, for example) that the body uses to heal itself. All cells in your body absolutely require these natural substances for life. Sick bodies need more nutrients, not more drugs. Not one cell in your body is made out of a drug. Detoxification, known to past generations as naturopathy or natural hygiene, involves body-cleansing techniques, such as vegetable juicing and fasting.

Detoxification and nutrition eliminate symptoms from the inside out. The trick is to get at the basic causes of most disease: a chronically unhealthy lifestyle. Change your life and you change your health. The human organism is not an opponent to be fought against with drugs, but an intelligent, immeasurably complicated living system that seeks its own health automatically, given the chance.[2]

THE HEALING POWER OF NATURE

Perhaps you lack confidence that your body can heal itself, but think of how you got here in the first place. Your body is the result of the combination and multiplication of just two original half-cells called gametes. From this utterly unsupervised union of two microscopic bits came your present body—trillions of highly organized cells. And how much supervision do you give these trillions of cells daily? Do you oversee the absorption of nutrients into each cell? Do you control the proportions of carbon, hydrogen, and oxygen in each one? Do you have to remind yourself to breathe or check that you pump blood every second twenty-four hours a day?

Right now, where you sit, take a minute and try an experiment—try to stop living. I don't expect that you will have much success. This tendency of your body to stay alive is called homeostasis, the natural balance of life forces in you that keeps you going, whether you choose to or not. In that moment when you stopped to see if you could halt your body's work by intention alone, perhaps you felt a sampling of the power that carries on the work inside you. This is the power behind natural healing.

The healing power of nature (*vis medicatrix naturae* in Latin) is behind all cures, whether with the aid of natural therapies or in spite of medical ones. Your body will heal itself; this is the first rule of nature-cure. We have mentioned the importance of "listening" to your body's calls for aid, such as pains and discomforts, and not hiding or masking over such clues with drugs. We've seen that natural treatment gets to the root cause of symptoms through diet and nutrition. We have also said that the tendency of your body is toward health and this tendency is automatic and powerful. At this point, though, we can stop and ask, "If the body heals itself, why are there so many illnesses and so many sick, suffering people?"

OUR POLLUTED BODIES

For many centuries, many natural-healing advocates have insisted that most diseases are differing expressions of one root cause of illness, which is termed *systemic toxemia.* Systemic toxemia basically means "polluted body." The underlying factor of sickness is a body filled with wastes, or as Plato put it, "We have made of our bodies living cesspools, and driven doctors to invent names for our diseases."

One way we do so is by chronic constipation. Medical writers have commented on the uncomfortable truth of this for generations. Two twentieth-century colon-cleansing spokesmen were Henry Lindlahr, M.D., and the more famous John Harvey Kellogg, M.D. More recently, it was Linus Pauling, Ph.D., who said, "I read a statement by physicians that they should tell their patients not to worry about being constipated. I think they should worry;

it's so harmful to carry waste toxic materials around an unnecessarily long period of time."

Constipation means poor elimination. Your wonderful sportscar of a body has a big plug in its exhaust, causing toxin buildup. Constipation is well established as contributing to diabetes, cancer, heart disease, and other major chronic illnesses. It makes sense. A body filled with garbage may express its plight as this disease or that illness, each a desperate attempt on the part of the organism to throw off the accumulated junk and cope with its weakened, malnourished condition. Chronic illness is the result.

This is not about blaming the victim; this is about preventing more victims. And it is hardly just a matter of constipation. Eating junk foods, popping useless drugs, and sitting idle in front of the TV will not do anything to make us well. And over time, often many years, the body's strength is eroded and its natural defenses weakened so that it no longer seems capable of healing itself.

It is precisely at this juncture that the biggest mistake in disease management is generally made. The sick person is seen as even more helpless and is given all sorts of drugs and medicines to fight its diseases. Such a seemingly logical action is, unfortunately, completely wrong. The last thing that the body needs is more polluting foreign substances to contend with when it's fighting to stay alive. The body needs less of the wrong things (pharmaceutical drugs) and more of the right things (nutrients). This view, of course, runs headlong in direct opposition to the medical profession.

THE TWO LAKES ANALOGY

Let's assume that there are two identical lakes, Lake A and Lake B. Let's also assume that there is a city by each lake and that these cities are also identical. We'll cleverly call them City A and City B. Each city has sewage and other wastes that it dumps into the nearby lake. Each city has factories and houses and public buildings that for years have used the lake for their waste disposal, and as a result both Lake A and Lake B are quite polluted.

It is possible to tell how polluted a body of water is by testing for the presence of coliform bacteria. If such bacteria are present in large numbers, the water is unclean. Each lake is polluted and coliform bacteria turn up in both Lake A and Lake B. At this point, we can begin the analysis of why the lakes are unclean and what is to be done.

Doctor A (for the allopathic approach) studies the findings about Lake A and Doctor B (for the biological approach) studies the findings for

Lake B. Dr. A reasons as follows: "We know that Lake A is polluted because of the presence of coliform bacteria, for coliform bacteria and pollution are generally found together. Since this is so, it must be the bacteria that cause the lake to be polluted. Because the bacteria cause the pollution, we can kill the bacteria and thereby eliminate pollution. My prescription, then, is to add chemicals to the lake to kill all the bacteria."

In accordance with Doctor A's instructions, two truckloads of chemicals are dumped into Lake A. This surely kills all the bacteria, for the next time the water is tested for coliform bacteria, there aren't any. Dr. A then concludes that the water is now clean.

Doctor B takes a different approach: "We know that Lake B is polluted, and we know that there are coliform bacteria in the lake. Bacteria thrive in a polluted environment because waste matter provides their food. The reason there are so many bacteria is because there is so much sewage and other waste in the lake. So, the way to rid the lake of bacteria is to first rid the lake of wastes. Let's eliminate or at least greatly reduce the inflow of pollutants into the water. Then the lake will clean itself through natural processes that break down the waste materials, and without the addition of more pollutants, it will become clean again. As its food supply of waste decreases, the bacteria population will automatically decrease at the same time."

In accordance with Doctor B's instructions, sewage treatment plants are installed and other pollutant-reducing measures taken in City B. This greatly cuts down on the wastes flowing into Lake B and the population of bacteria falls. The next time the lake is tested for coliform bacteria, there are virtually none. Dr. B concludes that Lake B is now clean.

Here, then, is how things stand: Lake A contains a poisonous chemical in addition to the original wastes, plus the added pollution from continued sewage flow into the water every day. Dr. A says this water is clean because of the absence of coliform bacteria. Lake B contains little or no waste, for the inflow of pollutants was cut down. What little sewage does get by the treatment plants is easily broken down naturally and the lake contains no chemicals.

From which lake would you prefer to drink? Which lake do you consider to be cleaner?

Dr. A basically took a medical point of view, and Dr. B took a naturopathic point of view. Dr. A, like a good allopathic practitioner, set out to kill the "germs" or bacteria that "caused" the pollution or "disease" in Lake A. To back up his premise that the bacteria caused the problem, he cited the fact that the bacteria are always found along with pollution.

Dr. B also saw bacteria present with pollution; however, he did not conclude that bacteria cause pollution but that pollution causes bacteria. This is why naturopaths say that systemic toxemia, or a polluted body, is behind most infection and illness. Just because detectives are at the scene of a crime does not mean they committed it. And just because bacteria are present at the scene of disease does not mean that they caused the disease.

When we begin to see germs more as scavengers trying to clean up refuse, as opposed to being little deadly gremlins out to get us, we can begin to take confidence that nature does heal and that our body will clean itself of the roots of illness, if given the chance. If your body is strong and healthy, germs are largely irrelevant. After all, germs are everywhere, so why aren't we all sick? Right now, on your tongue and in your mouth, there are enough types of bacteria to wipe out your neighborhood, if they had their way. But they can't, and they don't. Usually, that is. It is weakness, and a weak immune system, that provides for the proliferation of germs.

So what does eliminate sickness? The promotion of health. Killing bacteria is not building health, it's just killing bacteria. Trying to kill viruses is even harder. When germs, like many agricultural insect pests, become resistant to the poisons being used against them, new drugs must be developed in an attempt to stay a jump ahead of the microbial world. Some strains of drug-resistant bacteria can survive whatever drug we throw at them. It simply does not work to pump human bodies full of drug after drug from doctor after doctor. Natural treatment offers a completely different approach: stop illness by building health. The sooner you start, the better. How about now?

A Quick Start to Better Health

Not only is example the best way to teach, it is the only way.
—DR. ALBERT SCHWEITZER

The widely accepted (but all too rarely practiced) starting points to reverse our national "un-health problem" consist of eliminating bad habits, reducing your dependence on drugs, improving your diet, and increasing exercise. These behavior changes are also generally very cheap to implement.

ELIMINATING BAD HABITS

If you are going to do something for your health, you should first stop doing bad things to your health. Just what are you willing to do to get better? If you limit your answer, you are limiting your success. We need to do whatever it takes.

It has been said that Mother Nature will not be fooled, at least not for long. If you are what you eat and you eat a lot of worthless stuff, don't expect good health. If you provide your body with good food and a healthful lifestyle, you will feel better and look better.

We all have something we can do to improve ourselves. Mark Twain tells of a doctor at the bedside of a very sick, elderly lady. The doctor told her that she must stop drinking, cussing, and smoking. The lady said that she'd never done any of those things in her entire life. The doctor responded, "Well, that's your problem, then. You've neglected your habits." Twain added: "She was like a sinking ship with no freight to throw overboard."

What are your bad habits? What is keeping you from feeling better? Below is a list of common bad habits that may be scuttling your health. Go through this list and see what freight you can drop overboard.

- **Smoking**—Smoking kills over 400,000 Americans each year. Each one of those deaths is completely preventable. This is, in my opinion, the most detrimental thing you can do to your body. Stop smoking today.
- **Alcohol**—Alcohol, even in moderation, damages brain and body cells. Alcoholic beverages generally contain chemical additives as well; most suicides are alcohol related. Skip the booze.
- **Lack of Sleep**—Sleep deprivation makes any problem worse. There's rarely any real need to stay up late. Turn off that TV and read until you are drowsy. A good sleep

each night beats most vacations for refreshing the body and mind.

- **Chemical Abuse**—Chemical abuse includes overuse of prescription drugs as well as addiction to street drugs. Excessive use of over-the-counter medicines is another, though less obvious, form of chemical abuse. Headaches are not caused by aspirin deficiency, nor are digestive problems due to insufficient antacids in your diet. Look for the real cause of illness; it's staring back at you from your dinner plate.

- **Obesity**—Overweight by more than 20 percent? Most of us are. You can expect many more health problems, including heart attack, high blood pressure, diabetes, cancer, sleep apnea, and arthritis, not to mention a shorter life. If you travel overseas, try playing "Spot the Americans": they are usually the most overweight people in sight. Lose that excess weight!

- **Caffeine**—Drinking coffee is not harmless. If you "have to have your morning cup of coffee," then you are dependent on caffeine, which is a stimulant drug. In some people, even moderate caffeine use causes sleep disorders, heart arrhythmia, and symptoms that closely resemble bipolar disorder.

- **Chocolate**—Eating chocolate negatively affects more people's moods than you might think, and you may be one of them. Theobromine and other chocolate chemicals may set off what have been called "cerebral allergies" in chocolate-sensitive people, resulting in otherwise unexplainable fits of sleeplessness, anxiety, and rage. Try eating something else instead.

- **Sugar**—Sugar is not your friend. Avoid it and feel better right away. You will notice fewer mood swings. Presently, you will notice the numbers on the bathroom scale go down. In time, you will notice your dental bills go down. But mostly, you will notice that you don't feel as "down."

- **Worry**—Worrying is useless. A one-hundred-year-old lady was once asked to give a single bit of advice to help a person live a long time. She said, "Well, I think that people should not worry: 95 percent of the things we worry about never happen, and the 5 percent that do you can't do much about anyway." Worry, stress, and anxiety are contributing factors to host of health problems.

- **Soft Drinks**—If you are going to drink something, why not have something that is good for you? Carbonated drinks erode tooth enamel (because they contain carbonic and phosphoric acids) and also appear to promote kidney stones.

- **Artificial Sweeteners**—Artificial sweeteners add chemicals instead of sugar to your body. What kind of an improvement is that?
- **Meat**—Eating meat is a tradition, not a necessity. You need protein; you do not need to kill animals to get it.
- **Junk Foods**—Eating junk foods gives you extra calories and gives the big food corporations extra profits. Salt, sugar, and grease are bad for your ticker, blood vessels, and everything else in you as well.
- **Chemicals and Additives in Food**—Are you eating anything with a chemical ingredient that you can't pronounce? Why? Your body is not a chemistry lab! You need to read those food labels more carefully.
- **Overwork**—You may be working too hard. Henry David Thoreau said that, after years of hard work, the farmer really didn't have a farm, the farm had him. We should work to live, not live to work.
- **Not Chewing Your Food Properly**—Not chewing food results in an enormous variety of health problems, ranging from simple indigestion to chronic acid reflux. We are not wolves; slow down.
- **Constipation**—Constipation turns your body into a plugged sewer. Eating a raw food diet, one-half cup of molasses, or a can of sauerkraut will put an end to it.

- **Eating Too Fast**—Hurrying your meals almost guarantees poor digestion. Put on some music and relax and forget those high-pressure business lunches.

REDUCING THE AMOUNT OF DRUGS IN YOUR LIFE

The best doctor gives the least medicines.
—BENJAMIN FRANKLIN

Another way to put that is, "The best patient *needs* the least medicines." Anything that you can do to be healthier is likely to reduce the number and amount of drugs that your doctor prescribes for you. A good doctor is certainly willing to see that you are taking as little medication as possible.

All drugs carry a risk of side effects, so reducing your dependence on pharmaceuticals as much as practicable can help you avoid unnecessary suffering. You could say that everything in life carries some risk. You could, but that would obscure the real point that drugs carry a higher-than-average risk, and they are regularly used by a large number of people.

Vitamin supplements have an especially high margin for error; drugs do not. The biggest reason drugs require a prescription is because they are dangerous. Doctors and pharmacists try to carefully figure just how much of the medicine you can take without excessive danger. The information that they rely on is generally provided for them by the drug manufacturer. You might find this information in a leaflet included inside the box with your prescription. You will also find this information in the *Physicians' Desk Reference (PDR),* which is available at bookstores, pharmacies, and libraries. The PDR is basically a three-thousand-page "who's who" of every drug. Inside of the *PDR* you will find drugs classified under type, generic name, and brand name. It is easy to look up any drug that you or a family member takes. Be ready for some unpleasant reading—most drugs have many more precautions than uses; that is, more dangers than benefits.

Then why are drugs still used? Several hundred years of medical tradition is one reason. Physician unfamiliarity with therapeutic nutrition is another. Money—multibillion-dollar drug company money—is another. Pick your reason and consider another: Patients accept drug therapy, with the risks and the side effects. Patients practically demand a wonder drug. Saying "Cure me, doc" puts the physician on the spot. She has to do something, and since her background is in drugs and surgery, that's what she selects from. If the only tool you have is a hammer, you tend to see every problem as a nail.

What can you do, then, to reduce the potential harm from taking drugs?

- Ask the doctor to fully explain the risks and side effects of the drug. Then, ask for justification as to why you should let your body take those risks. If you do not get a full and straight answer, or if the doctor is "too busy" to discuss this with you, then it is time for a new doctor.
- Ask for the absolute minimum possible dose.
- Consult your doctor right away if there are any negative effects of the medication.
- Ask for an alternative instead of the drug. Some doctors are happy to work with interested patients who want to avoid medicines when they can. If your doctor is not interested, then you can find a doctor who is.

If you are already taking a medication, consider the following steps:

1. I really do *not* think it is a good idea to suddenly stop taking medication. This is especially true if you are taking something more than a pain-reliever or other nonessential drug.
2. Inform the doctor that you are interested in getting off your medicine. If that is not realistic, then tell the doctor that you

would like to gradually decrease the amount that you have to take.

3. It is best to work with the physician who prescribed the drug for you in the first place. After all, the doctor that put you on the medicine should be the one involved with taking you off of it. The doctor should give you a schedule to follow that gradually reduces your drug dose.

4. If the doctor wants to see you for monitoring your progress, then do it. That's only fair, plus it provides you with documented evidence that you are succeeding without taking the medicine.

5. If your doctor believes that you cannot reduce the level of your medication at all, you can honor that viewpoint without agreeing with it. A second medical opinion might be in order next. If you find a whole string of doctors saying, "Don't you dare stop taking your so-and-so," then you need to stop and do some serious reconsideration. Some people will then begin on their own to reduce or eliminate their medicines. No doctor is so naive as to think this doesn't happen. It is an individual's right, and an individual's risk, to do so. I cannot recommend it.

Drugs and surgery are options that do exist and should be considered. They are widely regarded as severe measures, though, and may not be necessary for your well-being. If proper nutrition and healthy living bring you good health, there is no need for medication. A prescription too often represents a guess; a guess with a risk of potentially serious side effects.

Therapeutic nutrition is a serious option, and a safer one too. Ask for it, or better still, insist on it.

A HEALTHIER (AND CHEAPER) DIET

Nothing will benefit human health and increase the chances for survival of life on Earth as much as the evolution to a vegetarian diet.
—ALBERT EINSTEIN

When in doubt, eat like a gorilla. Gorillas are very strong, very smart, and very vegetarian. The strongest and longest-lived animals are all vegetarians. You may think that the lion is "king of the jungle," but lions get out of the way of passing vegetarian rhinos and elephants. And vegetarian tortoises live up to 150 years. Vegetarian animals do not get excess protein, fat, or sugar. Humans pig out on all three.

- The average American eats enough fat every day to very nearly equal a stick of butter. Ugh!
- Sugar is the number-one cause of tooth decay. The level of sugar consumption at which most of the population will not get dental caries is 33 pounds (15 kilograms per person per year; the average American eats over 120 pounds annually).[1]
- Americans consume two to three times as much protein as they need. Worldwide, 30–40 grams of protein daily is usually considered adequate. The U.S. government recommends about 60 grams of protein a day for a man and about 50 grams daily for a woman. We generally eat over 100—or even as much as 120—grams of protein daily, mostly derived from meat. High-protein dieting is unwise. Chronic protein excess overloads and irreversibly damages the kidneys by middle age.[2]
- Cornell University's extensive nutrition studies in China have shown that people eating little or no animal protein are less likely to get cancer or heart disease. "These diets are much different from the average American diets, containing only about 0 to 20 percent animal-based foods, while the average American diet is com-prised of about 60 to 80 percent animal-

based foods. Disease patterns in much of rural China tend to reflect those prior to the industrial revolution in the U.S., when cancers and cardiovascular diseases were much less prevalent."[3]

This is a well-studied problem and we have a serious solution right at hand—the near-vegetarian diet. We are in error and need to change our way of eating. If we don't, we are going against Nature and sooner or later it will catch up with us.

By moving toward a vegetarian diet, you automatically reduce your high intake of protein, fat, and sugar. It is just that simple. There is no diet plan to buy. I think dairy products and eggs and fish must remain occasional options for most of us. One reason is that the healthiest, so-called "primitive" cultures tend to eat *some* animal products. Also, my kids did so well as lacto-ovo-vegetarians (eating dairy and egg products) that they never had an antibiotic. Nope, not even one dose. Plus, I'm a realist and know that more people will be willing to live for decades as near-vegetarians rather than as strict ones. I will compromise with anyone, if it will help them be healthier.

In addition to being healthy, high-fiber, low-fat foods are among the least expensive in the supermarket and the least labor-intensive to prepare. Opening a can of beans is a perfect example. They are precooked, loaded with fiber, the amount of fat is almost microscopic, and nothing could be cheaper to buy. Beans (including peas and lentils) also contain many beneficial plant compounds that fight cancer.[4]

Another example of a cheap, versatile food is rice. I'd like to read you your rice. You have the rice to remain silent. And you have a lot of nutrition in good old brown rice. Of course, rice is extremely low in fat and is a great source of complex carbohydrates, which are good for balancing blood sugar levels. But there's more: brown rice is surprisingly high in protein, fiber, B vitamins, and trace minerals. It is versatile, tasty, and sells for about fifty cents a pound.

Rice is actually a "complete" vegetable protein, for it contains all ten of the essential amino acids. It is not quite a "perfect" protein, for it has only small amounts of histadine and tryptophan. But rice added to practically anything else makes for a nutritionally complete meal.

Here are some hints if you are not yet a rice fan:

1. Go to a good Chinese restaurant and have rice as it should be cooked. Okay, it's probably going to be white rice, but that's close enough for starters and it will help you to appreciate how tasty rice can be when correctly prepared.

2. Try rice flour pancakes. Any health food store has, or can order, some rice flour. Rice flour pancakes are great for kids, especially really little kids. In fact, a finely minced and thoroughly cooked rice cereal is a preferred first solid food for babies. But all ages love rice flour pancakes.

3. If you are sensitive to wheat products, try rice. It is the ultimate hypoallergenic food.

4. If you must hurry a meal, make it rice, as it is easy to digest. Sure, it takes time to cook it or you can try Chinese take-out. Forget the fried foods. Forget the sugar drinks. Don't eat a McNothing meal when you can have no-fat, fresh, stir-fried vegetables in a yummy sauce, and plenty of rice.

The fact is if people ate more simply, they'd be more healthy. I sometimes go for six weeks without grocery shopping. I live out of my garden, fresh picked or from last year's haul in my freezer. Cheese and yogurt keep for weeks. If refrigerated, so do nuts and seeds. Rice, lentils, dried peas, and dried beans keep for years.

None of this stuff is expensive, and none of it is complicated. I have not seen my doctor for so long that if I passed him on the street, I wouldn't know him. Yes, I'll see him if I need to and, yes, I do have the occasional physical to tell me how I'm doing. But the *Fire Your*

Doctor! secret is not that you don't have a doctor, it's that you do not *need* your doctor.

THE FIRE YOUR DOCTOR! INSTANT HEALTH CLASS

There are a number of steps you can take immediately to improve your health.

- Encourage someone you know to stop smoking. Tobacco kills more Americans in one year than all U.S. soldiers killed in World War II. Nine out of ten smokers say they'd like to quit. Nine out of ten who have quit simply stopped smoking—no meetings, no techniques, no products; they just stopped.
- Regularly practice an organized form of stress reduction. From meditation to yoga to music to prayer, you have much good to gain (and much tension to lose) by taking some time to let it all go and center yourself. I've meditated twice a day for decades and it's been time well spent. People who de-stress daily have greatly reduced risk of heart disease, cancer, nervous disorders, and mental illness. They also have fewer hospital admissions and require fewer visits to the doctor.[5]
- Eat less fat. Better still, eat less meat. Even lean meat is 10 percent or more saturated fat. Vegetarians have far less cancer and

heart disease. Dean Ornish, M.D., put patients on a vegetarian diet and stress-reduction program with exercise: his patients *reversed* heart disease in one year. There are over 12 million vegetarians in America. Join up today! Learn by doing and see how much better you feel.

- Lose excess weight effortlessly by vegetable-juice fasting. It is easy and it works. Vegetables are low calorie and very nutritious. If you don't want to juice them, just eat them as salad. You can't hurt yourself with produce, and you can't get fat on it, either. It is simple to learn and to do.

- America is constipated, and this is no joke. The average American gets only about 10 grams of fiber daily. A vegetarian gets 50 grams or more. Meat has no fiber whatsoever. More fiber reduces the risk of bowel cancer as well as colitis, diverticulitis, spastic colon, and hemorrhoids. Give a diabetic more dietary fiber and she will require less insulin. No need to buy fiber in a jar—eat a diet largely consisting of salads and raw vegetables to guarantee a good supply. That's what gorillas do, and you'll never meet a constipated gorilla.

- The less you spend on food, the healthier your diet is likely to be. Packaged, processed, and pricey foods are the least nutritious. Read the label and marvel at the wonderful ways chemistry is used nowadays. You can eliminate those additives, save money, and eat better by avoiding 95 percent of what is in a supermarket. Buy rice, beans, nuts, yogurt, fresh produce, and check out.

- My family of four spent way less than half of what most families pay to eat. Remember that the protein in dairy products is just as good as meat protein. Any grain plus any legume (peas, beans, and lentils) together make a complete protein that is equivalent to meat. It is difficult to believe that you can be healthier and save money doing it. An even bigger surprise awaits you: simple, real-food-meals taste better as well.

- If you don't have the money or the time to go to medical school, you tend to become way too dependent on the pronouncements of a doctor. Medical education is not for the privileged few. Obtain a copy of the *Merck Manual,* the "Cliff Notes" of medical school: nearly everything most doctors do is in this single volume. To assist with any deciphering of medical terms, have a good medical dictionary handy, such as *Taber's Cyclopedic Medical Dictionary.* For a second opinion, it is wise to read books on natural healing. Alternative health techniques are well proven and nonprescription. A health food store, library, or bookstore will have many titles to help you.

These books elevate your health education to a whole new level of confidence and competency. You don't have to know everything. You can still go to the doctor, but now you can better judge the value of medical services rendered. Remember that your doctor works for you and not the other way around. Getting a doctor's opinion does not mean you have to follow it. It is your body, and how you want a health concern handled is your decision. You can only make a good decision if you are fully informed. Knowledge is power, and health knowledge is healing power.

CHEAP, HEALTHY EXERCISE

I'd like to interest you in becoming a budget behemoth through weight training. This is all you need to do:

1. Put up about sixty dollars and buy a cheap set of cast-iron weights. You can even go cheaper, with sand-filled vinyl weights, but cast iron doesn't break.

2. Take an old pair of leather gloves and cut the fingers off. There, you have weight-lifting gloves (or you can buy a pair for less than ten dollars).

3. For lifting advice, watch one of those fitness programs on TV or borrow a video from your library. Here is their advice, condensed:

a) Start with a really small, almost ridiculously easy amount of weight.

b) Do ten to twenty repetitions (reps) each of curls and squats.

   • Curls—Hold the weight bar in front of you, knuckles out. The palms can be up or down; try some each way. Draw the bar up near your shoulders, slowly, and then let it slowly down.

   • Squats—Squats involve putting the bar on your shoulders, behind your neck. Keeping your back straight, bend your knees, and squat down. Then push back up. It is best to have a "spotter" (stand-by helper) for assistance in lifting the bar off when you are done.

c) Increase your weight only when you hardly notice the increase at all. Gradually increase the number of reps and slowly add weight week by week. Rest between sets of each exercise. These steps help eliminate any chance of injury.

d) Do your full workout every other day. "Off" days reduce strain and soreness that might come from over-training.

e) It is beneficial to stretch before your workout. Put on some music too. Music you like will improve your mood, give you a good beat, and you will appreciate how quickly the workout time passes.

f) Do some push-ups and some crunches (abbreviated sit-ups) every day.

g) Hold a long broom handle behind your neck and on your shoulders, with one hand grabbing near each end. Stand, leaning forward about thirty degrees, with both knees slightly bent. Twist to each side, trying to pass the middle with each swing of the broom handle. You can move the handle down your back to exercise different muscles. This is also a great way to trim down while watching TV. Give it a try for even 5–10 minutes, twice a day, and watch what happens to your waistline. Don't like exercise? Me neither, but do it anyway.

FAST RELIEF FROM MALAISE

You can feel it coming: the blahs, the dull headache, the achy body, the weakness, the get-up-and-go that got up and went. Maybe you feel a chill or sneeze a few times. It is often called the "malaise" of approaching, encroaching illness. When you detect it, it is time to do three things.

First, you can thank your body for working correctly. Symptoms are hardly an unmitigated delight, but they are as valuable as stop signs are to a motorist. Just as we need to know when we are sitting on a hot stove, we also need to know when our resistance is down and sickness is imminent. Pay attention. Symptoms are advance notice and should be heeded promptly. The second-best way to deal with illness is to deal with it in its earliest stage (better still is prevention).

The moment you feel the malaise, you should take a teaspoon or two of vitamin C powder. That is known as a "loading dose," and it is a very powerful immune-booster and detoxification tool. Even that much vitamin C is easily buffered with a meal, snack, or calcium-magnesium tablet. Rinse your mouth with water after drinking an unbuffered vitamin C solution. Even unbuffered, a good strong solution of ascorbic acid is no more acidic than Coca Cola.

Why does vitamin C need to be taken immediately and why in such high quantity? Vitamin C builds the immune system. In high doses, it kills viruses and even cancer cells, without harming normal body cells.[6] And vitamin C is an extraordinary antitoxin, partly because it is a free-radical scavenger and partly because it has a laxative effect. It therefore well serves the naturopathic purpose of "cleaning you out." If all this "toxin" stuff seems like nonsense, it is time to call in two experienced medical doctors.

In his book *Vitamin C, Infectious Diseases, and Toxins,* Thomas E. Levy, M.D., specifically focuses on vitamin C as an antitoxin. The effects of alcohol, barbiturates, carbon monoxide, cyanide, a variety of environmental poisons including pesticides, and even acetaminophen poisoning in cats, as well as mushroom poisoning and snake venoms, are all shown to respond to vitamin-C megadose therapy. The effects of mercury, lead, and radiation are also alleviated by vitamin C. "The three most important considerations in effective vitamin C therapy are 'dose, dose, and dose'," states Dr. Levy. "If you don't take enough, you won't get the desired effects."[7]

Robert F. Cathcart, M.D., has been treating patients with high doses of vitamin C for thirty-five years. "The reason ascorbate ameliorates so many conditions is that it functions as the premiere free-radical scavenger," states Dr. Cathcart. "This function is not because it is the most powerful free-radical scavenger, but because it is possible to saturate every cell of the body with more molecules of ascorbate than any other free-radical scavenger. The reason it takes such massive doses is because high concentrations of ascorbate must be driven into the cells affected by the disease process sufficient to neutralize all of the free radicals. This premiere free-radical scavenger function has little to do with nutrition but is a pharmacologic effect."[8]

Vitamin C taken immediately knocks out an oncoming cold, flu, or grippe in a matter of hours. I have seen this so many times that I have lost count. Critics of this method, and the studies they try to cite, invariably make one fundamental error: they use too little vitamin C to do the job.

If you do not want to take megadoses of vitamin C, you can fall back on a tried-and-true alternative—get out your juicer and use it. Begin a vegetable juice fast and you will feel better and heal sooner. Personally, I recommend both: veggie juices and vitamin C together, because people who drink a lot of fresh vegetable juice need less vitamin C to feel better. If you will not juice, then take vitamin C to saturation or bowel tolerance.

And what is the best all-around exercise program? The one you will regularly do. I have heard a lot of excuses for not exercising, and I don't care about any of them. The only reason to work out is this: you want to feel and look better.

It is wise to check with your doctor before beginning any exercise program. Your doctor will probably be very pleased that you are willing to work at your health by working out.

CHEAPSKATE OUTDOOR EXERCISE HINTS

Some people buy expensive athletic footwear. Here is how to get all the benefits of exercise on a shoestring.

1. Adopt a dog. Even if you don't like to exercise, dogs like to. Here's an excuse to walk, jog, or run: blame the dog. A dog has to go out several times daily; it's automatic exercise for both of you.

2. Buy a pickup truck instead of a car. All your friends will want you to help them move. Guaranteed weight-lifting opportunities await you, not to mention how alluring trucks can be to the opposite sex.

3. Better yet, don't have a vehicle at all. Two bags of groceries looks like nothing, until you have to carry them home.
4. Always choose a house on top of a hill or choose a top floor apartment. It is quieter and you have daily exercise on the stairs.
5. Many couples already know that making love can be good aerobic exercise. (Whoops! Did I say these were outdoor exercise hints?)
6. Start a garden. Turn over the soil by hand (yes, using a shovel) and you will get real exercise. Then the planting, weeding, watering, and harvesting activities are also good exercise.
7. Get a wood-burning stove. Not only will you likely save money heating with wood, but you will get exercise in supplying the stove with the wood it burns. Henry David Thoreau said that wood warms us three times: once in cutting it and hauling it in, once from the heat it provides as it burns, and once more from the warm glow you feel as you watch the fire.

Curiously, many of the above exercise ideas were life's regular activities for our pioneer forefathers and mothers. They did not need health spas and gyms. They got exercise in keeping warm, feeding themselves, and taking care of their family.

I saw a bumper sticker the other day that said, "Ignore your health and it will go away." Health is a lifestyle, lifestyle is a choice—it is doable, and you can do it.

LET'S GET REAL

Most people who want to can and will improve their health given the information, motivation, and opportunity to do so. But you won't always be perfect in adopting a new health regimen, so give yourself a break. Be realistic in your expectations. Here are some hints for sticking with the program:

1. Daily health progress may fluctuate or plateau; just relax and stay with it. Sometimes it is useful to be reminded that "We are not in a hurry. After all, how long did it take to get in this condition in the first place?"

2. People may lose confidence in their ability to break a habit or lose confidence in getting better. They may quit. That's okay. Just restart yourself, like you do your computer. If you fall off the wagon, hey, who hasn't? We've all been there. Climb back on.

3. You might wish to keep this thought in mind: I'd rather you do half of what this

book offers for a decade than do all of it for a week.

4. On the road to self-reliance, family support is nice to have, but neither require it nor count on it. To fire your doctor, you simply must take an honest look at yourself and look inward. If there is anything more profound than the task of making lifestyle and diet changes, I do not know what it could be. Consistently walking the walk is always harder than occasionally talking the talk. That's why we have to be realists and, with our friends and relatives, moderates.

5. Can you stay well while eating wrong? Probably not, but you can cut your losses with intelligent supplementation. For those days when you are a junk food junkie, broiling the beef and chowing down the candy, well, here are some utterly shame-less ultramoderate hints to help you stay well even if you and yours are bound and determined to eat wrong now and again.

• If you are going to overindulge on dairy products, especially milk and ice cream, be certain to drink a lot more water. You'll experience less congestion, breathe easier, and, if you are dairy sensitive, have fewer headaches. If headaches persist, knock off the dairy completely.

- If you are going to eat sugary desserts and candy, be sure you take chromium, niacin, and the B-complex vitamins.
- If you are going to drink alcohol, take a lot of extra vitamin C and the B-complex vitamins. And please let someone else drive.
- If you are going to drink caffeine, take extra niacin and B vitamins.
- If you are going to eat fried or fatty foods, eat a couple of tablespoons of lecithin granules with them.
- If you are going to eat meat, chew it thoroughly and eat extra salads, beans, and other major fiber sources.
- If you are going to eat processed foods, then at least drink a lot of water and take a lot of vitamin C.
- If you are going to eat late in the evening, chew your food extra well, take multiple digestive enzymes, and eat papaya, mangos, kiwi fruits, figs, or fresh pineapple (all of which contain enzymes) along with your snack attack.
- If you are going to eat too much in general, then get off your duff and exercise (work out and walk).
- And, finally, if you will not exercise, then at least eat less.

To be a successful health homesteader, you need to be an extremist, but moderately so. This does not so much mean, "In all things, moderation," as it means, "In unimportant things, flexibility." Hold to what is important: eating right pretty much every day; exercising regularly; taking supplements; avoiding chemical additives and pesticides; reading, learning and seeing for yourself; and especially, taking charge of your own health. Stick to the main points; compromise on the minor points. Health is and always will be about balanced living.

Three Steps to Health

Disease is the censor pointing out the humans, animals and plants who are imperfectly nourished.
—G.T. WRENCH, *THE WHEEL OF HEALTH*

You cannot mistreat your body for twenty, fifty, or seventy years, and then expect a doctor to give you a wonder drug to cure your ills. You cannot expect that any more than you could drive your car recklessly, missing stoplights and breaking speed limits for years, and expect the judge to let you off. There is only one basic cause of disease and that is unhealthful living. Unhealthful living leads to un-health; this is so simple as to be routinely overlooked. How, then, can we help nature and help ourselves? It's easier than you might think. Here are three basic steps you can take for better health.

STEP ONE: STOP EATING MEAT

"I thought you said it was easy!" you might be thinking. "I like steaks, chops, and hamburgers." Maybe you do, but perhaps you are just accustomed to the seasonings, condiments, and habitual eating of the muscles of dead animals (and that's what meat is). After all, you were probably raised on meats. Most of us are; just check the baby food shelves at the supermarket and see the jars of processed meat that children are given before they have a chance to say "no." It's because we think, or believe, that meat is a good thing to eat.

However, humans do not have a carnivore's anatomy. A meat-eating (carnivorous) animal has sharp ripping-and-tearing teeth, like a cat's. Ever put your finger in a cat's mouth? Twice? A meat-eating animal does not have to cook, tenderize, and employ a steak knife to eat its meat. A meat-eating animal invariably eats its food raw and eats the internal organs of its prey, especially the brains, liver, and intestines. The first thing a lion does with its kill is open the belly and start eating there. Steaks, roasts, and chops are only the muscles of a dead animal and that's all that most people care for.

A meat-eating animal has a short digestive tract, about twice the length of its body. A vegetarian animal has a digestive tract about four times the length of its body. A longer digestive tract gives the vegetarian animal's system a chance to more fully utilize plant material, with the help of beneficial bacteria that help break it down.

Where do humans fit in? First of all, our total intestinal length is about 20–25 feet, roughly four times our body length. That's good for plant-fruit-vegetable digestion but not good for meat digestion. Meat will putrefy more easily in such a long digestive tract. That is a probable cause of constipation, diverticulitis, and perhaps worse in humans. Diabetes, heart disease, and cancer have all been clearly linked to constipation.

Second, we have to cook, tenderize, and cut up meat because we have a vegetarian's dental structure. Human teeth are mostly blunt grinding teeth for getting the most out of grains, vegetables, and fruits. Even our sharpest cutting teeth (incisors) in front are blunt compared to a dog's or cat's teeth.

Finally, we do not eat the whole animal. Farley Mowat, naturalist and author of *Never Cry Wolf,* observed wolves in northern Canada for months and discovered that through much of the year they feed on mice. It seemed so hard to believe that a large wolf could subsist on such small prey that Mowat also started to live on mouse meat. The diet of mouse meat seemed all right for him at first, but he developed a tremendous craving for fat, among other things. He then realized that he was not doing exactly as the wolves did: the wolves ate the whole mouse. Mowat began to do the same, eating the entire mouse, except for the fur and tail, and subsisted happily thereafter. Now a whole mouse means bones, brains, abdominal organs, skin and all that they contain: calcium, phosphorus, potassium, lecithin, fat, trace minerals, and the mouse's last meal of partially digested vegetation. That is a genuine meat-eater's meal. It is a far cry from a processed, cut-up, cooked, chemically treated, flavored, tenderized, steak-sauced, parsley-garnished slab of dead muscle that we call "steak."

If we ate the whole cow, the entire pig, or the complete chicken, we would be getting what natural meat eaters get in their diet. Also, we wouldn't be wasting two-thirds of the slaughtered animal that we waste now in butchering it. But the very thought of eating all an animal's innards repulses us and indicates a hidden revulsion to killing and gore, and therefore to eating meat the way it truly is.

American meat contains chemical, hormone, and antibiotic residues, and so much of them that the European Union countries will not buy it. So, we sell it to our own people. When I worked on a dairy farm, I saw healthy milking cows that got infection symptoms and were loaded up with penicillin and other antibiotics. These cows were always taken out of the milking line to avoid contamination from the milk. However, if the cow's health continued to fail, under the continued administration of literally millions of units of antibiotics, then the cow was sold at auction. The next stop would be the meat factory.

At least five days were supposed to be allowed from the time of the last drug dose to the time of the slaughter. But is five days, or even five weeks, enough time to get the residual antibiotics out of the animal's system? No. Most of the drug would be excreted, but not all. After five days, 3 to 5 percent of the antibiotic would remain in the cow's system. I personally administered individual doses of 2 million units of antibiotic to very sick cows. Three percent of 2 million is 60,000 units or so of residual penicillin. You can't tell me that some of that wouldn't be in the meat, cooked or not.

As if antibiotics weren't enough, there are even more chemicals added to our meat supply. Cold cuts, canned meats, and most hot dogs contain fillers, fat, salt, and nitrites. Sodium nitrite is a more potent preservative than sodium nitrate. It is a chemical sister to potassium nitrate, known as saltpeter. Saltpeter was given to soldiers to restrain their amorous proclivities while on liberty; in other words, it is a sterilizing agent. It's difficult not to chuckle when someone says, in a deep booming voice, "I'm a meat-and-potatoes man!" If we think that eating meat makes us virile, we've fallen for the same falsehood that leads some to think that smoking is glamorous or that drinking is cool. How can embalmed animal tissue, loaded with chemical odds and ends, possibly contribute to the quality of life?

Fresh meat will last in a refrigerator for perhaps a week; this assumes no additives and a temperature of about 40°F. Keeping this in mind, check the "freshness" or expiration date on a package of bologna, salami, or other refrigerated cold cuts: the shelf life of cold cuts is usually many weeks and may run into months. Same with bacon. For a meat product to last weeks and weeks, the meat literally has to be embalmed.

There is, of course, a simple solution to the food-preservative, food-additive, food-color, and food-chemical problem: simply do not buy, and do not eat, any food that contains any preservative, additive, color, or chemical. That will help tremendously to reduce the 10 pounds of chemicals that the average, FDA-reassured American eats each year.

In case you don't think that there will be any foods left after you reject the adulterated ones, let me suggest a trip to the health food store, a public market, food co-op, or organic garden supply store. You can even get a lot of good, everyday, additive-free foods at the supermarket. Just read the label and if you can't pronounce it, don't eat it and don't buy it. This "voting with your dollars" will do more to get additive-free foods on the shelves than just about anything else you can do.

STEP TWO: EAT WHOLE, NATURAL FOODS

People continue to ask, "If we don't eat meat, then what will we eat?" The answer is everything else, basically: vegetables, grains, fruits, nuts, salads, cheese, ice cream (if you must), yogurt, berries, juices, breads, pasta, beans, mushrooms, soups, nuts, healthy snacks, and homemade desserts—do I have to go on? The list is as long as Mother Earth's supply of whole, life-supporting harvest.

"What about getting complete protein, like in meat?" one may ask. Here's the answer, and it's important and easy to remember: corn, beans, and squash together form a complete protein. The amino acids provided by these three foods are fully equivalent to those from meat.

You should have a serving or more of these each day, preferably at the same meal. Now this can include any form of corn, beans, and squash. For example, cornbread, corn muffins, corn chips, corn-on-the-cob, corn relish, corn fritters, corn tortilla shells, corn in soups or vegetable stews, even corn flakes; these are all corn. Beans may be baked, refried, in three-bean salad, green beans, yellow beans, lima beans, pinto beans, kidney beans, chickpeas (garbanzos), and also peas, pea soup, lentils, and all other legumes. Squash may be fried, steamed, or baked, like in pumpkin pie, pumpkin bread, or zucchini bread. Summer squash can be sliced into soups or casseroles; eat winter squash like you would mashed potatoes. Corn, beans, and squash together in one dish makes succotash, one of the most nutritious, filling, and low-calorie dishes there is.

Additional meat alternatives include high-protein combos such as brown rice and practically anything served to accompany it; nuts with greens in a salad; and cheese with whole grains. If you really crave a steak or a burger, try these first and see if you are still hungry. "Vegetables just don't fill me" is a common complaint of the prospective vegetarian. In most cases, the person saying this has not eaten a balanced (corn-beans-squash) meal. Perhaps you've been brought up on mostly meat-and-potato meals and other foods are not a big part of your menu. There's no problem there, for your appetite is just bored. Your tastes will expand as you depend less on meat to fill you.

"Vegetarian dishes are tasteless and bland" is another groundless but often heard comment. That's only if you choose to prepare and eat bland and tasteless dishes. It all depends on how the foods are prepared. (Remember, an inept cook can just as easily ruin a good steak or wreck a lobster.) Good, whole, fresh foods prepared with simple care are appetizing and attractive. The more you eat them, the more your real, dormant appetite will be aroused again for the foods that you need the most and enjoy the best. Condiments, artificial flavors, salt, sugar, and spices are a big part of the flavor that people are used to, and often these are the flavors we seek when we elect to eat meat.

If you make vegetarian pea soup and add some ground cloves and a little vegetable oil, you will taste the "ham" that isn't there. Add some chopped pineapple to baked beans and again you might look for pork that isn't there. For ideas, recipes, and all-important confidence in cooking, there are fortunately many excellent vegetarian cookbooks, available at any book-seller or library. I personally like the *Deaf Smith Country Cookbook: Natural Foods for Natural Kitchens* by M.W. Ford, S. Hillyard, and M.F. Koock (Avery, 1991).

It is easy to cook without meat. *You just don't buy it.* Good diet starts at the checkout.

You cannot eat what you do not have. Don't let an obsolete meat habit keep you from something you truly like to eat that your body likes, too. When they try them, most people really enjoy whole, natural foods. I often have people tell me that they feel they could practically live on fruit or feel they could be happy eating just salads. Those are foods they love, but they rarely eat them! Why? If you would feel better after having a salad for lunch rather than a burger and fries, why not have the salad? Are you a person who rushes into the fast food restaurant feeling good and hungry and strolls out feeling a little worse, bloated, and stuffy? Why persist in eating things that don't make you feel good? Maybe it's all the advertising; maybe it's time and convenience; maybe it's because of never trying anything different.

Whole, good foods are very rarely advertised—there's no need to advertise really valuable products, for they sell themselves. Lettuce, peaches, carrots, sprouts, beans: when's the last time you saw ads for these? It's the junk food that is heavily promoted coast to coast and all the time. My mother told my brothers and me from an early age that if we saw it on TV, we probably didn't need it. *The advertising of a given food product will be inversely proportionate to its nutritional value.*

Or, the more it's pushed, the less your body needs it.

Nature produces a food from the first bud cells or seeds to its final, ready-to-eat form. Commercial food processors come in at the last steps of a food's development and purposely interfere with it. This interference may be removing part (or most) of what makes a food of value in the first place. For example, whole wheat has been a staple food for millions of people over thousands of years. They would eat the wheat grains without cooking or grind the grain into wheat flour for baking. Whole wheat made bread the "staff of life" and real whole-wheat bread still is; even store-bought whole-wheat bread has 15 to 20 percent of your daily protein requirement in just four slices. Today's commercial, spongy white bread would not be called the "staff of life" by anyone with common sense. That's because it's made with bleached white flour, which is so incapable of supporting life that even ants, bugs, and mold can't live on it.

White flour is basically nothing but starch—it has great baking qualities and almost zero nutritional value. That's why it is "enriched" with a few synthetic vitamins so the big baking companies can at least say something on the label under "Nutrition Information." White flour once started out as whole-wheat flour, which is just ground-up wheat grains. But whole-wheat flour is a nutritious food, and like any other nutritious food, it will support life. That is why it doesn't keep that well: the wheat germ is loaded with vitamins, minerals, enzymes, and oil that will spoil if not consumed within a fairly short time. For miller, baker, wholesaler, and storekeeper to get any kind of shelf life out of their flour, these nutritious but perishable food factors need to be removed. That is exactly what milling does. The wheat bran and germ are removed in the milling process and uniform, easily stored white flour remains. As if that isn't enough, the flour is bleached chemically to ensure a pure white color. Then chemical preservatives are added to bread on top of all that. Whew!

This is an example of fairly intense food processing. Things are taken away (bran, germ, oil) and something is added (bleach) to fashion a commercially useful substance from what started out as simple, nutritious whole food. Similar things are done to corn when it is made into cornmeal or cornflakes. Cornstarch is analogous to white flour. Rice is "polished" to make it white and pretty, and pretty valueless nutritionally. Sure, the rice grain's hull has to come off, like the shell of a seed, but rice "polishing" goes further and mills off the rice's outer layer, including the high-protein, high-vitamin germ. White rice is the result, and it stores a long time. But it doesn't support life much better than white flour. Millions of people worldwide live on rice, but the healthy ones live on whole grain rice.

We can take a highly processed or refined substance and add to it all the vitamins, minerals, and other factors recognized as important to good nutrition and still not have a food as good as nature makes it. Why? Because we can put back what we know we took out, but *we can't possibly put back what we don't know we took out.* The "enriching" process is only as good as our limited ability to analyze what a food contains. How can government scientists decide that only certain minerals and vitamins should be added to bread? We may think that individual food factors are important to health and life; nature knows what factors are important, or they wouldn't be there in the first place. For that matter, neither would we. That's why we should eat whole, natural foods.

STEP THREE: A CLEANSING FAST

Eating is one side of the coin; proper elimination is the other. Your body, like an automobile engine, consumes its fuel (food and air) and also produces exhaust wastes (carbon dioxide, urine, sweat). Quite a few organs in the body are involved in filtering, reclaiming, and excreting waste materials. These organs include the kidneys, lungs, liver, colon, spleen, bladder, and skin, your body's largest organ. If these organs of excretion are "clogged up" by years of junk foods, meat eating, food chemicals, additives, cosmetics, liquor, smoking, being overweight, vitamin deficiencies, and chronic stress, they will surely not be functioning properly.

You know what a "backed-up" septic tank or sewer system can do to a home. A backed-up bowel does the same to a body; so does a toxin-filled liver or an overworked kidney, or a cosmetic-covered, antiperspirant-coated skin. If the body wastes don't get out, they stay in. Naturopaths believe that this is the basic cause of all mankind's various illnesses: the polluted body or systemic toxemia.

A cleansing fast means not eating for a meal, a day, or a week. The longer the fast, the more detoxification the body can accomplish in that time. Naturopathic theory holds that considerable body energy goes into digestion, and if you rest the digestive process for a while, energy can go into internal healing.

Fasting a sick body is just as sensible as not putting any more gasoline into a burning automobile. First put the fire out, then repair the car, then fuel it up again. In the human body, the fast puts out the fire: fasting is known to eliminate fever, inflammation, infection, and other symptoms from the inside out. "From the inside out" means that fasting breaks down and eliminates the diseased tissues that are the root cause of the symptoms. The repair work is done naturally and thoroughly by the body. When the repair is done, then it's time to eat again, and eat right this time.

Most cleansing fasts need to go for four to seven days. Some people fast for weeks at a time, although generally in nature-cure spas or resorts. Such spas are found all over Europe, but are hard to find in America. For this reason, many people undertake a fast at home, with the aid of careful reading, common sense, and naturopathic advice.

"Won't I starve to death?" one might ask. No, you won't. Most of us eat far more than our bodies require for health. Too much food in a body is like too much wood on a fire: it doesn't get used efficiently. Either it burns quickly and wastefully or it smolders and smokes wastefully; either way, there's a lot of ash left over. This buildup of "ash" forms the grounds for disease. Fasting is the great fireplace clean-out. The right amount of food for most people is far less than they think, which is one of the reasons why the United States has so many overweight people.

If we miss more meals, or days, of eating, we will not starve. The body can go for weeks without food. Marathon walkers trotted all over Europe, covering 300 miles in just ten days, on nothing but water in 1954 and 1964. The doctors that monitored them found that they were just fine.[1]

Right now, there is enough food in your digestive system so that if you ate no more, your alimentary canal (stomach, intestines, and colon) wouldn't be empty for two days. Even then, your reserves of glycogen in the liver will last days longer and you will have fat reserves as well. A person doesn't really begin to starve for weeks, and doesn't really begin to "fast" for at least four days.

You might think that fasting would weaken a person, but the exact opposite is true—fasting strengthens. How strong do you feel right after a roast beef dinner? Pretty stuffed and wanting to just sit are common feelings after a big feed. Now: how do you feel on a camping trip before breakfast? Hungry, certainly, but with the strength, drive, and energy to gather wood, make a fire, and cook some pancakes. This is only a mild degree of fasting, but it is invigorating.

A long fast should always be conducted under the supervision of a naturopathically oriented doctor; going to a nature-cure establishment is ideal. However, many people fast over a weekend or for four or five days during the flu, severe colds, or other common ailments without any special arrangements. During a fast, it is important to drink water or vegetable juices regularly. You need to take in quite a lot of fluids because your body excretes fluids in urine and sweat, and balance must be maintained. In fact, you may find that you need extra water or juices during a fast, because your excretory organs are working overtime to clean out your system. Fluids also help flush out bodily wastes and will give you some feeling of "fullness" in your stomach and curb your appetite during the early part of the fast.

It is common to be hungry for the first few missed meals, but as the fast continues, the appetite diminishes. Vegetable juices contain minerals, vitamins, and other trace substances that are good for you and aid in cleansing. Also, the complex carbohydrates in vegetable juices may make work or other activity more comfortable if you are unable to take time off to fast. Some authorities feel that there is no need for consuming anything but water on a fast and that energy and blood sugar levels are not seriously affected by fasting. This probably

varies from person to person, and I would suggest doing whatever is comfortable for you.

Anyone with a medical reason why they should not fast simply should not fast. For example, *fasting is not for pregnant or nursing women, nor is it appropriate for growing children. Check with your doctor before fasting, especially if you are on medication.* Stay in touch with good books, experienced "fasters," and a naturally minded doctor for your first time at it.

Remember also that the hardest meals to miss are the first two or three, and after that it's easier. If you're really sick, it will be easy to miss the first meals, too. The first thing a sick animal does is "go off its feed." That is fasting, and we'd all do well to take our example from nature. Fasting is a great experience, and experience can be a wonderful teacher.

Go Meatless

Here are some good reasons to consider becoming more of a vegetarian:

• **Life Span**—Real meat eating is neither easy nor is it any guarantee of longevity. The cheetah is just about the fastest land predator there is. Fewer than one-half of cheetahs reach adulthood and those that do live only about seven years. Vegetarian elephants and tortoises live between 70 and 150 years.

• **A Close-up Look**—Here's what really did it for me. Back in 1974, when I was in West Africa, I was watching a flock of blood-soaked vultures attack an enormous pile of intestines and skin at an open-air meat market. The sight was horrific; the smell was unforgettable.

• **Mad Cow Disease**—Ever hear of "mad vegetable disease"? Enough said.

• **The Slaughter**—I think I know why all those cows are so mad: we kill 100,000 of them for food every single day, just in the United States. And it is far worse for turkeys and especially chickens: we kill millions of them daily. Chicken is America's favorite dead-animal flesh (only slightly decayed by the time you buy it), easily eclipsing dead cow (beef) and that "other white meat," dead pig.

• **Guilty Conscience**—Every time I ate meat in front of my pets, they seemed to take it personally. Okay, I'm just projecting. Maybe. I mean, they walk on four legs, too. However, both cats and dogs are themselves carnivorous. Let's leave it at this: "Animals are my friends, and I don't eat my friends." (Attributed to George Bernard Shaw.)

• **Kids**—Research shows that children who eat hot dogs once a week double their risk of a brain tumor; youngsters who eat other cured meats, such as ham, sausage, and bacon, have been shown to have an 80 percent higher risk of brain cancer.[1] And kids eating more than twelve hot dogs a month (that's about three hot dogs a week) have nearly ten times the risk of leukemia as children who ate none.[2] But here is the good news: children who ate hot dogs and other cured meats, but who also took supplemental vitamins, had a reduced cancer risk.[3]

• **Workman's Comp**—Meat-packing plants are unsafe for humans too. Of 2,000 workers at one meat-packing plant, 800 had become disabled in just one year.[4]

• **Chicken Shades**—Hens by the thousands are raised in such claustrophobic, crowded cages that the birds will literally peck each other to death. To reduce "prison-yard" aggression in chickens, red-tinted contact lenses are now marketed for poultry workers to slip into the birds' eyes. It takes a trained operator just a few seconds per bird, the manufacturer claims. This is my nomination for The World's Worst Job.

- **Chicken Keesters**—There is so much colon bacterial contamination in chicken meat that there is now a product to close off the bowels of dead chickens. It is called "RecTite" and is essentially super glue for chicken anuses. I am not making this up. "Superglue Advocated for Preventing Fecal Leakage in Poultry," reported the *Food Chemical News* on April 24, 1995. The article specifically suggested, "using super-glue to seal the vents on poultry before slaughter to prevent the birds from reflexively excreting fecal material at the time of death." Bon appetite!

- **Baby Cows**—Spend a while with a baby calf. Once one of the little critters sucks on your finger, you will think twice about your next pot roast.

- **Veal**—When I was a dairyman, I got to know a lot of calves. One was born while his mother was on her way up the ramp into the milking parlor. Bossy just dropped that little guy onto the concrete and in less than ten minutes he was up and walking around. At the end of the day, I saw him across the pasture, silhouetted against the setting sun, following his mother. He took about ten steps to her one. I didn't want to be the one to have to tell him what the future was for male bovines. The females would live to become milkers—the boys would become veal.

"Veal" has beautiful, big brown eyes with long, delicate lashes. "Veal" will suck on your fingers thinking it is Mom. "Veal" gets kept in horrible, cramped pens. The metal mesh pens we used were so small that the calf literally could not even turn around. He could stand, or he could lie down. There was not even room for him to swat the flies off his own backside, the location of choice for all hungry insects. And there were always clouds of flies, since calves chronically have diarrhea. This is because calves are loaded with antibiotics to keep them alive. A day or two after birth, they are taken from their mother and never nurse from her again. They are fed nutrient-deficient artificial "milk replacer" and Mom goes back into the milking line. And her baby is sent to slaughter for your next order of veal parmesan.

There is a way to stop it: eliminate the demand. If we do not eat veal, calves will not be killed. If we do not eat beef, steers will not be killed.

• **Anatomy**—Whenever I mention in a lecture that folks drink cow breast milk, they wig out. Then, for an encore, we talk about eating the muscles of dead animals. I delight in telling them the anatomical names of the specific muscles they munch from their pig, chicken, or cow. People do not want to think too much about what specific body parts they are actually eating. Try it at your next family gathering or class reunion. You will not be invited to many more, but what a way to go.

• **Quality Assurance**—"19 Million Pounds of Meat Recalled after 19 Fall Ill" was the headline of a recent *New York Times* article (July 20, 2002). It seems that 19 million pounds of ground beef, believed contaminated by the *E. coli* bacteria, had gotten into supermarkets. That's bad enough, but the federal government's response was worse. The U.S. Secretary of Agriculture, Ann Veneman, said of the recall: "This action is being taken as a cautionary measure to ensure the protection of public health. Public health is our No. 1 priority." However, officials acknowledged that it was likely that much of the meat had already been eaten.

Does anyone think that the government's "slam the barn door shut after the bull got out" response is anything more than a bad joke? By the way, this was by no means the only, or even the largest, bacteria-laden batch of meat released to a blissfully trusting population of American carnivores. The largest beef recall ever was 25 million pounds in 1997. And in 1993, contaminated hamburgers killed four children and sickened hundreds more.

• **Proven for Decades**—I invite you to carefully note the year in which this next statement was made: "A vegetarian diet can prevent 97 percent of our coronary occlusions." This was published in the *Journal of the American Medical Association* in 1961.[5] That's considerably more than forty years that we've known that less animal meat equals fewer human deaths. Is it any wonder why doctors who are members of the Physicians Committee for Responsible Medicine advise their patients to go meatless?[6]

• **Whole Lotta Bacon Goin' On**—It's porcine genocide to be sure: pigs are slaughtered monthly by the millions. The pig population in North Carolina alone is so huge that the state's hog farms produce as much sewage as the entire human population of New York City.[7] Now think of all the other, and even larger, livestock all throughout the other forty-nine states, and breathe deep.

Bacon is loaded with fat and salt and additives. One of the principal chemical ingredients used to "cure" meats is sodium nitrate ($NaNO_3$), a compound functionally identical to potassium nitrate (KNO_3), commonly known as saltpeter, a male sterilizing agent.

I remember the very day I stopped eating bacon. I was opening a package of ordinary supermarket bacon. As I separated the slices for frying, I noticed an odd-looking area, about the size of a nickel, at the same relative location on each slice. Upon closer examination (and I have taught tissue biology at the college level), I saw that the funny-looking spots were actually neatly presliced sections of a tumor. The pig that had been killed for that particular one-pound bacon package evidently had at least one tumor, and who knows how many more. The government should know, but they all too obviously never looked: the opened bacon package had the "USDA Inspected" seal prominently displayed on the front.

• **Moderation**—Just reducing your beef intake saves many lives. If we all simply cut out meat one day a month, we would prevent the murder of over 1 million animals annually. For every additional day per month that we refuse to eat meat, we will save a million more.

MEAT: LOTS, SOME, OR NONE?

Are humans really carnivores? We are revolted by the thought of eating live, bloody, still-moving meat. Carnivorous animals are never in a position to hunt a cooked meal. Additionally, "carnivores" are not strictly carnivorous: lions and similar predators gobble up the predigested vegetable material from an herbivorous prey animal's digestive organs in preference to any other part of the kill.

For humans, if a vegetable, fruit, or dairy food can be eaten uncooked, then it should be. As for raw meat, no thank you. The natural hygienists have always advocated the same message: eat fresh and raw. I seek to emulate such knowledge to the maximum practical extent, but I do not apologize for having a stove. A whole, good food diet, including legumes (peas, beans, lentils), grains, and potatoes clearly needs some cooking. But there is no need to make one's home on the range. We should emphasize whole, unprocessed, and, whenever possible, raw foods. In my opinion, some of these may be animal derived, but not many.

When in doubt, eat like other primates do: chimps and orangutans are very strong, very smart, and mostly but not entirely vegetarian. By moving toward a vegetarian diet, you reduce your too-high intake of protein, fat, and sugar. It is just that simple. There is no diet plan to buy. I think dairy products, eggs, and fish must remain occasional options for most of us. Again: my kids did so well as lacto-ovo-vege-tarians (eggs and dairy) that they never had to take a single dose of any antibiotic, not once.

To avoid all animal products makes one a vegan. I am most certainly not a vegan, and I do not universally advocate it. I have many good friends who utterly and totally reject animal products. I admire them, but I also observe that their conviction is, at times, more admirable than their health. Ethical issues aside, veganism truly is an excellent transition diet. As a short-term treatment for overweight, constipated, drug-soaked people, veganism cannot be beat. I think a few months without animal products is worth a therapeutic trial for most illnesses. But long term, for most people, I think some animal foods are necessary.

The majority of vegetarians are actually near-vegetarians, eating some animal products, such as eggs or milk products. I acknowledge that I am something of a cheese and yogurt fan. As a former dairyman, what do you expect? I also use eggs now and then for cooking. But I am not really much of a milk drinker and typically do not go through even half a dozen eggs in a month.

"Vegetarianism" is a process, not an absolute. The easiest way to facilitate an evolution to vegetarianism is to start when you're young. I personally think that cheese, yogurt, and some milk, has a place in a healthy natural diet for a child. For my children, their meatless lifestyle began in infancy. I regularly took my three-year-old son with me when shopping at the supermarket. We inevitably passed through the meat department. My son pointed to the blood-red packages and loudly asked me, "What's that, Daddy?" I replied, much more quietly, "That is meat." He then said, just as loudly as before, "We don't eat meat, do we, Daddy?" He was correct, of course, and I told him so. He smiled, and in a voice that could easily be heard in the produce department on the other side of the store, declared for all to hear: "We don't eat meat! We're not Italian!" Okay, he probably meant to say, "We're vegetarian," but I liked it better his way. And very few three-year-olds can say, "We're lacto-ovo-vegetarian, aren't we, Daddy!"

I also, on occasion, eat some seafood. Not often, and usually not directly in front of my aquarium. Fish and their aquatic companions are valuable sources of omega-3 fatty acids. After a millennia of changes to human civilization, the world's number-one animal protein source is still seafood. By the time we come up with a definition of "fishatarian," we are very close to the natural animal-products percentages that Dr. Weston Price found again and again in his travels amongst "primitive" cultures back in the 1930s.

NATIVE DIETS

In his book *Nutrition and Physical Degeneration,* Dr. Price found that isolated, healthy Swiss communities ate cheese and raw milk daily, plus a lot of whole-grain bread, but they only ate meat once a week. The basic foods of the islanders of the Outer Hebrides, Price wrote, "are fish and oat products with a little barley. Oat grain provides the porridge and oat cakes which in many homes are eaten in some form regularly with every meal."[8] Even traditional Eskimos, often held up as the ultimate example of human carnivorism, also eat nuts, "kelp stored for winter use, berries including cranberries, which are preserved by freezing, blossoms of flowers preserved in seal oil, and sorrel grass preserved in seal oil."[9]

In short, most vegetarians are not solely such, and neither are most carnivores. Optimum human diet is not to be found at either extreme. The issue is natural food more than where it comes from. Unprocessed foods, whether of animal or plant origin, are the healthiest. This is the enduring message. A fellow once wrote to a newspaper that healthy, robust meat-eating peoples were the most fit and, historically, had gained ascendancy over the rest. The writer used the mighty Roman army as an example. A professor of history wrote back and said that, actually, Rome's legions conquered the world on oatmeal.

When I visited rural Africa, I saw surprisingly healthy people. This was a slight shock to my Western expectations. I also saw what most people were eating: garden vegetables and whole grains, especially corn on the cob. In every village there seemed to be a big, rusty 55-gallon drum of boiling water containing, not a missionary, but steamed corn on the cob. Along the roadside, people sometimes sold a delicacy that looked like a dried, whole woodchuck nailed to a board. It's amazing how those little rodenty teeth stick out when the animal's skin shrinks in the hot sun. I passed on that. I also found bananas for sale everywhere. I could not get enough of them: though small, they were right off the tree and sweet as gumdrops. And nothing beats hot, peppery, delicious West African groundnut (peanut) soup.

As in China, rural Africans appear to eat what their poverty can bring them, mostly what they can catch and what they can grow. Practically speaking, subsistence agriculture is a more sure thing economically than subsistence hunting. It supports more people, and it is healthier. In my own neighborhood, backyard gardens continue to provide massive amounts of fresh, high-fiber, good-eating vegetables and fruits for practically nothing. I grow potatoes, lettuce, cabbage, tomatoes, beans, peas, beets, zucchini, apples, and raspberries.

As a biologist, I have seen too many internal organs of too many critters to want to chow down on them. Dr. Price noted that native peoples eat the fat that comes with the meat. That means viscera, organ meats, brains, and glands. And I forgot my spoon! The muscles of dead animals are simply not necessary for protein if you eat some dairy, fish, lots of legumes, and well-chewed, fresh nuts. Near-vegetarianism makes sense on all levels.

Vegetarians' health statistics even impress the U.S. Food and Drug Administration. At their website, you will find this statement by Johanna Dwyer, R.D., of Tufts University Medical School and the New England Medical Center Hospital: "Data are strong that vegetarians are at lesser risk for obesity, atonic [reduced muscle tone] constipation, lung cancer, and alcoholism. Evidence is good that risks for hypertension, coronary artery disease, type II diabetes, and gallstones are lower."[10]

TWELVE MORE EXCUSES TO STOP EATING MEAT

When you cut out meat:
1.   You'll feel better.

2. You'll save a *lot* of money on your food bill. My son calculated that the money our family saved by not eating meat equaled the purchase price of our house.
3. You'll have easier bowel movements and will not need to pay good money for extra store-bought fiber. Meat has no fiber at all and a vegetarian diet is fiber rich.
4. You'll lower your cholesterol levels. Dean Ornish, M.D., prescribes a vegetarian diet instead of coronary bypass surgery—it works as well or better, is much cheaper, and is immeasurably safer.
5. Your risk of cancer, as well as heart disease, will be cut in half. Cornell University conducted a ten-year study in China in which the diets of over 300,000 people were investigated. The more animal products eaten, the higher the incidence of cancer and heart disease; the less animal products eaten, the lower the risk.[11]
6. You'll have fewer dishes to do, and those that you do wash will be a lot less greasy.
7. You will save lives. There is plenty of food on Earth for each and every person. There is not enough for every person if we raise all those pigs and steers, too. If we all go meatless, or nearly so, famine will be ended.[12]

8. You'll save water (which is one of the reasons you stop famine). In the United States, half of our drinkable water goes to raising farm animals.
9. You will reduce pollution. Runoff from livestock farms is a major source of polluted water in America.
10. Your breath will smell better. I know this is pushing the point, so try this simple experiment. Let your dog breathe on you for a few minutes, then find a cow and compare. The vegetarian animal has different digestion and different bacteria, which result in different odors. I know: years ago, I milked 120 cows twice a day.
11. You will have less dandruff and your skin will look nicer.
12. You will automatically and effortlessly find your ideal weight. Meat, even lean meat, is 10 to 15 percent saturated fat. Cut that out and you start to drop the pounds. Your weight loss will be gradual but progressive. Most vegetarian foods are by nature lower in fat and calories, unless you become a "pudding vegetarian" and eat a lot of desserts and junk food.

HOW TO REDUCE YOUR MEAT INTAKE

Some flesh foods are clearly worse than others. You can start by eliminating the least healthful meats and gradually move toward a meat-free diet. Here is a continuum with the worst first and getting better as you go *down* the list:

• Cold cuts, such as pepperoni, salami, hot dogs, pressed ham, bologna, and so on. These meats are loaded with fat and chemicals and should be the first to go. All of the above would be a bit better if the animals were organically raised and their products were packed without preservatives and other additives.

• Pork, including bacon and sausage. Pork is notoriously difficult to digest.

• Beef, including hamburgers. Americans eat way too much red meat, particularly beef.

• Turkey and chicken. These animals are fed the remains of other animals that were condemned for human food, according to vegetarian cattle rancher Howard Lyman.[13] Organically raised turkey and chicken is the better choice. Ask your butcher if she or he can get these for you—the taste difference is incredible.

• Seafood. Avoid fresh-water fish unless you are sure that the lake or stream is not polluted. The oceans are pretty big and are generally pretty clean. Coastal waters are not as clean, of course. Still, seafood is not raised with chemically treated feed. Steroids are not given to whitefish and antibiotics are not given to flounder; this is more than we can say for animals raised on land.

• Eggs are a good source of complete protein. Since a typical (unfertilized) egg would not have developed to hatch anyway, many vegetarians consider this to be an acceptable alternative to meat.

• Dairy products are a good source of many nutrients, including minerals and protein. Cheese and yogurt are especially good for you. Avoid processed and orange-colored cheeses. After all, when is the last time you saw orange milk? Most store-bought yogurt contains a lot of sugar; it is better to buy plain yogurt and sweeten it yourself with fruit. In India, yogurt is diluted by half with water; you may find that your nose and throat are less "stuffy" if you try this.

Raw milk is probably better still because the nutritional value of milk is arguably higher without pasteurization. Some dairy farmers will sell you milk directly if you go to them in person with your own containers. They are generally not allowed by law to bottle their own cows' milk. You could perhaps say that the milk is for your pets if there is a question. When I milked cows, my wife and I drank raw milk all the time and raised my infant son on it as well.

Goats' milk (preferably raw) is perhaps the best dairy product of all. Goats' milk is very filling, but usually does not keep as long as cows' milk. It is therefore a good idea to purchase fairly small quantities at a time; fresh goats' milk may keep for up to a week.

• Tofu (bean curd), tempeh, miso, and other soy products are traditional sources of high-quality, nondairy protein. You may have tried these at a Chinese restaurant. Tofu is inexpensive and easy to use: just cut it up and toss it in any food you are preparing. Tempeh is like a soy "burger" when fried and miso makes a great soup base. "Textured vegetable protein" made from soybeans is also widely available and is an easy way to fortify any cooked food with extra protein. When eating, chew soy products (and all other foods) thoroughly for maximum benefit. Risk of cancer is reduced for those that eat moderate amounts of soy foods. [14]

• Sprouted beans and sprouted grains are sources of complete protein, just like meat. Vegans need protein just like anyone else, and sprouts are a great way to get it. Sprouts are loaded with other nutrients and dietary fiber as well and require no cooking. If they sound like an ideal protein source, well, they are![15]

STAYING WITH IT: HOW TO GET YOURSELF (AND YOUR FAMILY) EATING RIGHT

People who want to improve their health can be divided into two types: those who work at it daily and those who don't. Which are you? Are you ready for some power-packed, health-building, spirit-lifting, doctor-dodging ways to wellness? To help you get going and stick with a good diet, the foundation of any serious approach to better health, here are some pointers to ponder:

1. Remember that you are worth it. The time, expense and changes that go with a healthier lifestyle are an investment in yourself. The healthier you are, the more you can offer those you love. The time you spend each day on your health is not lost; rather, it adds to your productive years and you get it all back later, with interest.

2. Your entire family does not have to go along with you. It is wonderful if they do, but do not make it a condition for your own self-improvement. *Show* them that you feel great; living as an example is the best way to teach and encourage others.

3. Give a little. It is better to live an 80 percent natural lifetime than go 100 percent natural for just a week. Do your best to be as healthy as you can each day.

4. To make good health as easy and routine as possible:

    • Keep junk food out of the house. Simply do not buy it.

    • Have readily available good-tasting snack alternatives in the home at all times. Everybody likes to munch now and then, so make sure the only snacks around are good ones. Health food stores have aisles full of packaged goodies that are also nutritious. (Supermarkets do too, as you'll find if you make sure to read the label.) How about popcorn? You can make it fresh in an air-popper in no time at all for next to nothing. Without (much) salt or butter, it is very low in calories and an excellent source of fiber.

    • Have a cold veggie platter in the refrigerator at all times—a "party tray" with cut-up raw celery, carrots, radishes, broccoli, cucumber, and other vegetables. If they are already washed and cut up, they will get eaten.

    • Keep the freezer stocked with frozen juice pops instead of ice cream. You can buy plastic molds at discount stores and make your own natural version of juice-sicles. Use only 100 percent, unsweetened real juice.

• If the kids pester you for a sweet treat, give them a spoonful of molasses or honey. Both are as sweet as candy, but a lot more satisfying.

• Have a big bowl of fresh fruit on the kitchen table twenty-four hours a day. Then anyone can see that they can have as much fruit as they want anytime. There is no better snack.

• Fill a candy dish with dried fruit mixed with some unsalted nuts. Fill another with sunflower or pumpkin seeds. Place them on the table and they'll be eaten sooner than you think.

• Keep a pitcher of water in the refrigerator. Zero-calorie ice water is just as refreshing as a soft drink and a lot cheaper.

5. Build in rewards for eating right. These approaches work well with a family:

• Begin each meal with fresh vegetable juice or sprouts. Have nothing else in sight. Foods get eaten the fastest when you are the hungriest. We would tell our kids, "Eat your sprouts (or carrot juice, etc.) and *then* we will give you what you want."

• Each person gets a prize for staying on an all-natural diet each week. Something small will do, with a larger monthly reward. This is every bit as practical for adults as it is for kids.

• Give your children money if they trade in junk food from school, friends, or parties. Our kids made a pile on Halloween.

• Give each family member a share of the cash you save on doctor and dentist bills. J. Paul Getty said that such percent bonuses encourage "The Millionaire Mentality." If a filling costs eighty dollars, why not give a kid a few bucks for having no cavities? You are still way ahead. Make it worth their while and make it easy, and you will have a healthier family.

6. Tasty meals are very important. There is nothing worse than a good-for-you meal that tastes bad. Consult a good vegetarian cookbook.

7. More fresh, raw foods will get eaten if you serve more salads. Try fruit salad for breakfast. Begin each lunch and dinner with a large vegetable salad. Buy a dozen different bottled salad dressings for variety. The more natural the dressing, the better.

8. You can still go out to eat, but eat right. Go to restaurants where there is a salad bar. Many restaurants will prepare vegetarian dishes on request. When in doubt, call first.

WRETCHED EXCESS: DEVIOUS WAYS TO REFORM SOMEONE'S DIET

Do not forget the instructional power of overkill. Hell has been described as having to endure endless, relentless repetition of what you thought you liked to do. This principle constitutes a valid teaching tool.

When I was a freshman in college, and my stomach had its first opportunity for utterly unsupervised indulgence in alcohol, it was cheap beer that got there first. At a dorm party, my inaugural brewskis were dredged-up from the very bottom of the room-temperature aluminum keg, and they tasted awful. Ever since then, I've never quite met the recommended dietary allowance for beer.

When my mostly vegetarian preteen daughter wanted some hot dogs, I bought her several pounds of the cheapest, worst-tasting chicken-parts wieners I could find. Now don't panic: they were reasonably fresh, U.S.D.A. investigated, and lots of people eat them. Of course, she ate a few too many, and doesn't like them too well anymore. It is a bit like getting your first job in a doughnut shop. "Eat all you want," they tell you. That is possibly the best way on earth to reduce the amount the help will ultimately eat.

Try this same technique with candy, soda pop, and other junk foods. Abram Hoffer, M.D., lets his young patients have "Junk Food Saturdays": one day a week, kids can "garbage out" on all the colored, fatty, sugary junk they can hold. Of course, there is a reason why you only do this on a Saturday: they will be sick all day Sunday. Dr. Hoffer found that children were quite capable of drawing conclusions from the experience.[16]

If you find yourself up against some serious home-front resistance, here are some more shamelessly coercive ways to prod your kids away from flesh foods:

- If your child wants to eat meat, go right ahead and prepare some, and make a point to overcook it.
- If your child wants to eat hot dogs, buy the cheapest ones you can find and let the kid eat them to the point of nausea.
- Relentlessly serve meat and nothing but meat for dinner, lunch, snacks, and breakfast.

- Take your child shopping and pick out tripe, liver, brains, and tongue, so they can truly see what cattle are made from. Let them listen to a live lobster being steamed.
- Tour the meat-packing room at your local supermarket. You probably won't be allowed to tour a slaughterhouse, but that would be the consummate therapeutic trauma.

These are coarse techniques to be sure, but killing animals by the millions every day has got to stop. If the future is our children, let's tell them straight: Meat means dead animals and there is nothing pretty about it.

In the end, what really matters is living a healthier lifestyle every day. You have to actually *do* it, not just intend to. Vitamins do no good in the bottle; a juicer is valuable only when you use it; healthy foods help you only when they are in you. No doctor is going to follow you around all day and supervise your every mouthful—that part is up to you. One of the few true choices we have in life is to decide what we will or will not eat. Toddlers and even babies in highchairs do this all the time. As a grownup, you can do it right. And remember, your kids are watching what you do.

THE FIRE YOUR DOCTOR! TWOMINUTE CHECKUP

1. Look in the kitchen sink. The fewer greasy pots and pans you see, the fewer greasy foods you are eating. That is good. How long does it take you to wash your dishes? The longer it takes, the more fatty, cooked foods you are eating. Save time at the sink by becoming a near-vegetarian.

2. Look in the kitchen wastebasket. The fewer wrappers, plastic packages, and paper boxes you see, the less "convenience food" in your diet.

3. Look at your garden and compost pile. The bigger, the better. What, you don't have either? Grab a shovel and get outside!

4. Look at your multivitamin bottle. Vitamins C, E, and B complex should be provided in much, much larger than RDA/DRI quantities.

5. Not to be rude, but how long does it take you to have a bowel movement? The longer it takes, the more you need fiber in your diet. Instant fiber solution: be more of a vegetarian. Meatless diets usually contain at least three to five times more fiber than most carnivores

138

get from their McNothing meals. And while you are in the bathroom, hop on that dreaded bathroom scale! Read it, but don't weep: meatless menus are automatically lower in fat.

6. How long does it take you to fall asleep at night? High complex carbohydrate eating, with lots of nuts and beans, helps increase levels of calming tryptophan in your brain. A little bedtime niacin helps, too.

7. How many ashtrays can you spot in your home? If the answer is more than zero, you need to stop someone from smoking, immediately.

8. Let's go out to the garage. How many beer or soft-drink bottles do you have to recycle? That many, eh? You know what to do: recycle them and don't bother buying any more.

9. While you drive, are you drinking caffeine and/or eating sugary foods? Are you impatient in traffic? Pull over and buy some high-tryptophan cashews, nature's serotonin-laden alternative to SSRI psychiatric drugs, or to the feeling that you should be on them.

All of these self-monitoring methods can help you straighten up and fly right. It only takes a minute to check and lifestyle change gives you a lifetime of benefit. Don't let your grandchildren get to know you after you've gone: live longer and tell them your story in person.

"POBODY'S NERFECT"

Lifestyle change, the only sure way to prevent or cure anything, is not easy. Working on yourself requires flexibility, humor, and frequent renewal. If you fall off the wagon, just climb back on. We are in this for the long haul. Again, it is better you should be 80 percent vegetarian for a decade than 100 percent vegetarian for a week.

Tips for Healthier Eating

WHEN IN DOUBT, SPROUT!

Sprouts—you've seen them at salad bars and maybe at the supermarket. Now it is time to save money and improve your health in a big way by growing lots of those little high-fiber, high-protein sprouts at home.

One of the healthiest things you can do is eat a bowl of assorted sprouts each day. Sprouts are a complete protein, just like meat, but without the saturated fat and other negative aspects of dead animal muscle. Sprouts are loaded with enzymes, vitamins, and minerals. Eating different kinds of sprouts gives you year-round raw foods. Sprouts are inexpensive and really tasty when you grow them yourself. Sure, you can buy them in a store, but you will also pay more and get a much less fresh, and a much less flavorful, product.

To begin with, you will need six to twelve glass jars: mason jars are fine, as are mayonnaise jars or any other jars that hold about 1 1/2 quarts each. If you've not yet started saving your own jars, ask your neighbors for some. You will also need about a square yard of counter-top space, a small kitchen strainer that just fits the jar openings, tap water, fresh seed to sprout, a window, and ten minutes twice a day.

Place about enough seed in a jar to cover the bottom about three seeds deep. Too much seed gives poor results. Add about half a jar of cool tap water and let soak overnight (about six to ten hours). Next morning, fit the strainer into the jar opening to hold the seed back while you pour off the water that the seeds soaked in.

You now have a pile of damp seeds in the bottom of the jar. Wait until afternoon (or evening) and fill the jar nearly full of cool water again. This time, though, you should pour the water off (using the strainer) right away. There is no need for an overnight soak after the first night. You do need to continue to rinse and drain the sprouts twice every day; three rinses a day is even better. If you don't rinse the seeds, they will dry out and die out. If you add water and never drain it off, the sprouts will drown. They are not aquatic; they just need water like any other crop. *Rinse and drain twice a day!*

You can sprout several different types of seeds. Try alfalfa first; alfalfa sprouts are tasty, easy to grow, and ready in about six days. Most sprouts grow more quickly in the warm summer months and more slowly in cooler temperatures. You can also sprout wheat, whole (not "pearled") barley, clover, cabbage, lentils, mung beans, radish seeds, soybeans, and fenugreek seeds. If you sprout wheat or lentils, I recommend that you eat the sprouts quite early, such as on the second or third day at the latest. Wheat and lentil sprouts are rather hard to chew after that, although they are certainly still good for you and can be added in with vegetables you are juicing. I do not recommend trying to sprout mung beans or soybeans at first. Mung sprouts are fussy and soybean sprouts can have a rather strong odor. I am very partial to radish sprouts because they are a bit "hot" or spicy, just like a radish.

I also recommend sprouting sunflower seeds. There is no trick to sprouting sunflower seeds except one: you need to use some soil. Potting soil works great. I use a tray or lasagna pan (stainless steel or glass). Cover the bottom of the pan one seed deep in large, fresh unhulled sunflower seeds, then add enough soil to cover them about a half an inch deep. Sprinkle water liberally over all, two to three times a day. The soil should be moist, not soggy. Occasionally check to see if it is too wet by sticking your finger down in the dirt to the bottom of the pan. As soon as you see sprouts peeking up through the soil, place the pan in a sunny window. Sunflower sprouts take a while to grow to harvest size, which is 3–4 inches.

Cut off the lower seedy part, thoroughly rinse with water, and eat the tender white stem and little green leaves. Your local health food store or co-op probably has more information on seeds for sprouting. Delicious!

SPROUTING HINTS

It is important that you obtain unsprayed, *fresh* seed for sprouting. Stale seed does not germinate (sprout) very well. It is a good idea to smell the seeds that you are about to buy. Do they smell stale, old, or rancid? If so, shop elsewhere. Purchase your seeds someplace where they sell a lot of seeds to ensure freshness. You do not want to buy huge amounts of seed at a time, either. Start with perhaps half a pound or a pound at most. Keep your seeds in separate glass jars with tight-fitting lids and keep the seeds dry until you are ready to grow them.

Plain tap water is usually fine for rinsing your sprouts. If your harvest is small, you might consider filtering your tap water, or letting it stand for a day or two before use. These ideas often help if you are having trouble getting the seeds to germinate. It is normal for some of the seeds to not sprout. Most should, or the seeds are likely too old.

When you sprout in jars, your sprouts do not need sunlight for the first few days. After all, seeds normally sprout underground. For the final couple of days, it is a good idea to put them in the window to get sunlight. This will "green up" your sprouts and help them grow more quickly. Continue to rinse and drain the sprouts right up until you eat them.

In order to have sprouts to eat each day, you need to start sprouts each day. This is why you need all those jars that we mentioned earlier. If you start two jars daily, and the sprouts take six days to be ready to eat, then you need twelve jars. Starting three jars each day means eighteen jars, and so on. It does sound like a lot to eat two jars of sprouts per day. Remember, though, that each jar will not be full. Normally, the sprouts will only fill the jar half to two-thirds full.

Common reasons why seeds rot but do not germinate:
1. Old seed. Use fresh seed; buy from a store that sells a high volume of seed specifically for sprouting.
2. Excess chlorine in the rinse water. Take a hint from amateur aquarists: draw gallon jars of cold water and let the water sit for several days before you use it for rinsing and draining your sprouts.

3. Inappropriate use of light. Start seeds in low light; only for the last two or three days do they need daylight.

4. Failure to rinse and drain your sprouts at least twice daily. Once a day is not enough for taking vitamins, brushing teeth, feeding babies, or rinsing sprouts.

How should sprouts be eaten? Raw, that's how. (Soy and mung sprouts would be the exception; they are better cooked.) When you make a salad, use sprouts for a base instead of lettuce. Then add the cut-up vegetables that you like best on top of the sprouts. Feel free to use different salad dressings if you wish. Any dressing is good if it gets you to eat a lot of sprouts.

Should you find that you have too many sprouts ready on a given day, you can refrigerate them. I suggest loosely covering the jar opening with an upside-down plastic sandwich bag to keep the right moisture level inside. Avoid storing the sprouts in the back or bottom of the refrigerator where it is coldest. Frozen sprouts do not appeal to most people, and thawed-out frozen sprouts appeal to no one!

If I had just one piece of health advice to give to a person, it would be to try eating a substantial amount of raw food, especially a wide variety of sprouts. People who do are so much healthier. There's only one way to prove this and that is to try it for yourself.

DAIRY PRODUCTS IN MODERATION

I am a former dairyman who used to milk a hundred head twice a day. From the experience, I learned something that I am told Native Americans learned long ago: Have empathy and respect for the animals that feed you.

On the farm where I worked, we very much respected our cows. Admittedly, one aspect of such respect was purely about economics: cows are a valuable commodity to a farmer, and high milk producers are worth a lot of money. You simply must keep them healthy. All our cows were kept well vetted, very clean, and very well fed. Like most dairymen, we grew our own feed and made our own silage, which is a highly nutritious, fermented, stored grain. Unlike most dairymen, we gave preventive doses of cider vinegar to cows prone to mastitis. I put vitamin E on their teats when they got injured. Udder injury is a fact of life for cows bred for milk production.

On the farm, one of my weirder jobs was early-morning cow reveille. I'd go out to a pitch-black pasture and have to round up the entire herd for the 4a.m. milking. To do so, you first have to wake up the cows. To wake them, you have to find them. They were not hiding from me; it's just that the camo-coloration of black-and-white Holsteins, tan Jerseys, or the brown Swiss happens to make them remarkably hard to spot before the sun comes up. I usually did not bother to take a flashlight with me, and as a result the project could become quite interesting. As I ran about like a nut hollering "Come, bossey!" the pattern I traced would have looked pretty erratic to anyone equipped with infrared goggles and daft enough to be attempting to watch. Every time I sensed something looming in front of me, it was usually a cow. I was constantly altering my direction like one of those toys that backs up and pivots when it gets to a wall.

I just happen to like cows. I was eating my lunch by the pasture fence one day and a cow sauntered over to me, looked me straight in the face at close range, and literally said, "Moo." It was not a question; it was a statement. And it was not some guttural animal sound that I chose to anthropomorphize into the word "moo," either. The cow clearly enunciated, unmistakably, "Moo."

I am telling you this to give you a taste of what really goes into your milk. I personally choose to use cultured dairy products, primarily cheese and yogurt. I am not much of a milk drinker, possibly because I miss the real thing: fresh, raw milk, just hours old, right out of the farm tank.

FARM LIFE IS NOT ALL "OLD MACDONALD"

There is a largely hidden and brutal cost to milk. Although we appreciated our cows, every one of their male offspring was marked for execution. Since lactation follows childbirth, to obtain the milk you drink, some cow had to have a baby. When it is a male baby, it will be killed sooner (veal) or later (beef) or very much later (fast-food hamburger beef).

Years after I left farming, the dairy industry began the widespread use of bovine growth hormones. I object to this and have lectured for years against it. Farmers with brains know that cows are not warm-blooded milk spigots. You cannot get something for nothing: pushing too hard for higher milk production means a longer teat-contact time with the milking machine and that means more mastitis. That is not good for the cows or for the farmer. Increased insulin growth factor in milk, a result of the hormone injections, is not good for people. Pharmaceutical companies and their dubious products should stay out of food production.

If you are a milk user and if you possibly can, find a farmer (or better yet, a dairy) that agrees with me, refuses to trade in medicated milk, and will sell you the good stuff. And later, I am going to show you how to save money making your own yogurt, even if your choices are limited to supermarket brands.

But first, I owe this to my many vegan and otherwise nondairy readers: if you are not a milk user, I am in your corner more than you might think. I am absolutely certain that a dairy-free existence is the healthiest lifestyle for some people. I know folks whose headaches, earaches, allergies, or other ailments promptly go away when they avoid dairy foods, and come roaring back when they drink milk. The *Fire Your Doctor!* philosophy is "Do what works."

MILK AND MORALITY

One of the most influential vegetarians in history was Mahatma Gandhi. A meat eater during a brief part of his early life, Gandhi wanted to be a complete vegetarian (vegan) and even a fruitarian, having written, "It is my strong conviction that the human being doesn't need milk, except for the mother's milk he gets as a baby. His diet should consist exclusively of fruits and nuts."

Gandhi's stated position on diet was an extension of his advocacy of nonviolence far more than it was a health recommendation. To Gandhi, violence to animals was identical to violence to humans. And in fact, life really is all one. When I taught biology, I'd ask my students to examine the red blood of an earthworm and the red blood of a human. Then I asked them to tell me the difference. They could not, and the lesson began. Not only is our DNA 98 percent identical to a chimpanzee, but the basic physiology of our bodies is virtually identical with the physiology of a mouse, a frog, or even a gnat.

Consequently, to promote harmlessness to all life, Gandhi selected the vegetarian lifestyle, with no milk. However, experience led him to include milk products in his diet. Gandhi, who had previously vowed not to consume any animal product, went six years without eating any dairy foods. "When he became very emaciated, his doctor suggested goat's milk. Gandhi drank it, and after regaining his strength, decided to continue taking it."[1]

To make it as nonviolent as possible, and make up for the philosophical inconsistency, Gandhi only drank the milk of a goat that he personally took care of. I find more humanity in such a humble compromise than in a strict vow inflexibly followed. I raised my children from infancy on raw goat's milk and raw cow's milk. I think that such foods' value—great enough to have changed the Mahatma's mind—is good enough for me. Gandhi's mind was famously difficult to change. While the combined might of the British Empire could not do it, truth always persuaded him. The truth is that judicious use of dairy products, at least for some, makes good health sense.

Milk is a moral issue, but it is also a matter of what works. The solution may be as simple as a nutritional-ethical compromise, like Gandhi's, resulting in an overall decrease in consumption of animal products and an increase in ethical farming. In the United States alone, an astounding 10 billion animals are killed each year.[2] I do not ask anyone to reduce that number to zero; just try to lower it.

MAKE YOUR OWN YOGURT

A quart of plain yogurt costs about three dollars. For that money, you can buy a gallon (4 quarts) of milk and culture it yourself. You will also need some plain yogurt to use as a "starter" culture, and that's about it. All you have to do is heat the milk to the scalding or "frothing" point, and then let it cool to room temperature or just above it. Such cooling is the most important step, for if you add your yogurt bacteria to hot milk, they are toast. Let the milk cool down before you gently stir in a tablespoon or two of plain yogurt. I then place the preparation dish (I like to use glass or Corningware) into an oven that is off, and remains off, except for the little what's-in-my-oven light in the back. The heat of that lone light bulb is just right to incubate your yogurt. Leave your culture for about eight hours, or overnight, and in the morning put it in the refrigerator.

CULTURED AND RAW MILK

Cultured milk products, such as cheese or yogurt, are easier for many people to digest than fluid milk. Bacteria work milk over in a big and generally beneficial way. Cheese and yogurt, even if made from factory-farm, nonorganic milk would therefore be better than non-cultured milk from the same place. Not only are they easier to digest, but cultured milk products are, in a manner of speaking, a raw food. The beneficial microorganisms are alive in cheese and yogurt when you eat it. That's a raw food, and a good one.

If it isn't cultured, milk should be fresh and raw, not the skimmed, pasteurized, hyperallergenic white water that passes for "milk" nowadays.

"Raw milk? Good heavens, is that safe?"

Remembering that I do not think that bacteria are the primary cause of most diseases attributed to them, I support the use of scrupulously clean, unpasteurized ("raw") moo juice. When I was a dairyman, my breakfast was fresh milk, ten minutes old, right from the collecting tank. I raised my family on unpasteurized milk, from cows I knew rather intimately. I kept their quarters clean, their udders clean, and their milk clean. Clean, healthy cows give clean, healthy milk.

There are some farms that I would not knowingly drink milk from, cooked or not. Since most consumers have no choice and no information as to just whose milk is in the carton, pasteurization is an after-the-fact attempt to reduce bacteria count from the sloppiest farms. Pasteurization temperatures are not hot enough to do the job properly, and high-temperature auto-cleaving destroys nutritional value. I think we would do a lot better to focus on farm sanitation. But we don't. That is why it is so difficult to find certified raw milk for sale.

KIDS AND DAIRY

My ovo-lacto-vegetarian kids are now tall, strong adults. My no-milk critics have been revving up their word processors, so let me immediately add the following: elephants never eat eggs or dairy and they are even taller and stronger.

Kids can get protein and calcium (the usual reasons, aside from taste, that people choose to eat dairy products) from foods other than milk and eggs. If you check a nutrition textbook or online nutrition tables, you will see that beans, whole-grain breads, and even vegetables have significant amounts of protein. Nuts and sprouts are also excellent sources.

It must be rightfully emphasized that some people do much better with no dairy or eggs whatsoever. For example, pasteurized-milk allergies appear to be very common in children. They have been linked with sinus problems, constipation and diarrhea, chronic ear infections, behavior problems, and asthma.[3] Having worked with sick people for nearly thirty years, I think in many cases those symptoms are often due to an overall lousy diet and to vitamin deficiencies and that they are more aggravated by milk than caused by milk. An unusually restricted diet for your kids can backfire on you. I have indeed seen a few scrawny, strictly vegan children in my time. I have also seen a very large number of obese meat-fattened children. The path is yours to make.

155

START A GARDEN, AND STEP BACK!

You'll have more fruits and vegetables than you know what to do with when you start a garden. A few yards of soil and a couple of dollars for seed produces more veggies than you can eat. You'll save a lot of money, too. The average gardener puts less than forty dollars into a vegetable garden, with a typical return valued at many hundreds of dollars in fresh produce.

The money you save by not buying meat, milk, and medicine will buy a lot of fruit. Want to save even more? You do not have to live in a warm climate to grow fruit. I live in upstate New York, right off of Lake Ontario. Just across the lake is Canada, to one side Buffalo, to the other side Rochester. Does the word "cold" mean anything to you? Yet even I grow my own fruit.

CHEAP AND EASY LEGUME RECIPES

For those of you who are muttering under your breath that you'd rather take your chances with salami and Cool Whip than eat a diet like the one I've mentioned so far, please be encouraged with the following recipes. Many a person raised by meat-and-potatoes cooks is now a wonderful vegetarian cook. Most of us have learned by experience, reading, trial and error, and economic necessity to make and enjoy the following dishes:

BAKED BEANS

1 pound dry navy (pea) beans

1/2 teaspoon salt (to taste)

1 1/2 tablespoons unsulfured molasses

1/4 cup packed brown sugar or scant 1/4 cup honey

1/2 teaspoon paprika

1 tablespoon vegetable oil

Inspect beans and remove bad ones, stones, etc. Rinse well and allow to soak overnight with water about 2–3 inches above depth of beans. Next day, rinse beans again. Cover with water 2 inches above beans and cook for about 1–2 hours. Drain off most liquid from cooked beans, leaving some. Mix in salt, molasses, sugar or honey, paprika, and oil.

Pour beans into a large casserole dish and bake 45 minutes, covered, at 350°F, then 25 minutes uncovered.

LENTIL AND RICE SOUP

1 pound lentils (dry)

5 cups water

1 onion, chopped

1 carrot, sliced

1 stalk celery, sliced (use leaves, also)

1 or 2 bay leaves

1/2 teaspoon garlic powder

1 teaspoon salt, to taste

1/2–1 tablespoon cayenne pepper hot sauce

1 tablespoon unsulfured molasses

1/2–3/4 cup brown rice (uncooked)

Place lentils in a large saucepan. Inspect and pick over, then rinse well and drain. Add water, onion, carrot, celery, bay leaves, garlic, salt, hot sauce, molasses, and rice. Cover and bring to a boil. Reduce heat and cook for about 1 hour, or until lentils are tender. Add water while cooking as necessary. Note: You may wish to specify a primary (or "sweet") molasses for a sweeter soup or more hot sauce for a more spicy soup. Try your own ideas and create a new taste.

SPLIT PEA SOUP

1 pound split peas

5 cups water

1 medium onion, chopped

1 carrot, sliced

1 teaspoon or more salt

1 teaspoon dry parsley flakes

1–2 tablespoons vegetable oil

Inspect and pick over peas. Rinse very well, until "suds" stop forming, and drain. Add water, onion, carrot, salt, parsley, and vegetable oil. Cover and bring to a boil. Reduce heat and simmer for two hours or until peas have all broken apart. Do not undercook; the peas have to disintegrate to be done. Check your soup occasionally to add water, if needed. Stir frequently. Some fresh or dried garlic can be substituted for the onion. Also try adding 4–5 whole cloves.

LENTIL HASH

The truth is, I was trying to make lentil burgers, and they kept falling apart. Well, waste not want not.

1 pound cooked, drained lentils

1/2 cup wheat germ

1 cup soft whole-wheat bread crumbs or crumbled-up whole-grain bread

1 onion, chopped

1/2 teaspoon salt

1/2 teaspoon celery seed (optional)

Vegetable oil for frying

Starting with thoroughly cooked and mostly, but not entirely, drained lentils, mix with other ingredients in mixing bowl. Heat oil in frying pan (a large cast-iron frying pan is ideal), and brown and serve. If you like, lentil hash can be served with fried onions on top. Optional ingredients include cooked, diced potato, chopped green pepper, or whatever else you have on hand.

Homeowners, remember that fruit trees give food as well as shade and beauty. In cooler climates, try apple, plum, and cherry trees. You can buy specially tolerant fruit trees that will even grow in Montana or Maine. As a boy, I remember all the plums and cherries and apples that we got from nearly wild trees near our home. I never saw any of those trees get sprayed. You plant, you water, you wait, you get fruit. I've planted apple trees from seed and we now have a tree that produces well. Cost? Nothing. If a botanical underachiever such as myself can do this, then you certainly can expect success.

Apartment dwellers, "fruit" does not necessarily mean big trees. Tomatoes are a fruit, as are green peppers, green beans, cucumbers, and zucchini. (A "fruit" is any seed-bearing structure that develops from a flower.) Tomato, bean, pepper, and squash plants need very little space. If there is any spare corner, try to grow one of these really productive food sources. If yard work is out of the question, try a window box. If that is impossible (and it rarely is), you can grow sprouted seeds and sprouted beans in jars by your kitchen sink.

During World War II, rationing made Victory Gardens popular and necessary. We need them again, now. Today, we are at war with two great enemies: ignorance and disease. To paraphrase Charles Dickens, beware more of ignorance, for it is all too often the source of disease. It is time again for neighborhood Victory Gardens to overcome sickness and degrading poverty.

Following this approach to healthful, economical eating will reduce everyone's food bills, doctor bills, and tax bills. Simple eating saves dollar bills, and lots of them. And who can measure the value of being healthy? We've been told, for too long, that the more money you throw at a problem, the better it will get. Look at what you are spending on hospitals and prescriptions. If you feel that you've not gotten your money's worth, then spend less. After all, it is about the only approach we have not tried.

"OREGANO DOESN'T HAVE LEGS, DAD"

That's what my ten-year-old daughter said. She's right and she should know. At harvest time, I bring in bushels of wholesome vegetables from our garden. You might think that "bushels" is a figure of speech, but just ask my laborers: my son and daughter. They will confirm every basketful.

Mounds of produce piled on our kitchen counters, table, floors, and hallways has inspired me to many great culinary adventures. For instance, take my beets. Please. We have clay-laden soil that beets evidently love, and they show us their affection annually. The only problem is that nobody in the family really likes beets. I've planted them because they grow so well. I'm a cheapskate, and free food by the hundredweight really appeals to me.

There are not a lot of ways to prepare beets: boiled served with vinegar; cold in beet salad; and in borscht. I'm sure my children rue the day I learned to make borscht.

To make borscht, you also need cabbage, onions, some spices such as basil (fresh if possible), oregano, a bay leaf, pepper, and salt. I add a little olive oil for flavor, plus a cup of tomato paste. This improves not only the taste but the color of the borscht, reducing the soup's otherwise intimidating purple to a rather inviting magenta. If you are unusually inexperienced in the kitchen, I will add that you also need water. Boil all this up, and there you are: cheap, healthy, ethnic, and plentiful.

My particular variation on the borscht theme is to add broccoli, another vegetable my soil will yield in quantity. There are zillions of ways to cook broccoli and don't forget raw, with dips or in salads. Still, when you fill an entire freezer with broccoli and there is still more a-comin', you have to use this green stuff up somehow. I toss it in the soup, which includes my minestrone, pea soup, and lentil soup as well as borscht.

But nobody but me makes Aphid Borscht. I do not use pesticides. No need for any chemical bug-killers with broccoli or beets, or for that matter, anything else I grow: lettuce, green beans, peas, squash, tomatoes, potatoes, apples, or raspberries. Nope, just good-old-fashioned cow manure, grass clippings, compost, or some cheap fertilizer.

If you do not spray broccoli, you do get some wildlife living in it. Broccoli caterpillars, always quite small, happen to be exactly the color of broccoli itself. They are thus quite invisible to the casual eater. Fortunately, or not, depending on your point of view. My daughter wishes to share with the world a great secret: broccoli caterpillars turn yellow when cooked. So, the simple way to get rid of them is to lightly steam your broccoli, and the now-yellow critters will be easy to spot.

At this juncture, you must think that I wantonly fed my family half of the world's insect species. That is only partly true. We did eat the aphids. Not intentionally, mind you, it's just that aphids are extremely tiny, and they stick to broccoli stems, up under the florets where they know you are not looking. Even cooking fails to dislodge them, for their little boiled corpses are to be found in the hundreds, still clinging to broccoli spears. Some will fall off, and float in, say, your borscht. And this brings us to the day when my daughter insisted that there were bugs in her soup.

"No," I asserted with all my science teacher authority. "Those are not bugs. That's oregano."

My daughter was utterly unconvinced, and upon looking very closely, said, "Oregano doesn't have legs, Dad."

So she was right. Big deal! Well, yes. I realized that in my organic zeal, I had failed to be fair to my family. It is not right to feed your kids bugs. I came up with a chemical-free solution, though: a week or so before the broccoli harvest, I drop one of my many idle and hungry spiders onto each broccoli plant. As soon as the next day, there are no more aphids to be seen. Yes, I like spiders. When anybody finds a spider roaming about the house, they stick an upturned glass over it to save it for me. I put these spiders in the garage and basement, where they quietly prosper, waiting to be called up to the big leagues outdoors.

I'd like to add that the vast majority of spiders are basically quite harmless. Even tarantulas are incapable of doing any serious harm to a person. If you are very sensitive to bug bites, have a known medical condition, or handle black widows, the rules are, of course, different. But even I do not actually handle the spiders. You can move them about to your heart's content with a cup, a scrap of cardboard, or gloved hands.

Spiders in your garden do your bug-killing with precision. They eat insects, and they work cheap. Your broccoli will no longer shelter the bugs. And you will save a pile of money, and feel like a million bucks.

HOW TO MAKE YOUR OWN CIDER

If an apple a day keeps the doctor away, making your own cider should be the ultimate health plan. The trick to making cider is to realize that whole apples cannot be pressed; you must grind them up first. This can be done with a masticating ("chewing") type of juicer (such as a Champion), with all parts in place except for the juice strainer. This enables you to quickly run a large quantity of apples through it. First, cut the apples into quarters, both to check for critters and so that the apples will fit through the juicer's intake.

The coleslaw-consistency apple mash that the screenless juicer produces should be placed onto a good-sized cloth. I place the mash onto old but scrupulously clean fabric salvaged from my worn-out rugby shirts, and then fold it over into a nice, soggy football-shape and place it in my cider press.

Given the source of my straining cloth, you know that I was not about to spend any money on a cider press. I use a five-gallon, plastic, well-scrubbed, drywall compound bucket. I cut a piece of solid one- by twelve-inch pine-plank scrap into two discs, which fit loosely inside the bucket. The bottom one has a few dozen quarter-inch holes drilled in it. The top disc is solid. The cloth-wrapped apple mash goes between the boards, with a couple of cement blocks on top for weight. Gravity does the rest. To prevent such applied weight from jamming the lower wood disk down into the bucket, I place three stout plastic beverage tumblers, upside down, inside the bucket. The lower perforated wood disk sits on top of them. The cider collects in the chamber formed below.

Do not use plywood or composition wood for your pressing discs. In addition to contain-ing some rather unpleasant chemicals in the glue used to make them, plywood and chipcore products soak up liquid and will swell, distort, and quickly become unusable.

I can put about half a bushel of apples into this press at one time, if I prepare two large individual cloths of apple mash. I then get about 1 1/3 gallons of cider per pressing. That's better than 2 1/2 gallons per bushel. You can let your press sit overnight, or you can perch yourself on top of those cement blocks, read your favorite natural health book, and finish pressing in fifteen minutes. Kids love everything about making cider. If you are any kind of a Tom Sawyer at all, you can get them to literally line up to be the ones sitting on top of the press.

When pressing is complete, remove the cement block weights carefully and set them aside. Then take the now-flattened apple parcels out of the press slowly: it is important that they do not open, or your cider will instantaneously be transformed into extra-chunky applesauce. As you lift them and lighten the load on the bottom wood disk, the disk will tend to float up on the inverted tumblers and try to sharply tilt off to one side. Watch for it and you'll have no surprises. Using a large funnel, pour your cider into storage jugs and refrigerate (or, perhaps, ferment!).

Juice Fasting

Americans eat way too much fat, sugar, and protein. In fact, Americans simply eat too much of everything, more than ever before.[1] The way out of this dilemma is so easy that we usually miss it: consider occasionally fasting. I can almost hear the sound of yet another one of my books being slammed down, put back on the shelf, or quietly incinerated.

Look, nothing succeeds like success. We could spend all day talking about the value of fasting, but why not find out for yourself what it can do for you? Experience is your best teacher, and improved health is always the best proof. A fast will cost very little money and may be one of the best things you've ever done.

Fasting should be with your doctor's approval and is not for growing children or for anyone pregnant or nursing. People who are taking certain medications or who have other compelling medical circumstances should not fast. Diabetics and persons on medication requiring meals should check with their physician.

A common "scientific" argument against fasting is that it is inherently unsafe. Truly the pot is calling the kettle black when drug-based medicine—which kills over 200,000 Americans each year[2]—criticizes the safety of the therapy that all animals naturally use, namely fasting. The following is one approach to safe, comfortable fasting.

THE TWENTY-ONE-DAY GOOD-HEALTH JUICE CYCLE

What I call a "cycle" is made up of an eight-day juice fast, three days to come off the fast, and then ten days on a three-quarters raw food diet. This really works.

Eight days may seem like a long time to go without food. Actually, for the first day or two of a fast, your body uses up the food remaining in your digestive tract from previous meals. For the next couple of days, your body uses stored food reserves from your liver. This means that a fast doesn't really begin until about the fifth day. So, an eight-day fast is closer to a three-day fast and attainable by nearly every-one.

Since "fasting" conjures up visions of starva-tion, it is important to realize that we are talking about juice fasting here. Freshly made vegetable juices, taken in quantity, are not a beverage—they are a raw, highly digestible food. It is ideal to have all the juice you want, without forcing yourself to drink it. The rules:

When you are hungry, drink juice. When you are thirsty, drink juice also.

When juice fasting, it is generally a good idea to dilute juice 50/50 with water. If you can afford filtered water, use it. If not, don't worry—the goodness of the juices will carry you. Some people, including me, do not like the taste of diluted juice. An alternative is to drink a glass of water, then drink a glass of juice. This gives the same effect and tastes better. Be sure to drink the water first, for after the juice you may not want the water as much.

When we say "juice," we generally are referring to fresh vegetable juice. Fruit juice tends to be too sweet. However, there is nothing to stop you from experimenting and coming up with your own best regimen. As long as you get good results, how you get them is secondary.

GET A JUICER

You cannot buy freshly prepared vegetable juice in any store at any price, unless they literally juice the vegetables right in front of your eyes and you drink it down before they make you pay for it! Virtually any juice in a carton, can, or bottle has been heat treated and was certainly packaged at least a few days, weeks, or even months ago. This means that you will need one essential and somewhat expensive appliance: your own juicer.

A juicer is not a blender. A juicer makes juice; a blender makes raw baby food. To make juice, you need to extract the fluid part of the vegetable along with the vitamins, minerals, and enzymes it contains. Therefore, you need a juice extractor. Incidentally, I do not sell juicers, nor do I have any financial connection with any juicer brand, manufacturer, or distributor.

Be sure to get a really good juicer. Good juicers make tastier juices, faster, and also clean up more quickly than cheap juicers. There are many cheap juicers and also many dissatisfied folks who thought they'd save a buck and now regret that they bought a "bargain" juicer. If you spend too little, you will be disappointed with your purchase within weeks.

Here's a secret to easy cleanup: The moment you have finished making (and drinking!) your juice, just rinse the washable parts with water and set them in a dish rack until the next use. Soap will rarely be necessary as long as you don't mind the plastic parts of the juicer gradually becoming the same color as your favorite vegetables.

If your juicer has a metal screen that filters out the pulp, sooner or later that metal screen will become clogged. Prompt and thorough rinsing under the tap gets rid of most of the residue on a day-to-day basis, but over time a hardened material builds up in the screen and reduces output and efficiency. I have tried a variety of methods to combat this, including mild solvents, industrial hand cleaner, lime and rust removers, brushing, soaking, and even poking out the crud with a needle, spot by spot. Let me save you a whole lot of trouble: simply use bleach. Soak the strainer in undiluted chlorine bleach overnight (as much as twelve hours) and you will find the bottom of the soaking dish full of little dots that have eroded and fallen out of the strainer.

HOW MUCH JUICE TO DRINK

Drink as much juice as you wish. Remember that it is a food, not a beverage. There is little fear of overdoing it. It is, after all, hard to hurt yourself with vegetables! A good rule of thumb is to drink three or four eight-ounce glasses of fresh juice a day (for an adult). The best time is right before a meal or between meals, because absorption of and benefit from the juice is highest then.

You will probably find that you will be urinating more as you drink more juices. That figures, doesn't it? You are taking in more liquid. You may also notice that you have more bowel movements now than you were previously accustomed to. This, too, is to be expected. Your body may well respond to all this nourishment by "cleaning house" a bit. More excretory symptoms would be the result. Ever notice how many trash cans you fill when you clean out the attic or garage? You hardly noticed all the rubbish you had stored there until you went to clean it out. The same is true with your body. It's better out than in.

WHAT TO JUICE

You can juice almost anything you can eat raw. Vegetables are best, especially carrots, cucumbers, beets, tomatoes, zucchini squash, romaine lettuce, sprouts, celery, and cabbage. You may juice fruits too: freshly made raw apple, grape, and melon juices are delicious. Personally, I think fruits are so juicy anyway that they might as well just be eaten as is. It is not generally a good idea to juice potatoes, eggplant, or lima beans (not that you'd want to). The rule is *you can juice anything you can eat raw.*

It is wise to peel produce that has been sprayed or waxed, such as store-bought apples or cucumbers, before juicing. Carrots and other root vegetables often do not need peeling; instead, give them a good scrubbing with a nylon-bristle vegetable brush while rinsing under tap water. Beets are an exception—since beet skins are very bitter, peel beets before juicing. A hint to save time: dip the beets for about twenty seconds in boiling water and peel them; it's much easier.

Your juice will taste best if you drink it right after preparing it. I mean within moments! Fresh juice contains a great amount of raw food enzymes and vitamins, many of which are easily lost as the juice sits. Drink it right down, along with the satisfying thought that this is unbelievably good for you.

HEALTHY JUICE CHOICES

• Carrot juice is tasty and popular, and a few glasses of carrot juice per day are highly beneficial. Remember, there is no need to peel your carrots if you first scrub them well with a tough brush while rinsing them under water. This is quicker than peeling, and is less wasteful. Carrot juice is high in vitamin A; actually "provitamin A" or carotene. Carotene is completely nontoxic, no matter how much you consume. The worst thing that can happen if you drink a huge amount of carrot juice is that you will turn orange. You see, beta-carotene is a natural pigment or coloring. Excess carotene is stored in your skin until your body wants it and then turns it into active vitamin A as needed. This condition is called "carotenosis" and is harmless. To get rid of the color, simply back off the carrot juice (and other orange vegetables) for a while and it will go away. Naturally, you don't have to turn orange to enjoy the goodness of carrot juice. You can drink just enough to feel great without looking like a pumpkin!

• Celery juice is very tasty, but a bit high in sodium. Use small amounts of this juice to flavor the others. Juice celery leaves right along with the stalks for the most benefit.

• Cucumber juice is remarkably tasty and rather different from a cucumber itself. Perhaps you will find that the taste reminds you of watermelon. Again, peel cucumbers before juicing to avoid the waxes applied to their skins to enhance their shelf life.

• Kale, leaf lettuce, or bean sprouts will make an especially nutritious juice with a taste that is well worth acquiring. This "green drink" is loaded with minerals and chlorophyll.

• Zucchini squash juiced tastes better than you'd imagine. Peel first, and enjoy. Zucchini also helps keep your juicer from clogging on higher-fiber vegetables. After every few root vegetables you juice, run some zucchini through the juicer to keep it humming free and easy.

• Beet juice is traditionally considered a blood builder: in days past, herbalists looked at the blood-red beet as a tonic—more for its effectiveness than for any color similarity. Beets must be peeled before juicing, as beet skins are very bitter. The beets, on the other hand, are quite sweet and make great juice. They will also permanently stain your juicer, so don't try to remove that color by washing. Beet juice will also color your bowel movements. When you have beet juice, remember not to be alarmed the day after. It's just those beets!

• Cabbage juice was used by Garnett Cheney, M.D., to cure bleeding peptic ulcers back in the 1950s.[3] Dr. Cheney's patients drank a quart of cabbage juice a day and were cured in less than half the usual time, with no drugs whatsoever. Since then, cabbage juice has successfully been used for a variety of serious gastrointestinal illnesses.[4] Colitis, spastic colon, indigestion, chronic constipation, idiopathic (unknown origin) rectal bleeding, and other conditions seem to respond well to the nutrients in cabbage juice. The American Cancer Society has long urged people to eat the cruciferous (cabbage/broccoli) family of vegetables because of their protective effects against cancer.[5]

Yes, you can also juice kale and broccoli. All these, including cauliflower and Brussels sprouts, contain a highly beneficial plant chemical called sulforaphane. They are easier both to juice and to drink if you mix them with carrots. And, of course, you can just eat them, too.

• Tomatoes are easily juiced and really good for you. They are our primary source for the powerful antioxidant lycopene. By the way, the tomato is properly considered a fruit. And, yes, you can mix and match fruits and vegetables in the juicer, just as you can in any meal.

WHAT ABOUT HUNGER?

You need a juicing attitude. The first thing to remember is that fasting is a choice; starving is a sentence. We instinctively fear hunger, and with reason. I've gone hungry a few times in my life and there is nothing ennobling about it. Let's start by banishing the fear: Unless you have a medical condition to the contrary (check with your healthcare provider first), you'll be fine.

That brings us to appetite, the real problem. Like dogs and teenagers, we are always hungry. But for what? If you have a hankering for salty, sugary, greasy "foods," then I say you are not really hungry. Appetite is partly physiological, but largely learned. While the normal human body can go days or even weeks without food, your appetite is not about to let you do that without putting up a fight.

Appetite is linked to low blood sugar, a desire to chew, and an empty stomach. We can fix them all. First, the blood sugar. Water-only fasting tends to crash your blood sugar, and fruit juice-only fasting tends to make it (and you) a little hyper. Vegetable juice is more toward the middle, containing a natural mix of some but not too many simple and complex carbohydrates. If you are pooped out, drink more juice. For a picker-upper, have some fruit juice after you first have two glasses of plain water. If you are buzzing, try drinking more plain water. Otherwise, drink freshly made vegetable juices.

Now for the chewing part: simply snack on raw vegetables, any kind, any time, day or night. Chew them very, very well. Is this cheating? How can it be, if you were going to put those same vegetables through the juicer anyway? Relax! This is about good health, not distracting technicalities. If you need to, then munch; just munch on the right things.

As far as having an empty stomach, well, don't. If you have an empty stomach you are doing it wrong. When you are hungry, drink juice: all you want, any kind, any amount, any time. There is absolutely no need to have an empty stomach. Juice it up!

In summary, *if you can eat it raw, you can juice it. If you can juice it, you can eat it raw. If you are hungry, immediately do one or the other.*

COMING OFF THE FAST

Coming off the juice fast is best done by eating lightly for a while. Fruit, fruit salads, vegetable soups, cottage cheese, and other light foods are appropriate at this point. A good rule of thumb here is to eat only half as much as you want at any one time, but eat twice as often. This stage lasts for about three days.

For the next ten days of 75 percent raw food diet, you can eat all you want as long as three-quarters of it is uncooked and well-chewed. For the uncooked part of the diet, eat fresh, raw vegetables and fruits. And don't forget about nuts: if they are raw, they count. Chew all foods thoroughly.

Begin each meal with a large salad; perhaps try a fruit salad for breakfast. Then, when you have finished the salad, have whatever you want within reason. The 25 percent cooked portion could include whole-grain breads and pasta, brown rice, cooked beans, lentils, and cooked vegetables (including potatoes, sweet potatoes, yams, and squash). Meat is not recommended, nor is chicken or turkey. If you need to eat flesh, eat fish, which is a major source of important oils and other nutrients in addition to protein. Avoid fat-laden breaded or fried seafood and avoid eating a catch from questionably polluted waters.

If you don't want to eat seafood, eggs (in moderation), cheese, unsweetened yogurt, raw cow's milk, goat's milk, tofu, miso, tempeh, nuts, and especially beans and bean sprouts are all good protein sources. The issue is not where you get your protein but are you getting *enough* protein. The simple truth: vegetarians get plenty of protein; everyone else eats too much. If you are not yet a vegetarian, now is the time to move in that direction.

When you go out to eat, it's easy (and economical) to stay right on this program by eating at salad bars. This is a fun way to be sure you make three-quarters of your diet fresh and raw.

Supplements and How to Use Them

Nutritional supplements are essential for maintaining good health. Naysayers claim that taking supplements is wasteful and unnecessary, because all the nutrients you need are found in food. The sad truth is that most people's diets are utterly inadequate for providing proper nutrition.

Supplements make any dietary lifestyle, whether good or bad, significantly better. They are an easy, practical, entry-level, better-nutrition solution for nearly everyone. Media scare stories notwithstanding, taking supplements is not the problem; it is a solution. Malnutrition is the problem.

Research continues to prove the value of supplements for staying healthy and treating a variety of health conditions in a safe and effective manner. Remember, it is not enough to "say no" to medicines. You have to say "yes" to something else. Switch to what works—the intelligent use of supplementation. (And remember, I have no financial connection whatsoever with any supplement manufacturer or distributor.)

MULTIPLE VITAMINS

High-potency multiple vitamins are probably the most economical means of getting most of the whole team of essential nutrients for the lowest cost. Because people so often ask, what follows is what I personally take every day. The asterisk (*) indicates a large increase over current U.S. government standards such as the Recommended Dietary Allowance (RDA), or Daily Reference Intake (DRI), which are usually way too low. The following opinion specifically does not apply to children or pregnant or lactating women. As a general rule, calculate a child's dose as a percent of adult body weight (for example, think of a 40–50 pound kid as one-quarter the weight of an adult). For pregnant or lactating women, consult your doctor.

So, if you were to ask me what should be in a multivitamin (assuming it would fit!), this would be it:

Fat-Soluble Vitamins

- Vitamin A, as carotene, 20,000 International Units (IU)* (or 10,000IU if taken as fish oil)
- Vitamin D, 800IU*
- Vitamin E, 600IU*

Water-Soluble Vitamins

Note: The dose of the water-soluble vitamins should be divided throughout the day. I do this automatically by taking a multivitamin with every meal.

- Vitamin C, 6,000mg* (many people need far more than this amount)
- Vitamin B1, 65 mg*
- Vitamin B2, 65mg*
- Vitamin B3, 200–500mg*
- Vitamin B6, 65mg*
- Vitamin B12, 125 micrograms (mcg)*
- Biotin, 200mcg*
- Pantothenic acid, 65mg*
- Folic acid, 500mcg

Minerals

- Calcium, 1,000–1,200mg
- Magnesium, 400–600mg*
- Iron, 18mg for nonpregnant women (most men do not need to supplement with iron)
- Iodine, 200mcg
- Zinc, 50mg for men*; 20mg for nonpregnant women
- Manganese, 10mg*
- Copper, 3mg
- Chromium, 200mcg
- Selenium, 100mcg

Related Nutrients

- Phosphatidyl choline, 2,000mg
- Phosphatidyl inositol, 1,200mg
    (Note: Two rounded tablespoons of lecithin granules would provide both of these.)
- Omega-3 fatty acids, 500mg

It is not possible to find all of the above in a single tablet (unless it is nearly the size of a hockey puck). You don't want to take all your vitamins at once anyway. Your body absorbs more and wastes less if you divide the dose throughout the day.

Why so much and why so many? Because most people's diets are so rotten that higher levels of nutrients result in recognizably better health. A person wanting to take fewer supplements should eat more salads, have a lot of sprouts, and drink a great deal of fresh, raw vegetable juices each day. It is better to get as many of your nutrients as possible from good foods than from bottles. A really good diet will reduce but not eliminate one's need for supplements. Vitamins C, E, and B complex are especially important to supplement.

WHY MEGADOSES?

Why vitamin megadoses? First of all, because they work. But another interesting way to look at it is this: each individual cell in your body contains six feet of DNA, which, if unraveled, would stretch 11 billion miles. And your body contains several dozen trillion cells! If there ever were an obvious argument for large vitamin doses, could this be it?

Two questions must be asked of the methods of all physicians: are they safe, and are they effective. Vitamins are both. Isn't it odd, really, that small amounts of vitamins are known to be absolutely essential for life itself, yet large doses are routinely denied therapeutic usage in hospitals?

There is a recurrent problem with vitamins being perceived as "too good to be true." Frederick R. Klenner, M.D., found ascorbate (vitamin C) to be an effective and nearly all-purpose antitoxin, antibiotic, and antiviral. One vitamin treating polio, pneumonia, measles, strep, snakebite, and Rocky Mountain Spotted Fever? Layperson and professional alike certainly struggle with that. The root explanation may be as simple as this: *The reason that one nutrient can cure so many different illnesses is because a deficiency of one nutrient can cause many different illnesses.*

This has led to something of a vitamin public relations problem. When pharmaceuticals are versatile, they are called "broad spectrum" and "wonder drugs." When vitamins are versatile, they are called "faddish" and "cures in search of a disease." Such a double standard needs to be exposed and opposed at every turn.

People often ask, "If vitamin therapy is so good, why hasn't my doctor told me about it?" I do not know the answer to that question. Quite frankly, over time, I have grown to be less and less fired-up about even wanting to know why your doctor does not know. This is because there are too many sick people that need positive help.

SAFETY OF VITAMINS

A lot of people go through life trying to prove that the things that are good for them are wrong.
—WARD CLEAVER TO HIS SON, BEAVER, IN *LEAVE IT TO BEAVER*

If you have been told that vitamins are harmful, then keep reading. The number-one side effect of vitamins is failure to take enough of them. Vitamins are extraordinarily safe substances.

As a contributing editor to a medical journal, I have learned that it is easier for most researchers to get a negative vitamin study published than to get a positive one published. As with the evening news, where the policy is usually "If it bleeds, it leads," the scare story sells. There is strong economic inertia at work.

Successful vitamin therapy is a triple threat to the medical cartel. It threatens physicians because they know practically nothing about it, and it represents real competition. It threatens the pharmaceutical industry because vitamins cannot be patented to be sold at huge profits. I believe it also threatens most dietitians because the fallaciousness of the food groups—always, supplements—never dogma will be exposed. In all three cases, it is the very success of vitamin therapy that is cause for such alarm.

The only sure way to quash the popularization of vitamin therapy is to try to discredit it by claiming it to be dangerous. This is the world's oldest way to stop progress: just declare it a fraud. Condemnation without investigation.

So, right up front, these important reminders:

There are over 106,000 deaths from pharmaceutical drugs each year in the United States, even when prescribed correctly and taken as prescribed.[1] In addition, there are an estimated 150,000 more people killed by other aspects of medical care, including botched and unnecessary surgeries (12,000); hospital-caused infections (80,000); medication errors

(7,000); and other medical mistakes (20,000). That makes a total of a staggering quarter of a million deaths caused by the medical profession. Per year.[2]

There is not even one death per year from vitamin supplements.[3] Therefore, "The attack on the safely of vitamins is really an attack on the efficacy of vitamins," says Abram Hoffer, M.D.

VITAMIN A

Vitamin A, as carotene, 20,000 or more International Units (IU)* (or 10,000IU if taken as fish oil) gives you healthy mucous membranes and a strong immune system, and helps prevent cancer. It's a myth that excess carotene consumption is dangerous. The fact is that your body makes vitamin A on demand from carotene. Excess dietary carotene causes the skin to turn slightly orange, once succinctly described as resembling an artificial suntan. The medical name for this condition is hyper-carotenosis, or just carotenosis. Both are harmless. Excessive ingestion of carotene does not cause a toxicity of vitamin A. It is singularly difficult to kill yourself with carrots.

In one review of fifty years of vitamin studies, researchers noted that "approximately 10 to 15 cases of vitamin A toxic reactions are reported per year in the United States, usually at doses greater than 100,000IU. No adverse effects have been reported for beta-carotene (a vitamin A precursor)."[4] After first noting that this review confirms that carotene is indeed safe, some explanation is necessary. First, a "toxic reaction" is very different from a "fatality." Had there been any fatalities, the authors would have said as much. Unfortunately, "toxic" may erroneously imply "deadly." That is not the meaning of toxic as it properly applies here: toxic means "makes you sick." American poison-control statistics fail to show even one death from vitamin A in a given year.

One reason there are no vitamin A deaths is that occasional high doses of vitamin A do nothing. It generally takes long-term, chronic overdose of vitamin A oil to even cause headache, nausea, and other symptomatic warnings that occur before serious problems can arise. Pregnancy is a special case, because prolonged intake of too much preformed oil-form vitamin A might be harmful to the fetus, even at relatively low levels (under 25,000IU per day). Interestingly enough, you can get over 100,000IU of vitamin A from eating only 6 ounces of beef liver. I have yet to see a pregnancy overdose warning on a package of liver.

It is vitamin A deficiency during pregnancy, and in infancy, that poses a far greater risk. Deficiency of vitamin A in developing babies is known to cause birth defects, poor tooth enamel, a weakened immune system, and blindness. Megadoses of vitamin A are considered sufficiently safe to be given to newborns to prevent infant deaths and disease.[5]

This is not to say that vitamin A, as the preformed oil, should be taken recklessly. Too much vitamin A oil is not good; too little vitamin A is worse. And, you can eat all the carotenes you want. Fruits, vegetables, and vegetable juices are the absolutely safe answer to vitamin A megadosing: they are all high in carotene.

B-COMPLEX VITAMINS

The safety record of the B-complex vitamins is extraordinarily good. Since their discovery, beginning with thiamine (B1) in 1911, many thousands of studies have verified an unequaled therapeutic value of these essential substances. Side effects have been rare, and toxicity is nearly nonexistent, even at the highest doses.

Vitamins B1, B2, B12, Biotin, Folate, and Pantothenic Acid

Regulating blood sugar, nourishing your nerves, improving mood, and preventing cardiovascular disease are just a few reasons to take 50–100 milligrams per day of the B-complex vitamins. They are cheap and safe. I have seen no scientific evidence of toxicity for thiamine (B1), riboflavin (B2), cobalamin (B12), biotin, folate, or pantothenic acid. The American Association of Poison Control Centers' Toxic Exposure Surveillance System reported zero problems with these nutrients.[6] Furthermore, there are no toxicity reports published for these vitamins in the *Merck Manual,* generally regarded as a particularly authoritative medical reference.

Vitamin B3 (Niacin; Niacinamide; Inositol Hexaniacinate)

Nutritional (orthomolecular) psychiatrists have used niacin (vitamin B3) in doses as high as tens of thousands of milligrams per day for more than fifty years. It is an effective treatment for obsessive- compulsive disorder, anxiety, bipolar disorder, depression, psychotic behavior, and schizophrenia.

Most physicians have ignored niacin's usefulness until recently. Niacin has finally gained popularity as one of the cheapest and safest ways to lower cholesterol. Persons truly seeking to lower their cholesterol need to eat more fiber, vegetables (especially carrots), and vitamins E and C, and to exercise more. They also need to eat less sugar, fat and meat, and to reduce stress.

The government's daily recommendation for niacin is less than 20 milligrams, yet half of all Americans will not get even that much from their diets. Niacin's special importance is indicated in that even the RDA/DRI for niacin is nearly twenty times higher than the other B vitamins, and that's just for everyday, healthy people. As niacin is one member of the team of B vitamins, it is logical to back up megadose niacin therapy with a moderate quantity of the rest of the B-complex vitamins.

The discoverer of niacin therapy for lowering cholesterol, Abram Hoffer, M.D., says that niacin is very safe. "No fatalities have ever been shown for humans," Dr. Hoffer says. "For animals, it is about 5 grams per kilogram." This means that for an animal that weighs what an average human does (165 pounds or 75 kilograms), a fatal dose would be about 375,000 milligrams per day. Most people, healthy or not, would never exceed a fraction of that. Physicians frequently give patients 2,000–5,000 milligrams of niacin to lower cholesterol. The safety margin is large.

The most common side effects of niacin therapy include flushing, skin itching, and, with a large overdose, nausea. Such symptoms vary with the dose, the body's need, and volume of food consumed with the vitamin. Changes in liver function tests will sometimes be found in niacin users, especially those with a history of alcohol abuse. Dr. Hoffer, with over fifty years of experience using niacin, says that those changes in liver function merely indicate liver activity, and not underlying liver pathology. Taking supplemental lecithin (2 tablespoons per day) and vitamin C diminishes the side effects of niacin; take at least twice as much vitamin C as niacin—more vitamin C works even better.[7]

Do not be dissuaded from taking niacin if you are taking statin drugs for cardiovascular disease. If an underinformed physician has told you that the two don't go together, it may be because she is not up-to-date.[8]

Vitamin B6

Vitamin B6 (pyridoxine) improves mood, reduces risk of cardiovascular disease, and has been shown to be clinically effective against carpal tunnel syndrome. Occasionally, it has also been reported to cause temporary neurological symptoms such as heaviness, tingling, or numbness of the limbs in persons taking very large doses. It is very important to realize that such cases are not common, and when they do occur, almost always result from huge doses of pyridoxine taken alone. The B vitamins are a team and work best as a team. No single B vitamin can do the job that the whole team can do.

B6, by itself, in doses of 2,000–6,000 milligrams daily (that's at least a thousand times the standard U.S. dietary recommendation!), can produce side effects and is therefore way too much to take. Very few persons report symptoms on 1,000 milligrams daily, and only rarely are there reports of symptoms with any lower doses. When taken with, or as part of, a complete B-complex supplement, B6 side effects, other than a harmless deeper-colored urine, are virtually unknown.

Premenstrual tension symptoms often improve dramatically with only a few hun-

194

dred milligrams per day of extra B6 taken in divided doses throughout the day. At least 50–100 milligrams of supplemental B6 daily is a virtual necessity for women taking oral contraceptives. The "pill" causes some abnormal physiological changes that create a deficiency of B6, as well as lower blood levels of thiamine (B1), riboflavin (B2), niacin (B3), folic acid, B12, and vitamin C.[9]

VITAMIN C

Vitamin C is the world's best natural antibiotic, antiviral, antitoxin, and antihistamine. This book's recurring emphasis on vitamin C might suggest that I am offering a song with only one verse. Not so. As English literature concentrates on Shakespeare, so orthomolecular (megavitamin) therapy concentrates on vitamin C. Let the greats be given their due. The importance of vitamin C cannot be overemphasized.

Vitamin C has been shown to be helpful for over thirty major diseases, including pneumonia, herpes zoster (shingles), pancreatitis, hepatitis, arthritis, some forms of cancer, leukemia, atherosclerosis, high cholesterol, diabetes, multiple sclerosis, and chronic fatigue.[10] Many well-designed studies show that large doses of vitamin C improve both quality and length of life for cancer patients.[11] Supportive megavitamin-C therapy also reduces hair loss and nausea from chemotherapy, enabling oncologists to give maximum strength treatments.

Individual needs for vitamin C vary greatly, especially during illness. A relatively small amount of vitamin C (a few thousand milligrams per day) is often sufficient for normal health, whereas tens of thousands of milligrams may be absorbed during viral or bacterial illness, particularly if the dosage is divided during the day. When sick, you should take the minimum that gets you well, and you can expect that level to be very high during illness. Doses should be measured in grams, not milligrams, up to bowel tolerance (saturation).

If you are currently in good health, beginning at whatever level of vitamin C you are already taking, increase your intake by 1 gram (1,000mg) each day. Keep increasing your daily consumption of vitamin C by an additional 1,000 milligrams per day until a slight looseness of the bowels is felt. This may take many days or even a few weeks. At that point, decrease the dosage by a gram or two, and that is your level of vitamin C saturation. This saturation principle also works with kids. Simply adjust the dose by body weight: an 80-pound youngster is 1/2 the adult dosage; a 40-pound child is 1/4 the adult dose.

Your saturation level will vary with illness. As a dry sponge soaks up more milk, so a sick body holds more vitamin C. When sick, follow the above plan, only faster. Instead of an increase of a gram a day, try a gram every hour. Or every half hour. When I am ill, I take 4 grams (4,000mg) every ten minutes until my symptoms go away. I generally see dramatic results within the hour.

Vitamin C is best absorbed when taken in divided doses, spread throughout the day as frequently as possible. Better absorption reduces urinary waste and therefore saves money. There will also be fewer potential discomfort symptoms, the most common of which is a sensation of stomach acidity. To comfort all sensitive tummies, divide the dose and buffer any excess acidity with any combination of calcium, food, and liquid.

WAYS TO COMFORTABLY TAKE A LOT OF VITAMIN C

There are two principal side effects from taking vitamin C. The first is a failure to take enough. The second is the chance of gastrointestinal upset from taking too much. You can maximize success by heeding the following hints:

• Take smaller doses, but much more often. Because you need vitamin C all day, you should take it all through the day. Especially when sick, take it frequently.

• Take vitamin C with a beverage, snack, or meal whenever you can.

• Buffer the vitamin C with a calcium-magnesium tablet or two.

• Purchase a buffered vitamin C supplement. Your stomach is many times more acidic than ascorbic acid is. Still, if the buffered form works best for you, then use it.

• Try the new ascorbyl or so-called "esterified" forms of vitamin C. They are the most expensive nonacidic kinds of vitamin C, but are easiest on an especially sensitive tummy.

• Calcium ascorbate, magnesium ascorbate, or potassium ascorbate are also nonacidic forms of the vitamin. Calcium ascorbate is the cheapest and easiest of the three to find.

• Try a different brand. Sometimes it is just the tableting materials that need changing and not the vitamin. Try vitamin C powder, which is free of any extra ingredients.

• Sweet juice is the way to get little kids to take lots of sour ascorbic acid. Of course, you can simply use children's chewable vitamin C. Many kinds are really delicious, but they can be pricey. Select the nonacidic variety.

• Start low and work up: gradually increasing the dosage enables you to discover the amount that is most comfortable for you.

• Sprouts, especially sprouted wheat and wheatgrass, are extremely high in vitamin C. If you eat more of these excellent foods, you will reduce your need for a supplement.

• Regular supplementation with even a moderate quantity of vitamin C prevents disease and saves lives. Just 500 milligrams daily results in a lower risk of death from any cause.[12] For best results, make taking vitamin C part of your daily routine, like brushing your teeth and regular meals.

You can stop taking vitamin C at any time, but why would you want to? If you are taking very high doses, you should lower your dose gradually rather than just suddenly stop taking the vitamin. The human body likes gradual change. Saturation loose stools is a marker, not a goal. Still, drink more water (as you should be anyway) and back off when you get to bowel tolerance.

It is a myth that your body doesn't absorb extra vitamin C and all that you get from taking vitamin supplements is expensive urine. Urine is what is left over after your kidneys purify your blood. If your urine contains extra vitamin C, that vitamin C was in your blood. If the vitamin was in your blood, you absorbed it just fine. It is the *absence* of water-soluble vitamins such as vitamin C in urine that indicates vitamin deficiency. If your body excretes vitamins in your urine, that is a sign that you are well-nourished and have nutrients to spare.

"Vitamin C," wrote board-certified chest physician Frederick R. Klenner, M.D., "is one of the safest substances you can put in the human body." Vitamin C is remarkably safe even in enormously high doses. Compared to commonly used prescription drugs, side effects are virtually nonexistent. It does not cause kidney stones.[13] In fact, vitamin C increases urine flow, favorably lowers urine pH, and prevents calcium from binding with urinary oxalate. All these features help keep stones from forming.[14]

VITAMIN D

Vitamin D was first isolated from tuna fish oil in 1936 and synthesized in 1952. It is a pro-hormone sterol that your body manufactures, given sunlight, from 7-dehydrocholesterol. Vitamin D3 (cholecalciferol) is the form we and other animals make and is found in fish liver oil. Vitamin D2 is made from ergosterol, not cholesterol, and consequently is called ergocalciferol. This is the form found in plants; it also can be man-made by ultraviolet irradiation of ergosterol; it is usually added to milk and found in most American supplements. Vitamin D3 is more commonly used as a supplement in Europe.

Although D2 and D3 differ by a single carbon atom, there is evidence that D3 is more efficiently utilized in humans. There are two commercial sources of natural vitamin D3: fish liver oil and an oil extracted from wool. If a label lists "vitamin D3 (cholecalciferol)," then it is from wool. This is considered a vegetarian source. Fish liver oil will be listed if it is the source of the vitamin D.

As with all vitamins, there is ongoing and protracted debate about vitamin D's safety and effectiveness. In the end, the issue really boils down to dosage. Because vitamin D can be made in the body, given sufficient sunlight, it has been considered more of a hormone than a vitamin. This terminology is likely to prejudice any consideration of megadoses and that is unfortunate. Government-sponsored "tolerable" or "safe upper limits" for vitamin D have been established, perhaps based as much on speculation as on available facts. For babies under one year, that "upper limit" is 1,000IU (25mcg) per day. For everyone else, including pregnant and nursing women, it is 2,000IU (50mcg) per day.[15] However, these "safe upper limits" may be excessively conservative.[16]

In 2003, the *British Medical Journal* published a double-blind, controlled trial of 100,000IU vitamin D3 given orally to over 2,000 elderly patients once every four months for five years. The authors reported, in addition to greatly reduced fracture rates, that the high-dose therapy was "without adverse effects in men and women."[17] It may readily be conceded that huge but occasional doses are insufficient to produce toxicity because vitamin D is fat-soluble, stored by the body, and it takes many months of very high doses to produce calcification of soft tissues, such as the lungs and kidneys.

With the exception of oily fish, foods do not contain a significant amount of vitamin D. Because of concern over mercury levels, eating the flesh of some fish may not be practical advice and, while it contains no mercury, there is widespread dislike for cod liver oil. Since the 1930s, vitamin D has been added to fluid milk but not to other milk products.

It is cheap and reliable for people to get their vitamin D from enriched foods. Iodine, iron, and some of the B vitamins are other examples of nutrients that have been added to foods for decades. That action should be seen for what it is: a national policy effectively acknowledging that people eat so inadequately that they are otherwise unable to avoid the most obvious clinical ramifications of nutrient deficiencies, including iodine-deficiency goiter, iron-deficiency anemia, and pellagra. In the case of vitamin D, it is a tacit statement about safety as well. With 400IU added per quart, it is simple for many a milk-drinking teenager to easily quadruple the DRI of 200IU per day. Few dieticians appear worried that many people are routinely and substantially exceeding government DRIs for vitamin D.

An optimum health recommendation of 1,000–4,000IU per day, in total from all sources, is not unreasonable for the vast majority of healthy adults. Effective therapeutic levels for illness may be far higher. When high doses are used, appropriate testing and monitoring is recommended. It would be unreasonable to deny a therapeutic trial of vitamin D in cases of multiple sclerosis, scleroderma, psoriasis, congestive heart failure, hypertension, and various forms of cancer.

VITAMIN E

A prevailing myth is that you do not need to take vitamin E supplements because you get plenty of it in vegetable oils. Well, you don't, not even close. According to research, only 8 percent of men and 2.4 percent of women in the United States met the average requirements for vitamin E intake from foods alone. And this amount included vitamin E–fortified breakfast cereals.[18]

While vegetable oil contains natural beneficial cofactors, count the number of IUs of vitamin E in it. The amount of vitamin E that is preventive of cardiovascular disease is at least 200IU, probably 600IU, and an entire cup of olive oil contains less than 35IU. "Some doctors claim that vitamin E helps many heart cases, but the official view is that the substance has not been proved of value in treating heart disease." This sophomoric statement could have been taken verbatim from any of a number of recent news reports, but, in fact, this quote is from a 1953 article in *Maclean's Magazine* entitled "The Fight Over Vitamin E."[19]

Half a century later, it would seem that little has changed: "We do not support the continued use of vitamin E treatment and discourage the inclusion of vitamin E in future primary and secondary prevention trials in patients at high risk of coronary artery disease."[20] This statement is from a 2003 analysis that looked at studies employing daily treatment dosages between 50 and 800IU. Yet since the 1940s, clinicians have been reporting that vitamin E dosages between 450 and 1,600IU (or more) are required to effectively treat cardiovascular disease. Researchers and analysts know that high dosages will obtain different results than low dosages.

Vitamin E is the body's chief fat-soluble antioxidant. It is a powerful one indeed, when you consider that an RDA/DRI of 22IU is presumed adequate to protect each one of the tens of trillions of body cells in a human being. Even though there has been a veritable explosion in antioxidant research since 1968, the RDA for vitamin E has been decreased during that same time period. Vitamin E strengthens and regulates the heartbeat, like digitalis and similar drugs, at a dose between 800IU and 3,000IU daily. It reduces inflammation and scarring when frequently applied topically to burns or to sites of lacerations or surgical incisions. Internally, vitamin E helps to very gradually break down thrombi at an oral dose of between 800IU and 3,000IU.

Recent research has indicated that vitamin E normalizes high blood pressure.[21] In some hypertensive persons, commencement of very large vitamin E doses may cause a slight temporary increase in blood pressure, although maintained supplementation can then be expected to lower it. The solution is to increase the vitamin gradually, along with the proper monitoring that hypertensive patients should have anyway. High blood pressure has been called the "silent killer," and nearly a third of adults have it. It is all too frequently unrecognized and untreated. Nearly half of all deaths are due to cardiovascular diseases, and often the first symptom is death. Advocating daily supplementation with several hundred IUs of vitamin E would be good public health policy. Yet vitamin E, for decades lampooned as a "cure in search of a disease," remains virtually the "silent healer" for as much as the public has been advised of its benefits.

Vitamin E has an oxygen-sparing effect on the heart, enabling the heart to do more work on less oxygen. The benefit for recovering heart attack patients is considerable. Taking 1,200–2,000IU daily relieves angina very well. Vitamin E moderately prolongs prothrombin clotting time, decreases platelet adhesion, and has a limited "blood thinning" effect. Vitamin E is a modest vasodilator, promotes collateral circulation, and consequently offers great benefits to diabetes patients.[22] Vitamin E also works synergistically with insulin to lower high blood pressure in diabetics.[23]

In one study, states Emanuel Cheraskin, M.D., "The effect of daily vitamin E supplementation (800IU alpha-tocopherol for thirty days) on the immune responses of thirty-two healthy subjects (over sixty years old) was examined in a placebo-controlled, double-blind trial. The data suggest that vitamin E supplementation improves immune responsiveness in healthy elderly."[24] A recent study looked at patients with colon cancer who received a daily dose of 750 milligrams of vitamin E over two weeks. Short-term supplementation led to increased CD4/CD8 ratios and enhanced T-cell activity. This means a rough and tough immune system, and that is precisely what every oncologist wants to see. The authors concluded that "dietary vitamin E may be used to improve the immune functions in patients with advanced cancer." That improvement was achieved in only two weeks merits special attention.[25] (Table 8.1)

SOME WAYS AND WHYS OF VITAMIN SUPPLEMENTATION

	ADVANTAGES	DISADVANTAGES	SUGGESTIONS
Tablets or Capsules	Easy to carry and easy to use; excellent shelf life	"Pills" to take; tableting ingredients sometimes bother sensitive stomachs	Take higher potency tablets; divide doses; take with a meal or buffer with calcium
Chewables	Tasty; great for kids	Relatively expensive; unbuffered forms are tough on tooth enamel	Rinse mouth afterward with water; try powder instead, in tasty juice

	ADVANTAGES	DISADVANTAGES	SUGGESTIONS
Powder	Cheap; pure (no fillers); easiest oral-dose way to body saturation	Taste must be hidden in juice; awkward to take in public	Use powder at home; travel with tablets
Liquid	Convenient for babies	Potency quickly diminishes after opening	Add fresh vitamin powder daily to fortify the mixture
Injection or I.V.	Best possible absorption; ideal for the very sick or hospitalized patients	Just try to find an M.D. who will give them!	Frequent oral dosing simulates an I.V.; for serious illness, see a doctor
Intra-nasal	Excellent absorption; good alternative to B12 injections	Looks pretty strange; may irritate sensitive membranes	Limit use to B12
Healthy Foods	Food vitamins are natural; cost-efficient since you have to eat anyway	Low potency; many good foods are unpopular	Juice your vegetables; garden; sprout beans and grains, especially wheat and sunflower seeds
"Fortified" Processed Foods	Better than not fortifying a processed food	Too little fiber and trace nutrients; loaded with sugar and fat	Do not buy any food with artificial flavors, preservatives, or colors

Table 8.1

The most common reason for irreproducibility of successful vitamin E cures is either a failure to use enough of it, or a failure to use the natural form (D-alpha, plus mixed natural tocopherols), or both. Natural vitamin E is always the dextro- (right-handed) form. On the other hand, synthetic vitamin E is a mixture of eight isomers in equal proportions, containing only a fraction of d-alpha toco-pherol. The initial dose should be small and be gradually increased. If this is done, the fi-nal dose can safely reach 800–1,200IU or more.[26]

Another myth about vitamin E is that if you take too much, it will cause problems with prolonged blood-clotting time. Vitamin E will prolong clotting time, but beneficially. That's why it is such a competitor for Coumadin (warfarin). The solution is to gradually reduce the dose of Coumadin, while increasing the intake of vitamin E. Any doctor can help you with this. And any doctor should, because vi-tamin E is far safer than the drug.

Vitamin E is a safe and remarkably nontox-ic substance. Even the 2000 report by the Institute of Medicine of the National Academy of Sciences, which actually recommends against taking supplemental vitamin E, specifically acknowledges that 1,000 mil-ligrams (about 1,500IU) is a "tolerable upper intake level that is likely to pose no risk of adverse health effects for almost all individuals in the general population."[27]

A Columbia University study reported that the progression of Alzheimer's disease was significantly slowed in patients taking high daily doses (2,000IU) of vitamin E for two years.[28] The vitamin worked better than the drug selegiline. The patients in the Alzheimer's study tolerated their vitamin E doses well. Perhaps the real story is that 2,000IU per day for two years is safe for the elderly.

Children using anti-epileptic medication have reduced blood levels of vitamin E, a sign of deficiency. So, doctors at the University of Toronto gave epileptic children 400IU of vitamin E per day for several months, along with their medication. This combined treatment reduced the frequency of seizures in most of the children by over 60 percent. Half of them "had a 90 to 100 percent reduction in seizures." This extraordinary result is also proof of the safety of 400IU of vitamin E per day in children (equivalent to at least 800–1,200IU per day for an adult). There were no adverse side effects.[29] It also provides a clear example of pharmaceutical use creating a vitamin deficiency and an unassailable justification for supplementation.

MINERALS

Throughout this book we will be discussing dietary minerals, as well as the vitamins, on a case-by-case basis as we look at the *Fire Your Doctor!* approach to dealing with specific illnesses. But before we do, here's a brief overview:

Calcium and Magnesium

Calcium and magnesium are so important together that they are best thought of as one supplement. Look for about a 2:1 ratio of calcium-to-magnesium, around 1,000–1,200 milligrams of calcium to 400–600 milligrams of magnesium. The "citrate" forms are especially well absorbed, without being expensive.

Iron

It takes iron to make blood. Although this is certainly important for growing kids and women of childbearing years, most men do not need supplemental iron. If you have ever seen child-resistant caps on a supplement bottle, it is usually thanks to iron. While too much iron is not good, let's not obsess over iron issues. Since 1986, there has been an average of two deaths per year "associated with" iron supplements.[30] Small number? Yes, but it is two deaths too many. I choose multivitamins without any iron in them. Women can take their individual iron supplement separately, and of course, keep it away from any children. Veggie child hint: plentiful vitamin C helps kids efficiently absorb safe, plant-based "nonheme" iron from their meatless diet. Note to men worried about hemochromatosis: it is blood iron ("heme") that some adult males can overdose on. You cannot over-absorb nonheme iron. This is yet another good reason to stay away from meat.

Iodine

Your thyroid needs iodine, but not much. A drop of iodine tincture in a half-gallon of water or juice is a cheap, easy way to get your iodine without having to eat iodized salt.

Zinc

Men of child-making years lose zinc in every seminal emission. A healthy prostate gland has a tremendous preference for zinc, as does a healthy immune system. Move over, Fido: supplemental zinc (50–75mg per day) is one of man's best friends.

Manganese

Ligament and tendon strength is enhanced by manganese; along with vitamin C, it is like a "nutritional chiropractor." Your body's absorption of manganese is lousy, and supplements are good compensation.

Copper

If your tap water is delivered through copper plumbing, you are generally all set. Especially high zinc consumption (several hundred milligrams per day long term) requires a few extra milligrams of supplemental copper.

Chromium

Your body's natural insulin-balancing system works best when chromium is present. A couple of hundred micrograms (mcg) per day will ensure this. Divide the dose for best results.

Selenium

Preventing cancer, endometriosis, and recycling vitamin E are three of selenium's functions in the body. Two hundred micrograms (mcg) per day is enough to make up for our generally selenium-poor soils.

NATURAL VERSUS SYNTHETIC SUPPLEMENTS

I recommend "natural" vitamins with the following considerations weighed in:

• Can you can afford natural vitamins? If not, it's better to take synthetic chain-store vitamins than not to take vitamins at all.

• The differences between vitamin brands are usually not great. For example, almost all vitamin companies use ascorbic acid as their form of vitamin C. Since ascorbic acid is made from starch, it is technically "natural." There are a few exceptions. I have seen a vitamin C product concentrated entirely from beet tops; each tablet has 5 milligrams of natural vitamin C. If you have a 500-milligram vitamin-C tablet, you can be sure it is made with laboratory vitamin C, and that is okay too. Is the beet-top C better? I'm sure it is, but it is simply too cumbersome and too expensive to give to a patient who may require thousands of milligrams a day for prompt recovery.

• Natural products have stood a longer test of time and are generally recognized as safe. Synthetics may be only an approximation of the natural substance. But the best

214

way to get a supply of entirely natural vitamins cheaply is to eat only really good foods, leaning toward the fresh, the raw, and the near-vegetarian. Then, you also supplement for the extra quantity of vitamins that you do indeed need more of: vitamins C and E, magnesium, zinc, chromium, and the B complex.

RELATED NUTRIENTS

Phosphatidyl Choline and Phosphatidyl Inositol

Inositol is a relative of the B vitamins, and your body makes choline into an important neurotransmitter called acetylcholine. Eat lecithin granules and you'll get plenty of each. Clinical studies have shown that lecithin improves memory, even in Alzheimer's patients.

Omega-3 Fatty Acids

Omega-3 fatty acids are found in fish oils; you can also get them from nuts and veggies. A supplement of a few hundred milligrams per day is heart healthy and sensible. There is no mercury in fish oil, by the way. Mercury can't dissolve in oil.

COMMON ERRORS WHEN USING SUPPLEMENTS

It is extremely difficult to hurt yourself by taking vitamins and other food supplements. It is easy, though, to fail to achieve maximum benefit from them. Here are some things to watch for:

1. Supplement labels provide information on potency, or how much of this nutrient you are getting for your money. Check the label carefully to see *how many tablets* it takes to provide a single dose. Many people buy a product that states, in small print, that "six tablets daily provides" the label's nutritional claim, yet they take only one or two tablets daily.

2. Mineral supplement labels require some extra attention. The front label may say, for example, "Amino Acid Chelated Zinc." That is good, for amino acid chelates are very well absorbed by the body. However, the manufacturer may then state a per-tablet weight (in milligrams) that includes the weight of the chelate. The chelate (the carrier substance) may be many times heavier than the mineral it carries. You must look to see how much *elemental* mineral the supplement actually provides in each tablet. The mineral is what does

the job, so base your dosage on elemental weight. If this information is not provided, either write to the company or buy another brand.

3. The water-soluble vitamins are the B-complex vitamins and vitamin C. These should be taken in divided doses all through the day. If a person takes a lot of them at once, the greater part will be urinated out of the body within a few hours. That is a waste of money and of potential health benefit. People who take all their vitamins at breakfast often report that they are dragging by early afternoon. Lunch is an important meal, and vitamins enable you to release the energy from proteins, carbohydrates, and fats. The body's complex enzyme pathway for energy production (also known as the citric acid or Kreb's cycle) comes to a complete stop in the absence of vitamins. Vitamins do not themselves contain energy, but they are absolutely essential to enable you to get energy from your food. Taking them with each meal makes good physiological sense.

4. The fat-soluble vitamins, A, D, and E (K is almost never needed as a supplement), may be taken once per day be-

cause they can be efficiently stored. However, even they are absorbed better in divided doses, especially with meals.

5. Minerals need to be taken with each meal. Your body can only take in so much of a mineral at a time. Very large amounts of magnesium have a laxative effect. Taking zinc on an empty stomach can upset the tummy. Many complaints people have about supplementation stem from not knowing this, so always take zinc with some food.

FOODS THAT ARE ALSO SUPPLEMENTS

People that eat a Standard American Diet ("SAD") don't care much for the following unpopular foods. On the other hand, we'd need fewer supplements if we ate more of these:

Nutritional or Brewer's Yeast—Contains vitamin B12, other B vitamins, chromium, and selenium. Many people don't care for the taste of yeast, so try hiding the flavor in pineapple juice. You may prefer the taste of primary-grown nutritional yeast, as it is not a byproduct of beer making. Debittered brewers' yeast also offers a taste improvement.

Wheat Germ—Contains vitamin E, magnesium, B vitamins, and vegetarian protein. If vacuum packed in a jar, wheat germ is one of the best foods in the super-market. In bags, only buy very fresh, refrigerated wheat germ at a store where they sell a lot of it. The nose knows: smell to tell if it is fresh.

Sprouted Grains and Beans—are a complete protein containing all vitamins and minerals as well as fiber. Eat sprouts raw and often. Sprouts are the best food at the salad bar and probably the most complete food you'll find. They are low calorie and cheap to grow at home. If you had to live on only one food, your best choice would be a variety of fresh sprouted beans and grains.

Fresh, Raw Vegetable Juice—Contains carotene, a variety of minerals and vitamins, and fiber. Vegetable juice tastes great and is better for you than any beverage on Earth. Get a juicer and use it. No bottled vitamins can compare to an uncooked, concentrated extract of veggies. Drink some daily: start with a cup and increase. I down six or seven cups at a sitting.

Wheatgrass Juice—One way to get megadoses of vitamin C without taking supplements is by drinking wheatgrass juice. Wheatgrass (sprouted whole-wheat kernels) is very high in vitamin C. Wheat is very cheap, and you can sprout it right in your kitchen. On a flat tray or two, under a bit of soil, you can have an indoor sprout farm. When several inches high, harvest with regular scissors. Add a bit of water while putting the wheatgrass through the juicer. If you want to feel better fast, drink fresh wheatgrass juice.[31]

Yogurt—Contains calcium, phosphorus, beneficial acidophilus and bifidus bacteria, protein, and B vitamins. Yogurt is about the easiest dairy food to digest and absorb. Dilute it with water as an alternative to milk. Most "fruited" yogurts are sugar-laden, so buy plain and sweeten it yourself.

Lecithin—Lecithin granules by the tablespoon beat those horse pills that contain only 1.2g of the stuff. Lecithin is the cheapest, best source of choline, phospholipids, and inositol, and it is totally vegetarian. Start small and gradually increase your daily lecithin.

Whole Wheat, Barley, Oats, and Brown Rice—Contain fiber, vitamins and minerals, protein, and complex carbohydrates. Who needs extra bran or laxatives when you can just eat the fiber-rich whole grains in the first place?

Molasses—Contains iron. Avoid bitter blackstrap molasses and select a "primary" or sweet molasses as an alternative to sweet snacks.

Fresh Fruit and Raw Vegetables—Fruits and vegetables are loaded with fiber, potassium, and bioflavonoids, in addition to their well-known, if modest, quantities of vitamins and minerals. So, eat a lot of them. If you choose not to megadose with tablets, then "megadose" with low-calorie, high-vitamin raw foods, the best first source of natural vitamins.

If you are not enthusiastically chowing down on the above goodies, a regular supplement program is essential. When you are sick, supplements are needed even more. Diet alone cannot meet the nutritional needs of a sick body. In my opinion, supplements are also needed to properly maintain a healthy body. An ounce of prevention is worth a pound of cure. And at today's prices, probably worth a ton of it.

GETTING KIDS TO TAKE THEIR VITAMINS

Here are some hints to help parents get easy compliance and safe results with kids and supplements.

- Vitamin supplements are much safer than medicines, so it is not necessary to be that exact in figuring how much to give. With our kids, we found it convenient to think, "What fraction of an adult do we have here?" We figured an adult dose for an adult weight. If an adult weighed 180 pounds and took one tablet, then a 90-pound adolescent would take half a tablet and a 45-pound child would take a quarter tablet. You can safely round up and give more than this. Pound for pound, a youngster's need for vitamins is proportionally greater than that of an adult.

- You can't expect a small child to swallow a tablet or a chunk of a tablet. You can crush the tablet (or tablet fraction) and give the resulting powder in juice or mixed in a bit of food. However, hot food is not an appropriate choice for heat-sensitive vitamins. Applesauce or other pureed fruit works well; pineapple or other sweet juice is fine too. Pick a fa-

vorite food or sweet drink that hides the vitamin taste.

- For infants, the best way to give vitamin C
in antibiotic/antiviral high doses is to use
ascorbic acid powder mixed into sweet food
or sweet juice. As a quarter-teaspoon is
1,000 milligrams of pure vitamin C, this is
doable even for the highest doses.

- Giving "doctored" portions early in the meal
helps ensure they get down. Use as small
an amount of juice or fruit as possible,
rather than "taint" an entire portion. The
moment the dose is swallowed, immediately
follow it with a favorite "chaser" of some
sweet juice or fruit to take away any after-
taste from the supplement.

- With babies, all of the above preparations
may still result in the desired mixture ending
up on the floor, on the highchair, or on you.
Try it again. Just like learning to walk, as it
becomes routine, the child will accept it.
Start early and acceptance will come early.
Good habits thus formed will bring dividends
for years.

- Premixed commercial liquid vitamin preparations are fine, with a drawback. They do not
keep particularly well after opening and lose
potency quickly even in the refrigerator. Incidentally, vitamin tablets or capsules should
not be kept in a refrigerator. I know it says,

"Store in a cool, dry place," but a refrigerator is a cold, wet place. Moisture generally reduces supplement potency. Keep the bottles out of the sun, out of the car, and off the stove and they will be cool enough.

- Chewable supplements are tasty and convenient. Once a child is old enough to handle chewable tablets, he will usually take to them without complaint. Beware of artificial colors, artificial flavors, and especially artificial sweeteners. These potentially harmful chemicals are money-savers for the manufacturer and do no good for your child. Try a health food store and always read labels.

- Chewable vitamin C is handy for restaurants and traveling. Try to get the nonacidic ascorbate form of vitamin C in your chewables. This is easier on tooth enamel than the common ascorbic acid form of vitamin C. Ascorbic acid chewables can still be used occasionally. We always gave our kids a rinse of water or juice after chewing any tablet. Nonacidic vitamin C is more important for regular, repeated chewable vitamin C use, such as when a child is ill and taking a lot.

- Here is one way to tell if a child is old enough to swallow a vitamin tablet: offer a small cash reward if the kid can do it. Since chewable tablets tend to be more expensive than regular tablets containing the same amounts of nutrients, you will still save money if this works. Start first with a small capsule. Tell the child that it is okay if they can't swallow this like a big boy or girl. Pride and spending money seem to be an irresistible combination for kids.

- There are adults who cannot swallow a tablet. Many of these people, I've found, were forced as children to take a pill before they wanted to. Since honey is better bait than vinegar, you can try offering a teaspoon of honey after your child has swallowed the supplement.

- If all this seems like coercion, that's because it is. And why not? Supplements do no good in the bottle.

- When in public places, keep supplements low key. Likewise, when visiting relatives, there is no need to make a show or an issue over children's vitamins. You can give your child their vitamins before you leave home or when you get back.

- Technically, most schools require a letter from a doctor giving permission for a child to take supplements at school. If you can get such a letter from your M.D., it is handy to have. Try to avoid letting the school health people make a big production over it. Your child should not be pulled out of class or out of an activity to take a vitamin. There is no reason for any kid to be singled out at school just because supplements have always been a part of their good diet. Most principals are sensitive to children's feelings, and will respond well to your friendly parental note or phone call.

HOSPITALS AND VITAMINS

You've probably seen those golden-gilded replicas of sixteenth- and seventeenth-century world maps. They usually portray the twin hemispheres of our globe side by side, in gorgeous and strikingly incorrect detail. Truly beautiful and utterly unreliable—heaven help the explorer who tried to navigate by such maps, which amount to little more than freeze-frame representations of ignorance. They generally have nothing to say about most of the interiors of Africa, the Americas, or Asia. The old maps also may be entirely missing a continent or two, like Australia.

Columbus did not plan on colliding with the Americas on his way to the Indies, but there it was. Conversely, Australia was later discovered largely because it had been theorized that something should probably be down there, and some brave hearts just had to go and look for it.

I discovered Australia in 1973, when I went to study at the Australian National University for a year. One of the first things I did was get to a bathroom sink and see if the water gurgled the "other" way as it went down the drain. It sure did.

I was a fairly straight-laced and serious student, who happily went off in a cloud of premed preoccupation to the organic chemistry lab, whiffing benzene and virtually immersed in acetone. Didn't give it a second thought, not even when I touched my glasses with an acetone-dampened finger and it left a little fingerprint permanently etched on the plastic frame. Then it was over to the anatomy and physiology labs, where we sorted through heaped-up piles of various species of fish and cut formaldehyde-soaked specimens with ungloved hands. We hooked up live cane toads' hearts to cardiographs and dissected a very dead python. For a would-be doctor, this was all in preparation for doing this stuff to people someday soon.

As my studies progressed, I spent a considerable amount of time observing at the Canberra Hospital. I learned, among other things, that pathologists, those denizens of the hospital basement, have the best sense of humor in the whole place. They need it, because they get all of modern medicine's failures, the people who followed an incomplete map and fell right off the flat earth. I learned something of how bloody and barbaric medicine can truly be. I saw it close and personal: I scrubbed and then hovered over surgeons in the O.R. Some of their customers also ended up in the hospital basement.

Then there was the hospital food. At lunchtime, the house staff stuck a pager into the chest pocket of my white lab coat, passed me off as one of the interns, and I ate in the hospital cafeteria for free. The food was worth that price. The food patients got was no better and, in retrospect, that may well be why they often didn't get better.

Gaps in modern medical knowledge are much like gaps on old maps. The body of knowledge represented is considerable, technical, and impressive. Many would agree that what is not yet known is far greater. But what is already known *and not utilized* is the worst ignorance of all. Nutritional therapy and megavitamin treatments are prime examples of this. For decades, it has been known that high doses of vitamins cure disease.

Hospitals by definition are collections of sick people. I need no lectures on how necessary they are. I have seen the good along with the bad. But they could be immeasurably and immediately improved, in just three steps.

1.   All hospital patients should receive a multi-vitamin with each meal.
2.   Hospital meals should be near-vegetarian, fresh, and mostly raw. People that temporarily cannot eat raw foods should have theirs juiced or pureed. Health food in a hospital? What a concept!
3.   All pre- and postsurgical patients should be given an I.V. of vitamin C, 10 grams (10,000mg) every twelve hours.

Don't tell me that this cannot be done or that these measures are not safe, or that they are too expensive. These improvements are the most basic imaginable: they will reduce mortality and shorten hospital stays; they will reduce complications and lower costs; and they are all do-able, this very minute. If not done by legislation or by the hospital brass, then they can be done by you.

Hospital Reform How-To's

You can override the hospital dietician and head off the hospital food cart. Insist on bringing in your own food to your favorite patient, and do it. If you need to offer an explanation, I recommend a religious one. And, if you must, you can sneak in vitamins. I've done it myself with a family member or two. It is a bit silly that you'd even have to consider this, but the option remains.

Some day, health care without megavitamin therapy will be seen as we today see childbirth without sanitation or surgery without anesthetic. But can we afford to wait? As we don't navigate by five-hundred-year-old maps nowadays, likewise we no longer need to set our course to the profit-driven dictates of the commercial pharmaceutical industry.

A hospital, by definition, is a collection of the sick, the injured, the infirm, and the stressed. All these situations call for larger-than-normal quantities of dietary vitamins. When is the last time you saw a hospital or nursing home routinely give even a daily multi-vitamin, let alone specific high-dose therapeutic supplements?

This can immediately change and you can help do it. Prepare to stand firm on what is most important, and negotiate the rest.

- If you want to take your vitamins while hospitalized, bring them with you. A written statement from your doctor that you will be doing so can save a lot of fuss. Hospital staff often tell patients they may not take any-thing that the hospital didn't provide. You can hardly count on them to provide mega-doses of vitamins. So, it is a bit like a movie theater telling you that you can't bring in your own popcorn, but they won't sell you any either. Vitamins are vastly more impor-

87

tant to an enjoyable hospital stay than popcorn is to a movie.

- If you are given a plausible medical reason why you should not take vitamins, be bold and ask for written references. Look up each surgical procedure or medicine that you are offered. Is there really a problem with a vitamin? Complete information on drugs is contained in the *Physicians' Desk Reference (PDR),* found in any hospital pharmacy, library, or doctors' lounge. Your public library will probably even look it up for you if you telephone them from your room. The *PDR* lists all prescription medications (and there is another book for nonprescription medicines) with all their side effects, contraindications and any nutrient-drug interactions. It is quite rare for a vitamin to interfere with a prescription drug. Any such caution is in the *PDR* in writing.

By the way, any doctor or nurse who makes fun of you for being thorough probably should be more thorough themselves. Don't stand for harassment, especially when you are in the right. Tell a supervisor.

Yes, take supplements, not abuse. If you or a loved one must hospitalized, be sure to take your supplements while you're there. Do not be intimidated by hospital staff.

Unacceptable Reasons for Stopping Vitamins

- *"Vitamins will interfere with your tests."* Just have the words "takes vitamins" added onto any paperwork. Interpretation can readily be made. One physician friendly to vitamin supplementation told me of a good argument for continuing your vitamins while in the hospital: "I took them before and I'll take them after I get out, so wouldn't any tests be inaccurate (or symptoms be confused) if I stopped them now?" If there is a specific and essential test or procedure that clearly requires suspension of vitamin supplements, you can stop the day before and resume immediately after it is over, so you only lose a day.

- *"Vitamins will be dangerous after surgery."* Since all nutrition textbooks indicate a substantially increased need for vitamins during wound healing, this is illogical. Some patients have been told that their blood-thinning medications (like warfarin) are incompatible with vitamins, especially vitamins K, C, and E. First of all, your supplements probably do not contain any vitamin K, because your intestinal bacteria make it for you. Vitamin

C may slightly lessen clotting time and vitamin E may slightly increase it, so taking both typically enables the body to achieve a natural balance. If you are given warfarin, your clotting time should be monitored anyway. Instead of reducing your vitamins, doctor scan simply adjust the amount of their drug.

- *"Vitamins are unnecessary if you eat right."* Long hospital stays are unnecessary if you are fed right. Since they don't feed you correctly, supplements are the simple answer. If you find a hospital that feeds you a vegetarian, three-quarters raw-food diet, then I will lighten up. Until then, "hospital food" will continue to deserve its almost pathogenic reputation and supplements are completely justified.

It may be their building, but it is your body. Accept nothing without an explanation that is satisfactory to you. Hospitals provide essential services and save lives. They will save even more when they fully utilize megavitamin therapy. Until then, it is up to you to do it yourself.

Discovering the Nature-Cure

I would catch a little flak from my graduate students every time I'd punctuate a lecture by trotting out "old" research studies from the 1940s, 1950s, and 1960s. Now to really annoy them: may I introduce to you a pack of pre–Civil War era drugless doctors? When raw-food, simple-food vegetarians (often known as Natural Hygienists) speak of the 40s and 50s, you don't even know which century they are referring to. The natural hygiene lifestyle not only avoids drugs, but also involves neither supplements nor remedies of any kind. Its reliance on clean living, sunshine, water, unprocessed raw food, and therapeutic fasting is straight out of the 1800s. Its leaders include Dr. Sylvester Graham (born 1794), who is known for the crackers that bear his name. There's also John H. Tilden, M.D., the originator of the theory of systemic toxemia as the root cause of all illness, the inspiration for the later work of famed twentieth-century nature-cure author Dr. Herbert M. Shelton.

And there is my favorite, Russell Thacker Trall, M.D., who founded the first hydrotherapy facility in the United States in 1844, instituting a system of natural hygienics still followed to this day. So convinced was Dr. Trall that drugs were poisons, and that food and water would cure, that during the Civil War he wrote to various departments in Washington and to President Lincoln himself, offering "a system of the healing art which, applied to the treatment of the diseases prevailing in the camps and hospitals of our armies, would save thousands of the lives of our officers and soldiers."[1] Dr. Trall's successful patients included members of Congress. When he lectured at the Smithsonian Institution in February, 1862, he argued that Willie Lincoln, the President's teenage son, need not die from "a cold, pneumonia, or a fever," but to no avail. Subsequent presidents and Congress have yet to act on the advice of natural-healing advocates.

JACKSON AND MACFADDEN IN DANSVILLE

Joy, temperance, and repose Slam the door on the doctor's nose.
—HENRY WADSWORTH LONGFELLOW

Daylight was fading fast as I wriggled through a weed-covered chink in the metal fence surrounding the old Jackson Sanatorium. It was 1979, and I had been a natural health lecturer for only a couple of years. When I was promised a tour of what remained of this grand old five-floor naturopathic hospital in Dansville, New York, I jumped at it. I had little idea of what to expect. But fortunately Henry, natural hygienist, unofficial caretaker, and my guide this late autumn afternoon, was an enthusiastic scholar of the works of James Caleb Jackson, M.D. (1811–1895). He undertook my reeducation immediately. For like most people, I knew nothing of Dr. Jackson, though he was actually one of the most influential natural health practitioners of the nineteenth century. Jackson was a personal friend of both Frederick Douglass and Susan B. Anthony, and he was Clara Barton's personal physician. It was not by mere coincidence that the first chapter of the American Red Cross was founded in Dansville.[2] Jackson's nutritional health contributions have been largely obscured by his better known contemporary, John Harvey Kellogg, M.D.

As we fumbled our way toward a side door into the darkened hospital basement, my guide filled me in. Jackson, not Kellogg, was the true originator of the first dry breakfast cereal. Basically twice-toasted, crumbled whole-wheat graham crackers, Jackson's "Granula" was not flaked nor was it as successfully mass marketed.

We were inside the big building now. I looked around and there was just enough light to see that I was standing in what was once a hydrotherapy treatment room. There were assorted tubs, hot water tanks, sitz baths, and massage tables, some with neatly folded fomentation towels still hanging silently beside them. I asked if those towels had been hanging there since Dr. Jackson's day.

"No," Henry said, with a faint smile. "The facility was later operated by Bernarr Macfadden and, after his death in 1955, was kept open as a health resort and spa until 1971."

Bernarr Adolphus Macfadden, born in 1868, was orphaned by age eleven, and a millionaire by age thirty-five. He was the immensely successful publisher of long-running popular magazines including *True Detective, Photoplay,* and *Physical Culture.* At one time, Macfadden outsold legendary news mogul William Randolph Hearst on the newsstand. The archetypal "health nut," Macfadden personally led a mass health walk every year from New York City to Dansville. Dansville is upstate near Rochester, so that is quite a hike. The 300-mile health-food-powered marathon was dubbed the "Cracked Wheat Derby." Macfadden, a public relations genius, decided to try parachute jumping while in his eighties. He landed without injury, possibly due in part to the fact that he was used to routinely sleeping on the bare floor.[3] The "Father of Physical Culture" was eighty-seven when he died.[4]

We climbed upstairs into a cavernous, tiled lobby that looked the part of a once-elegant, formal ballroom. I found Macfadden literature and educational packets in a drawer, neatly mimeographed and slightly musty. We moved to the main hallway, at the center of which was a massive cast-iron stairway. "It is fireproof," Henry said, "because the first Jackson Sanatorium burned to the ground. This building was built in 1883, and built to last." And so it had.

On the fifth floor, we proceeded down a long, turquoise-painted hallway. To either side, each patient's room had a louvered door to improve fresh airflow. I stepped into a room and the first thing I noticed was that it was taller than it was wide, with an enormous window and exceptionally high ceiling. Such high ceilings were to be found on all floors of the hospital, said Henry, because fresh air and sunshine were as much a part of "taking the cure" as were mineral waters and fresh, raw garden foods.

One more flight of stairs upward and we were on the roof. Henry led me over to what looked like one of several playground merry-go-rounds, but these were different: each of the round platforms looked as if someone had placed a small, wood-framed, glass-paned greenhouse on it.

"Patients sat in one of these to sun themselves," Henry explained. "And every hour or so an attendant would rotate the thing so that the patient continually had the sunlight fully on him." The rest of the roof resembled a cross between a dance floor and a high-school gymnasium. "There were daily exercises up here, and people stood where these marks are. And, yes, there were dances, too. Over there is a bridge and pathway leading up the hill to a mineral spring, which opened after an earthquake here in 1798. That spring is the reason Dr. Jackson built here in the first place."

It was getting dark now, and time to go. Henry produced a flashlight and by its weak, yellow beam we managed to make our way back down and out the way we came in. As we left, I looked straight up the side of the massive brick building, now just barely visible in the twilight. I thought how great it would be today to have a true choice in hospitals like people had a hundred years ago. If there is a full-service, nutrition-based hospital somewhere in America, it is news to me. Even a natural-diet nursing home would be a genuine medical milestone.

THE FACTS OF FADDISM

Those who would speak only of the eccentricities of the health "faddists" marginalize their many lasting medical contributions. Too much of what the public hears today effectively distracts it from the real success nature-cure advocates have achieved. When we dwell less on the practitioners' personalities and focus more on their actual treatments, we see an ahead-of-the-times emphasis on physical activity and eating right. It is strikingly difficult to find any modern scientific basis for condemning the essential "health faddist" lifestyle. Regular exercise and eating high-fiber, nutrient-rich foods is urged by today's most respected health authorities. Long ago, Macfadden's "Physical Culture Creed" specifically called for "reasonable regular use of the muscular system" and a "wholesome diet of vital foods." Such advice is beyond reproach.

Poor health may result from consuming too much of the wrong thing as well as eating too little of the right thing. It was the health-food "faddists" who were first to promote abstinence from tobacco, alcohol, junk food, and overeating. What the "faddists" insisted on—from long before Jackson until long after Macfadden—is now universally regarded as part and parcel of good health.

WATER CURE

Even Dr. Jackson's emphasis on the curative powers of water has considerable merit. Jackson had been very sick as a young man, and attributed his dramatic reversal to hydropathy.[5] He was far from alone: in his century, the practice of water-cure was widespread. While the dietary doctrine that accompanies hydropathy almost certainly had a major role in the doctor's personal recovery and that of his patients, much of hydropathy has been quietly assimilated into conventional medical practice. Bathing, proper hygiene, Epsom salts soaks, sitz baths, hot and cold compresses, massage, and a keen appreciation of dietary trace minerals and the importance of proper hydration are now regarded as commonsense medicine.

President Ronald Reagan's personal physician, Ralph Bookman, M.D., has long been urging his patients with asthma or allergies to drink lots of water to relieve their symptoms. In an interview, Dr. Bookman said, "Unquestionably, the single most important element in the treatment of asthma and other bronchial allergy symptoms is hydration." He added that, without adequate fluids, bronchial mucous secretions are very difficult to bring up. "Liquids are medications," said Dr. Bookman. "Liquids make mucus liquid. I demand that my patients drink

10 full glasses of liquid every day. You must make a fetish of it."[6]

LEADING-EDGE DIET

Health-spa diets tended to be simple, fresh from the garden, and low meat or no meat. If not exclusively vegetarian, as were Jackson's, they were not far removed. Macfadden, regarded by traditional vegan natural hygienists as a milk-diet revisionist, nevertheless offered menus that were nutritious, low fat, low cholesterol, low sugar, and high fiber. Though Macfadden's expansive claims for such a diet continuously got him into trouble with regulatory authorities, this is a therapeutic diet no matter who puts it in front of you. Recently, rather strict vegetarianism has been shown by Dean Ornish, M.D., to be a highly effective way to prevent and even reverse serious cardiovascular disease. This is a therapy straight out of Dansville and, as Dr. Ornish acknowledges, far more ancient sources.

I think much of Ornish's diet prescription invites comparison with "Bernarr Macfadden's Culinary Creed," an original copy of which is in my possession. It makes the following recommendations:

- "Use lemon juice instead of vinegar for sauces and salad dressing. Use lemon in all salads, with fish dishes, and wherever possible. Do not discard the green outer leaves of cabbage or lettuce."

- "Do not use chemically bleached white flour or sugar."
- "Never discard left-over vegetable pot juices. They can be used in soups, or served as vegetable cocktails with lemon and tomato juice added. Place left-over juices and pot liquors in the refrigerator, in tightly covered containers, to prevent vitamin spoilage. Cook carrot and beet tops with your soups. They contain valuable minerals. Fresh beet tops can be used as a green vegetable. Add parsley, mint, pimento, watercress, and lemon wherever possible to salads and dishes. They are relishable and provide you with minerals."
- "Throughout winter months, continue to use as many fresh fruits and vegetables as possible to procure. They are the protective foods."
- "Watch fruits and vegetables for residues of insecticide sprayings containing poisons, which frequently account for diseases of an insidious kind, difficult to trace." (If there was a better foretelling of multiple chemical sensitivity, I have yet to hear it.)
- "Food must be thoroughly masticated and mixed with the saliva."

- "Use vital foods only, those that contain all necessary vitamins and minerals."
- "Use salt sparingly."
- "All raw vegetable juices are especially recommended."

The foods mentioned above are far better sources of vitamins and minerals than are highly processed factory foods, and before the advent of food fortification, they were the only sources. Compared to orthomolecular (megavitamin) medicine, food-based doses of many of the major vitamins are low. Nutritional supplements were completely unavailable a century and a half ago. Vitamins were not discovered until 1895, the year Dr. Jackson died, and they were not synthesized until the 1930s. Strict adherence to fresh, raw, or unprocessed sanatorium dining, extreme as it might superficially seem, was the only sensible orthomolecular regimen of the day.

Sanatorium diets were and remain quite high in vitamin C (from fruits, raw milk, and sprouted grains), relatively high in vitamin E (from nuts, seeds, whole grains, and wheat germ), and very high in carotenes (from fruits, vegetables, and vegetable juice). Macfadden emphasized all such foods, and the man loved carrots more than any person in history.

FASTING

Because Macfadden happened to be on a short fast when he died, his death has often been wrongly attributed to fasting. That he completed innumerable fasts throughout his entire long and doctor-free life is generally downplayed. As a matter of fact, for decades he routinely fasted every Monday, year after year, with many additional extensive fasts. Macfadden was known to all for his long work-days and notorious for his physical stamina. This is a man who could rip a deck of cards in half, twice over, and repeatedly lift 100 pounds over his head with one hand.[7] No wonder a young man named Angelo Siciliano became a Macfadden protégé and would later achieve his own fame as Charles Atlas.[8]

Upton Sinclair was another Macfadden supporter. After fasting for seven days, Sinclair wrote, "I have been about and busy every minute of the day and until late at night. I have walked miles every day and have felt no weakness to speak of. I shall continue the fast until I feel hungry." He did so, and after twelve days concluded: "The fast is not an ordeal, it is a rest."[9] The Pulitzer Prize winner, who fasted frequently, lived to be ninety.

Although he did suggest one- or two-week fasts in some of his writings, Macfadden primarily endorsed short fasts and, in particular, habitual undereating. In his creed, he wrote: "If no appetite at meal time, wait until the next meal" and "To prolong life, do not eat to repletion. Stop when you could enjoy more, or better still, fast on water alone or fruit juices for one day each week." These are hardly reckless recommendations. Indeed, widespread adoption of the overall mindset of therapeutic fasting ("when in doubt, leave it out") would do our overfed, overweight Western society much good. Gerontologist Roy Walford, M.D., recommends systematic undereating (with the addition of high doses of supplemental vitamins) in order to increase the human life span by as much as forty years.[10] Other physicians, notably Alan Cott, M.D., have authored how-to books recommending fasting for weight loss and also to promote general health and well-being.[11]

LAW OF CURE

The homeopathic pioneer Constantine Hering (1800–1880) formulated a "Law of Cure," which states that all healing begins from the head down, from within out, and in the reverse order that symptoms originally appeared. This concept, originally a homeopathic one, describes how the nature-cure works and it has several practical applications.

1. Feeling better is a most important step in getting better. That is not as thin a statement as it may at first seem. You can very often see recovery in a patient's face and attitude long before tests and technology confirm it. A healing state of mind is as least as important as juicing, eating right, and taking vitamins, and those three are extraordinarily important. When I fast during sickness, I "feel" fine even though I know I am sick. That's an odd thought, but then, why not feel good when you are sick? And when at the first blush of physiological trouble, I take a lot of vitamin C, I feel great immediately and the sickness does not get a chance to start.

2. With well-established chronic diseases, one cannot expect an overnight cure. In chronic illness, cure tends to be more of a process than an event. "Healing from within out" is a rough guideline meaning that deeper symptoms may clear up before all externally obvious symptoms go away. You might feel better before you look better. But feeling good (sleeping well, pain relief, positive mental disposition) for me remains a primary goal. Many naturopaths feel that outward symptoms such as skin outbreaks, temporary diarrhea, and mucus expectoration are evidence of beneficial

body cleansing, and therefore good signs of recovery.

3. Hering's "reverse order" healing postulate is like employment seniority at a layoff-happy factory: last hired, first fired. Or like stripping away layers of paint: down deepest is the oldest, and the oldest comes off last. Our longest-standing health problems take the most time for resolution; that is logical. Patients get impatient; that is inevitable. If you have a lifetime of lousy eating and bad health habits behind you, doesn't it figure that it may take some months to tidy (or "excavate") the mess in your cluttered anatomical attic?

Don't chase symptoms. If you wander about after every symptom, you will likely spend your life lost in the pharmaceutical aisles. Respect symptoms, yes. See them for what they are: lifestyle indicators. But the way to eliminate symptoms is to end their fundamental, underlying cause: change what's wrong in your life. Drop your bad habits and drop your excuses for keeping them. Instead, eat right, exercise, juice vegetables, and take your vitamins.

The rest is just a matter of details. Even the most conservative medical and dietetic professionals will admit that at least two-thirds of all illness is caused by poor health behaviors. I think it is far higher. Most people are understandably but narrowly focused on the particular symptoms of "their illness." They commonly want to know "What vitamin should I take?" for this or for that. It doesn't work like that, all-purpose megadoses of vitamin C notwithstanding.

The way out is to overhaul your way of life. Symptoms are a guide. Only living bodies have symptoms. Where there are symptoms, there is life. And something you can do about it. Life may be work, but consider the alternative.

MEDICAL POLITICS AND THE NATURE-CURE

While Macfadden endured harsh attacks from medical-political forces of the mid-twentieth-century, Dr. Jackson operated what his grateful patients affectionately called "Our Home on the Hillside" the century before, during a time when allopathic medical associations and the pharmaceutical industry were yet to gain the exceptional governmental and media influence that they maintain to this day. Between the end of the Civil War and the start of World War I, there was still freedom of choice in health care in America. Homeopathy, herbology, naturopathy, hydrotherapy, chiropractic, and, of course, all manner of patent medicine men competed shamelessly for the healthcare dollar. It was an ideological open season.

It is a great loss that most countries of the world have since invested so heavily, and often exclusively, in pharmaceutically based health care. Such a single-party system inhibits a patient's choice and, in my opinion, inhibits a patient's recovery far more.

How different things must have been when the "Home on the Hillside" was not only the health center of the Northeast, but was "the largest hygienic institution in the world."[12] The sanatorium even had its own rail spur. What made the nature-cure hospital so popular, even in a location as remote as Dansville? Perhaps it was Dr. Jackson's personality, which by all accounts was impressive, or the water, or the huge organic vegetable gardens. But perhaps it was simply the sanatorium's success rate that brought in the crowds. Nutrition-based therapy works—it worked then and it works now.

The times have changed since Jackson's and Macfadden's day. People no longer flock to grand health hotels to "take the cure." But there is nothing stopping us from making our homes into our own personal health retreats. Daily routines can include the same health-boosting program of whole-foods diet and life-affirming exercise that once led thousands to Dansville.[13]

Part Two

Natural Healing Protocols for All-Too-Common Health Problems

Acne

Let's "face" it—if there were an effective and safe magic bullet for curing acne, you'd already know about it. The drug companies are hard at work looking for a lucrative chemical cure to what remains fundamentally a dietary problem. In the meantime, they advertise and sell various notions, potions, and lotions. Slathering stuff on blemished faces is big business. And let's not forget antibiotics, for many a teen has seen tetracycline.

In promoting antibiotics to treat acne, we are trying to put the blame on bacteria. But bacteria are on every human face. Why do some people have much worse cases of acne than others? As a dental hygienist once told me, the bacteria that cause dental decay are just scavengers doing their job. What you have to do, she said, is brush and floss to remove their food supply. My question is, What is the facial bacteria's food source?

I think we have no choice but to look at the average teenager's terrible diet, containing too much of the wrong things and not enough of the right things. Too few whole grains, beans, fruits, and vegetables, and far too much meat, junk food, fast food, snacks, sodas, sugar, and chemical additives.

Modern medical fashion has excluded bad diet as the underlying, common problem behind the pimples. However, vitamin A and its derivatives are sometimes used to treat globular acne, according to the *Merck Manual,* which suggests that there is a diet connection.[1] Although vitamin A is effective, the high doses necessary put the patient at risk for vitamin A toxicity. Getting the kids to eat and juice vegetables makes more overall sense and is immeasurably safer. Vegetables are loaded with carotene; you cannot overdose on it, and the body makes it into vitamin A as it needs to.

One of the functions of your skin is to excrete wastes. Per square inch, it does not do the kind of job that the colon and kidneys do, but then you have so much of it. In cases of renal failure, when a person's kidneys cease to operate, the skin is called upon to excrete the wastes normally eliminated in urine. A white-silvery powder coating of urea crystals on the skin indicates life-threatening renal failure.

But there are lesser degrees of skin excretion, and a diet of junk food means excretory overtime. The first thing to try with acne is a complete dietary overhaul, something all too many teenagers have never been asked to do.

Some people want to believe that diet is not a factor. Dermatologists flatly state that chowing down on chocolate has nothing to do with acne. I think they are wrong. At the very least, candy displaces good foods in the diet. Even over-consumption of oily foods like French fries, some say, has no impact on the condition. Over-consumption of fries means underconsumption of wholesome vegetable foods. And let the dietitians and dermatologists answer this: What exactly is the positive value of greasy foods? There is no downside to forgoing the grease from any teen's table.

I speak from personal experience, having once been a teenage boy whose diet was typically awful. Yes, I had acne, though not as bad as some of my friends did. It peaked when I was seventeen. My passport photo from that year proves it. Then I went overseas to study, was more than a bit stressed, and took my already considerable chocolate, sugar, meat, and greasy-food eating habits to new heights. My broken-out skin broke out still worse. Eventually, having failed to see any improvement otherwise, I changed my diet, and the acne went away. This may have been coincidence; I think it was curative. To me, the test is this: to this day, if I eat wrong, my skin will break out. The theory that acne is all about overproduction of skin oils and blocked skin pores due to hormones fails to adequately consider why some teenagers get acne so bad and others don't. And acne can hit people in adult life and even in middle age. Why the variation in incidence and degree of symptoms? I think the answer, old fashioned or not, is connected to people's diets.

Nature-cure theory has long maintained that rashes, pimples, pox, and other skin outbreaks are attempts by the body to clean itself. The body will try, must try, to clean itself of toxins, foreign chemicals, and the residues of junk food. Nature eliminates wastes. If you want the body's natural clean-out process to stop, you have to first stop your unnatural knack for sending junk down the hatch in the first place.

I've known quite a few young people who have started drinking fresh, juiced vegetables and taken a simple multivitamin/mineral supplement twice daily, and their skin cleared up immediately. I challenge any young person to become a whole-foods health nut and fail to see results in the mirror.

AIDS

Question: What's the difference between most AIDS drug research and $500 hammers bought by the Pentagon? Answer: The public has received more honest value from the hammers.

Research and conferences open and close with still no AIDS cure in sight. So we go on spending vastly more money per patient looking for a cure for AIDS than we do even for cancer, even though cancer kills over ten times as many Americans. And cancer research itself has been largely inconclusive. After all, have you heard of a cure for cancer? But money isn't the problem. The billions spent in the United States on AIDS research has resulted in nothing that would stop people from dying.

Depressing indeed is the sentence of death implicit with the diagnosis of "HIV-positive." Go get medical treatment, yet expect to actually get little more than hope. Hope might be in the form of knowing that not everyone that is HIV-positive ends up with full-blown AIDS. AIDS-related complex (ARC) and "carrier" patients exist. Half of all HIV-positive individuals have remained free of disease after ten years.[1] Why?

Maybe it is because some people have stronger immune systems. In that case, it is logical to build up the immune system of any AIDS patient. The body's natural defense system, which is so weakened by the AIDS virus, is highly dependent on that individual's nutrition. Ordinary diet obviously won't cure AIDS. Concentrated nutrition research might. Just how much research has been funded to see how well large doses of vitamins do fighting AIDS? Too little. Ask yourself this: Can a weak immune system really be due to a bodily deficiency of antiretroviral drugs? No, but it might indeed be due to nutritional deficiency.

A seven-year study of 281 HIV-positive men at Johns Hopkins University showed that those taking vitamins had only about half as many new AIDS outbreaks as those not taking supplements. A 50 percent reduction in AIDS cases just from vitamins! The real wonder is that the dosages used were so small: only 715 milligrams of vitamin C a day and about five times the RDA of the B vitamins and beta-carotene.[2] Larger (orthomolecular) amounts would almost certainly save more lives. Even so, the research team concluded that "the highest levels of total intake (from food and supplements) of vitamins C and B1 and niacin were associated with a significantly decreased progression rate to AIDS."

After an astounding eleven-year delay, another low-dose vitamin supplement study was finally conducted in 2004. Reported from Harvard University as if it were original news, the new research *also* finds that vitamins cut AIDS deaths by 27 percent and slow the progression to AIDS by 50 percent. "Multivitamins also resulted in significantly higher CD4+ and CD8+ cell counts and significantly lower viral loads. Multivitamin supplements delay the progression of HIV disease."[3]

Clearly, nutrition supplement therapy for HIV-AIDS patients is well worth doing. Today, over 40 million of the world's people have AIDS. How many deaths have resulted from decades of nutritional inaction? In July 2004, the Joint United Nations Program on HIV/AIDS estimated the amount of money needed to treat the world's poorest AIDS patients will top $12 billion. This prediction contains two silent assumptions: (1) that the spread of AIDS will continue virtually unabated, and (2) that treatment efforts will continue to be pharmaceutically based. Yet drug treatment has been spectacularly ineffective in lowering either the spread or the mortality rate of AIDS. Any limited, medicines-only approach diminishes the humanity of AIDS sufferers to that of already-doomed pharmaceutical customers. Now, in 2004, we have research confirming what the Johns Hopkins study showed more than a decade ago: Even very modest doses of nutritional supplements slow, or even help stop, AIDS. To the tune of 50 percent. If there were a drug that did that, it would be trumpeted from every media rooftop.

Robert Cathcart, M.D., in California treats AIDS patients with up to 200,000 milligrams of vitamin C a day. His findings are that even advanced AIDS patients live significantly longer and have far fewer symptoms with vitamin C. Imagine what prompt, large doses of vitamin C might accomplish in a recently diagnosed HIV-positive individual.

According to Dr. Cathcart, "Massive doses of ascorbate (50–200g per 24 hours) can suppress the symptoms of the disease and can markedly reduce the tendency for secondary infections ... This clinical remission is achieved despite continuing laboratory evidence of helper T-cell suppression."[4] He states that AIDS patients are usually capable of ingesting extraordinarily large doses of vitamin C; the amount of ascorbate taken orally is to be maximized to bowel tolerance. Dr. Cathcart uses a "balanced ascorbate" mixture, consisting of a combination of approximately 25 percent buffered ascorbate salts (calcium, magnesium, and potassium ascorbate) and 75 percent ascorbic acid, dissolved in a small amount of water and taken at least every hour. "The usual amount tolerated initially is between 40 and 100g per 24 hours. Doses in excess of 100g per 24 hours may be necessary with secondary bacterial and viral infections." Sometimes intravenous ascorbate is necessary, because the patient's need exceeds their ability to take adequate amounts of ascorbate to scavenge all of the free radicals created by the AIDS infection.[5]

When nutrition succeeds where drugs have failed, it poses a tremendous threat to medicine and pharmacology. If supplemental doses of vitamins can do a better job than drugs, then it is an embarrassment to health professionals who have maintained, "You don't need vitamin pills; just eat a balanced diet." When vitamins outperform drugs, big money is at risk. Vitamin C costs less than twenty dollars a pound for pure crystals. Multiple vitamin pills cost just pennies each. And high dose supplements are vastly more economical than designer drugs. Safer, too. If these common nutrients work, they certainly cannot be patented by a drug company. No potential for profit? Then no interest or funding for research.

An example of this would be the medical profession's stiff reluctance to endorse or even do extensive clinical trials of University of Victoria professor Harold Foster's nutritional AIDS protocol of selenium, cysteine, glutamine, and tryptophan. Dr. Foster noted the work of E.W. Taylor,[6] which indicated that HIV might be selenium dependent. Then, Dr. Foster observed, in considering all of Africa, AIDS incidence is strikingly low in the country of Senegal. In Senegal, the soil is very high in selenium. Abundant dietary selenium, Dr. Foster thinks, prevents a fatal HIV-induced selenium deficiency. The rationale for adding the three amino acids as well is fully described in his book, *What Really Causes AIDS*.[7]

The medical profession considers giving selenium, cysteine, glutamine, and tryptophan to HIV/AIDS patients (if they consider it at all) to be too simple to work, and therefore too silly to even try. The medical profession has been wrong before, and here I think they are wrong again. The Foster therapy has been successfully field-tested in five countries in Africa. There is righteous need for urgency. With every delay, AIDS patients suffer and die, and so many do so unnecessarily. For those that have already died from AIDS, it is too late for us to apply yesterday's research. For those dying from AIDS right now, tomorrow's research is too late.

Only one thing matters, and that is results. Even the small amount of nutritional research done has shown more promise than heavily funded medical research for AIDS. The public has been told to line up, wait for, and try out exorbitantly expensive new drugs as they come along. That same public has been told to not try vitamins. There is a bolt loose here somewhere. For the HIV-positive individual, and certainly for the AIDS patient, it must be "any port in a storm." Nutritional therapy may prove to be a safe harbor for many with HIV.

Anxiety and Panic Attacks

When it feels like a jungle out there, don't you just want to hide up in your tree? This is a common response, and not the worst one. No one knows how many people are in prison because of destructive outbursts that normally should have been controlled. Millions of regular folks just barely manage to function within their "lives of quiet desperation" every day. Millions of prescriptions are written every year for emotional illness. Two out of three visits to family physicians are for stress-related illness, with an annual cost of at least $75 billion.[1]

So much can be done for so many of these people, including some good, natural remedies and regular practice of stress-reduction techniques. When I was an undergraduate at the Australian National University, my anxiety over schoolwork (and being 12,000 miles from home at age eighteen) caused me actual pain. The university physician did an appropriate examination, got out his prescription pad, and started to write. Here it comes, I thought, "Rx: Take thou a tranquilizer." Not so. This doctor had written down the name of a book: *Relief without Drugs* by Ainslie Mears, M.D.

I was being told to relax and I did not like it. To top it off, the doctor assumed (correctly) that I did not know "how" to relax, so he provided a reference so I could learn. The novelty of this educational, drugless approach is what persuaded me to try it. It worked and the pain went away. For the first time, I had a prescription filled, not at the drugstore, but at the bookstore.

While studying at the nearby Canberra Hospital, I learned other stress-reduction techniques such as imaging, self-hypnosis, and auto-relaxation from staff and consulting psychiatrists. Many people I knew and respected began practicing Transcendental Meditation, with evident beneficial results. Use of these techniques provides you with a proven solution to anxiety.

L-tryptophan—Nutritional therapy also shows positive results for anxiety and panic attacks. Melatonin can help you get a good night's sleep and serotonin can mean freedom from anxiety during the day. You cannot tell someone to relax unless they have the biochemistry to do it. It is safer (and cheaper) to let the body make the molecules than to use pharmaceuticals.

You provide the raw materials and your body does the rest. Your brain produces both melatonin and serotonin from the essential amino acid L-tryptophan. You can buy trypto-phan as a supplement, but it is quite expensive. There is little, if any, justification for such prices for something so safe and vital to life that it is put in liquid feedings for the elderly and is in all infant formulas.

The good news is that you can get plenty of tryptophan at the dinner table simply by eating beans, dairy products, and especially, nuts. A high complex-carbohydrate, mostly vegetarian diet helps your brain take up the tryptophan you eat.

Vitamin B6—In order to properly use tryp-tophan, your body needs vitamin B6 (pyridox-ine). B6 deficiency is very common in Ameri-cans and that deficiency is measured against an already ridiculously low RDA/DRI of less than 2 milligrams. It is unfortunate that some people have been wrongly warned off B6 supplementa-tion with scares of overdosing.

Large doses of B6 taken alone have pro-duced temporary neurological side effects. It usually takes between 2,000 and 5,000 mil-ligrams of B6 daily for symptoms of numbness or tingling in the extremities. That is an awful lot of B6. Some side effects have been reported with as low as 500 milligrams daily, but these are rare indeed. Therapeutic doses between 100 and 500 milligrams daily are commonly prescribed by physicians for PMS relief, so a few hundred milligrams of B6 a day are strictly safe. Higher doses are likely to be without side effects, if taken along with the entire B complex to ensure a reasonable nutrient balance.[2]

Niacin—Vitamin B3 (niacin) is so effective against psychoses that half of all mental ward inmates in the South were able to be released once a Depression-era dietary deficiency of this vitamin was corrected. Niacin in larger-than-dietary doses acts as a natural tranquilizer and induces relaxation or sleep. It is nonaddictive, cheap, and safer than any pharmaceutical product. Dosage varies with condition. Ortho-molecular physician Abram Hoffer, M.D., whose experience with niacin dates back to the early 1950s, routinely recommends at least as much vitamin C as niacin. Body saturation of niacin is indicated by a warmness of the skin and blushing or "flushing" sensation. Most persons will also experience a feeling of relaxation and ease. Unlike pharmaceutical tranquilizers, niacin simply feeds the body what it needs to internally and naturally provide relief.[3]

Lecithin—Lecithin is a food supplement that is high in phosphatidyl choline. Your body is able to make acetylcholine, a neurotransmitter, out of this, which has a wonderful "settling effect" on a person. A third of your brain, by dry weight, is lecithin. Feeding the organ what it is largely made of can help it to function better.

Lecithin supplements are made from soybeans. Each tablespoon (7.5g) of lecithin granules contains 1,700 milligrams of phosphatidyl choline. The lecithin that is available in capsules is the most popular. In order to get even one tablespoon of lecithin, you would have to take eight to twelve capsules. Since an effective supplemental dose is 3 or more tablespoons daily, that's a lot of capsules to swallow. Much less costly is liquid lecithin. However, liquid lecithin tastes, well, crummy. After taking liquid lecithin, it is wise to have a "chaser" of any dairy product. A bite of cheese will hide the taste completely.

Probably the best way to get a lot of lecithin easily is lecithin granules. Stir the granules quickly into pineapple juice or milk. They won't dissolve, but rather will drift about as you drink. Lecithin granules can also be used as a topping on any cold food. If you are really reluctant, try lecithin on some ice cream. Also, the granules are not bad if stirred into yogurt.

Chromium—Chromium may help even out sugar-induced mood swings and perhaps even sugar cravings. Chromium deficiency (daily intake under 50mcg) affects nine out of ten adults. An amount between 200 and 400mcg of chromium, in divided doses, substantially improves your cells' ability to use insulin.

Chromium polynicotinate or chromium picolinate are well-absorbed forms.

B-Complex Vitamins—B complex also helps with blood sugar regulation. In addition, the metabolism of just about everything you digest hinges on one or more of the B vitamins. Taken together, they are especially safe and effective. However, your body needs proportionally more niacin than the other B vitamins (the RDA for niacin is about twenty times that of other B vitamins). Therefore, extra niacin is appropriate.

Foods to Limit—Avoiding sugar reduces anxiety symptoms. If you don't know this, it's because you haven't tried it. The swings from low to high to low blood sugar result in corresponding mood swings. Eat complex carbohydrates instead. Chocolate or artificially colored candy can trigger what has been termed a "cerebral allergy" in some people. Such episodes can be so severe as to border on the psychotic. Allergist Benjamin Feingold, M.D., took people off colored foods and noticed them calm down immediately.

Caffeine, a xanthine chemical stimulant, is well known to provoke an anxiety response, which in some persons can be extraordinarily intense. Some forms of dementia may actually be caffeine allergies.[4] Even low doses can affect sensitive persons. Have trouble kicking the caffeine habit? Try megadosing on vitamin C.

A meat-dominated diet can result in a dramatic drop in your body's serotonin levels. Carbohydrates, on the other hand, assist absorption of the amino acid L-tryptophan into the brain.

Water—Some people have found that drinking more water calms their anxiety. How hard is that to try?

Homeopathic Remedies—Remedies such as *Aconite, Coffea Cruda,* and *Kali Phos* have been used to treat symptoms of anxiety for nearly 200 years. These very dilute, natural remedies are safe and can help significantly. I recommend that you get a copy of *The Prescriber* by J.H. Clarke, M.D. This very practical book concisely explains this healing approach and helps you easily select the most appropriate remedy. Homeopathic remedies are nonprescription. Many health food stores carry them. I know a number of people who carry a bottle of *Kali Phos* 6X tablets in their pocket or purse just in case: it is good first aid for a panic attack.

Herbs—Herbs such as chamomile and catnip make a soothing tea. There are certainly many other useful anxiety-healing herbs to consider, which a library search or Internet search will bring forward for you.

Exercise—Exercise reduces anxiety. Is it because you are too pooped to worry? Who cares—it helps. Exercise has many other health benefits, too, so there is no way you can lose by trying it. Walk, swim, chop wood, jog in place, lift weights, whatever works for you. Start easy, and gradually work up to really calm yourself down.

Arthritis

For decades, it was medical doctrine that there was little or no connection between arthritis and nutrition.

Nature-cure advocates hold that the etiology of arthritis parallels a history of bad diet. You will rarely see an arthritic patient that is not a cooked-food-and-meat eater. Animal evidence supports this. Francis M. Pottenger, M.D., did nutritional experiments on hundreds of cats over a period of many years. He found that cats fed our typical cooked diet did in fact develop many degenerative diseases, including arthritis. What is especially interesting is that Dr. Pottenger found you could reverse the condition by feeding the animals only fresh, raw foods.[1]

What should the arthritic person eat? I recommend the following protocol:

- Primarily a raw food diet, high in sprouts, and including modest amounts of cultured dairy products such as cheese and yogurt[2]
- Niacinamide every two hours, up to several thousand milligrams daily[3]
- Vitamin B6, 100 to 300 milligrams daily, preferably taken with a B-complex supplement and in divided doses
- Vitamin C to saturation

Vitamin C—Since 1753, deficiency of vitamin C foods has been known to produce scurvy. One of the chief symptoms of scurvy is profound joint troubles. Sailors with scurvy could be heard literally rattling as they walked on deck. At that time, no one believed that there was any connection between diet and joint disorders, either.

"Arth-" means joint and "-itis" means inflammation. It would be asking a lot of a few pieces of fruit to cure it. However, large doses of vitamin C have been shown to reduce all forms of inflammation throughout the body. The joints are no exception. The amount of vitamin C needed is the amount that will get the job done. You take enough C to be symptom free, whatever the amount might be.

In addition to reducing inflammation, vitamin C also helps form collagen, the protein "glue" that holds cells together. Collagen is especially important in connective tissue to ensure healthy ligaments, cartilage, tendons, and the joints themselves. Without sufficient vitamin C, collagen cannot be properly made, which may lead to joint deformities.[4]

The key is to use enough. Studies that show little vitamin C benefit for arthritis generally employed only a few hundred milligrams of vitamin C daily. Thousands of milligrams, at least, are required for clinical improvement. A person with arthritis seems to require vastly more vitamin C to correct the problem than the deficiency it took to cause it.

B Vitamins—William Kaufman, M.D., Ph.D., suspected an arthritis-diet deficiency connection and acted on it. One of Dr. Kaufman's primary tools was niacinamide (niacin, vitamin B3). He gave 250 milligrams of niacinamide (the form of niacin that does not cause a warm flush) every one and one-half hours for a daily total of ten doses. That is 2,500 milligrams a day. The results were improved grip strength and joint mobility.[5]

In a 1978 radio interview, Dr. Kaufman said, "I had one patient who was so severely arthritic that I could not bend his elbows enough to measure his blood pressure. He was one of my first patients. I gave him niacinamide for a week in divided doses, and then he could bend his arm. I took him off it and gave him a look-alike medicine (placebo). In a week, he was back where he was before: his joints were stiff again."

It was necessary to divide the doses so that blood levels of niacinamide were uniform throughout the day. Using frequent 250-milligram doses of niacinamide is more effective for arthritis than larger, but less frequent, 500-milligram doses. The greater the stiffness, the more frequent the doses. Severely crippled arthritic patients needed up to 4,000 milligrams per day, divided into ten doses. In one to three months, patients could get out of their chairs or beds. By the end of three years of treatment, they would be fully ambulatory, and even older patients would respond.

Dr. Kaufman treated close to 1,000 patients with niacinamide plus the B vitamins thiamine (B1), riboflavin (B2), pyridoxine (B6), and pantothenic acid. It will not surprise you that he also gave large doses of vitamin C. What will surprise you is that he started using vitamins to successfully treat arthritis as early as 1935, and niacin in 1937.[6] Niacinamide, alone or combined with other vitamins, caused no adverse side effects in Dr. Kaufmann's studies.[7] Nausea is the upper limiting symptom for niacinamide. Niacin, which although it causes a flush rarely causes nausea, may be substituted instead.

In 1983, John M. Ellis, a physician in Texas, published an entire book on vitamin B6 (pyridoxine) entitled *Free of Pain*.[8] Dr. Ellis found that B6 shrinks the synovial membranes lining the joints, which helps control pain and restore mobility.[9] While very large doses of B6 alone may cause transient neurological side effects, relatively modest doses of around 75 to 300 milligrams daily are very safe. The safety of one B vitamin is magnified by giving it with the rest of the B complex.

Behavior and Learning Disorders

I have taught at every grade level, from primary school all the way to the doctoral level. This experience has helped me to understand the essential role that nutrition plays in the education process. May you never have a class full of sugared-up, chemically fed, vitamin-deficient students. Regardless of age, they are too poisoned to pay attention.

Many, perhaps most, of the "difficult" pupils in schools today are not "bad" but are nutritionally impaired. School lunch programs attempt to provide calories and a full belly, but it would be much better to approve and fund only menu items free of artificial colors, flavors, preservatives, and added sugar. The addition of a good multiple vitamin and extra vitamin C to each meal would do even more. Large research studies confirm that American kids are not getting even the modest RDA/DRI levels of many vitamins and minerals. This no doubt affects their school performance.

Did you know that children are not allowed to take vitamin tablets in school without a doctor's written permission? Yet they can be fed cupcakes and candy right in class or the lunchroom.

There is reason to suspect that attention deficit hyperactivity disorder (ADHD) is really a vitamin deficit disorder. What is so difficult about giving schoolchildren vitamin supplements to make up their deficit? Don't tell me that vitamins would be too dangerous, expensive, or impractical to administer in school. They give kids the prescription drug methylphenidate (Ritalin) in schools everywhere, and it has numerous contraindications and side effects. Let's get safe food supplements into kids whose parents cannot afford them. Isn't that the logic behind school meals?

Omitting junk is even easier. Schools can easily avoid artificial chemicals in their menus. Here's an eye-opening field trip assignment for parents: Visit the kitchen of your local public or private school and read the labels on the boxes they get from their food distributors. Yet a school district has only to specify a standard and the suppliers will jump to keep their business. How about putting a little pressure on your Board of Education to go chemical free in their served meals?

The behavior benefits of subtracting food chemicals and adding vitamin supplements are elementary. Many children respond promptly to a chemical-free diet. Allergist Benjamin

Fein-gold, M.D., wrote *Why Your Child is Hyper-active* to help parents get behavior improvement through foods without drugs. It works for many, and it's safer than Ritalin. In 1990, more than 750,000 American schoolchildren were on Ritalin.[1] In less than ten years, that number had soared to over 4 million children.[2] Kids as young as age six line up daily, in school, for this drug. Let's line them up for vitamins instead.

We can begin with vitamin B3 (niacin or niacinamide). William Kaufman, M.D., Ph.D., describes the effect of niacin: "One patient wondered whether or not his vitamin medications contain a sedative. He recalls that before vitamin therapy was instituted, he had a great deal of energy and 'drive,' and considered himself to be a 'very dynamic person.' But his history showed that, prior to niacinamide therapy, he suffered from a type of compulsive impatience, and he was often careless and inefficient in his work, but was busy all the time. With vitamin therapy, he became unaccustomedly calm, working more efficiently and losing the feeling that he is constantly driving himself. If such a patient can be persuaded to continue with niacinamide therapy, in time he comes to enjoy a sense of well-being, realizing in retrospect that what he thought in the past was a super-abundance of energy and vitality was in reality an abnormal 'wound-up feeling,' which was an expression of aniacinamidosis (niacin deficiency)."[3]

Natural healing is very dissimilar to drug medicine: it's safer. The FDA classifies Ritalin (methylphenidate) as a Schedule II substance, a category that includes amphetamines and cocaine. Dangerous drugs are not for kids. Malnutrition needs to be considered first. ADHD is not caused by drug deficiency, but it may indeed be caused by nutritional deficiency. Many major symptoms of attention deficit hyperactivity disorder are very similar to those of niacin deficiency. Natural diet need not work for every child to still help thousands of them. It is safe to try it for all. There are no harmful side effects from avoiding added sugar and artificial food additives. Drug dependency isn't encouraged with good nutrition.

I know of case after case where a kid stops getting food additives and starts taking vitamins, especially C and the B complex, and is off Ritalin or similar drugs in two weeks or less. It is most effective to give vitamins in divided doses along with food. Breaking a B-complex tablet in thirds can cover all three meals. Frederick R. Klenner, M.D., recommended giving children their age in grams of vitamin C (one gram is 1,000 milligrams). We found that half of that was enough to keep our kids well; that is 4,000 milligrams daily for an eight-year-old, divided over three meals or snacks.

I was on my way out of a downtown building when a little girl (six years old at most) was on her way in, holding her mother's hand. I only heard the last moment of their conversation, which apparently consisted of a discussion of her brother's questionable behavior in a nearby store. As she looked up at her mother, the girl matter-of-factly said, "I think he had too much sugar." If a six-year-old can figure out the cause of problem behavior, why can't America's doctors and dieticians? Their food-processor-friendly party line has been, and continues to be, that sugar and chemical foods do not affect children's behavior.[4] Well, they do.

Bipolar Disorder (Manic-Depressive Disorder)

People who've suffered with bipolar disorder for years will find this next statement amazing:

"The manic/depressive state was assessed in twenty-four subjects who completed two generally accepted psychometric tests. Each patient was provided with either a three-gram (3,000mg) ascorbic acid effervescent tablet or a placebo. In the vitamin C–treated group, the severity of the bipolar state was reduced within the first hour and then declined even more rapidly between the second and fourth hours. No change occurred in the placebo subset."[1]

Improvement in a matter of hours? Take a look at the above study again. First, note that the study was placebo controlled, then focus on the dose. The patients took a dose of 3,000 milligrams of vitamin C. Not 500 milligrams, and not a glass of orange juice. If the vitamin C is continued in repeated doses, the improvement will also continue.

Here's more good news: if you add in megadoses of niacin, the results can be better still. Psychiatrist Abram Hoffer, M.D., has successfully treated bipolar patients nutritionally for fifty years with both niacin and vitamin C. He writes: "Not long ago, a man came up to me and greeted me as if he knew me. He told me I had seen him many years earlier. He was well and neatly dressed and buying groceries. He was still taking three grams (3,000mg) of niacin every day, which he thought was great. When I looked up his file, it showed that I first saw him in the intensive care unit of a psychiatric hospital. He was admitted to a chronic mental hospital years ago following abuse of amphetamines. He suffered from hallucinations, voices and visions, paranoid ideas, mood swings and was often hyperexcitable. He had been diagnosed as bipolar. He drank a lot and used street drugs. After I saw him, I started him on niacin, 1,000 milligrams after each meal, and ascorbic acid (vitamin C) at the same dose. When I saw him last, he was off drugs and liquor."

With another patient, Dr. Hoffer added the B-complex vitamins plus minerals. "A woman, age 32, had been diagnosed as manic depressive and had been on and off lithium for 13 years. She heard voices and had paranoia, poor memory, and difficulty with concentration." He started her on a dairy-free diet with vitamin C (ascorbic acid, 1,000 milligrams after each meal), B6 (pyridoxine, 250 milligrams daily), zinc citrate (50mg daily), selenium (200mcg daily), and a B complex once daily. After a few months, she was well. She had started to improve about ten days after starting on the program.[2]

Another possibility to consider is that a reaction to caffeine may be so profound as to be misdiagnosed as bipolar disorder. One woman wrote to me: "My entire life has changed since I started learning about how caffeine affects behavior. I was diagnosed with bipolar disorder, but medication didn't seem to help. I thought about suicide every day. I was ready to shriek with laughter or break into sobs at a moment's notice." Then she stopped using caffeine and consequently no longer needed her medications. Since then, she has not had any thoughts of suicide or a moment when she did not feel clear-headed and in control. She feels like a different person.

Eliminating caffeine makes sense, costs absolutely nothing, and deserves a therapeutic trial for all persons suffering from what seems to be bipolar disorder. I am certainly not saying that this is the answer for all, but it may be a significant part of the solution.[3]

Caffeine Addiction

Caffeine is America's drug of choice. I suppose if you are going to become dependent on a drug, it might as well be caffeine. Caffeine is certainly better than alcohol, nicotine, or narcotics. Consenting adults can have their blast of caffeine in their morning coffee if they choose to—that's their business. But an increasingly large number of children are having that same blast. "One-fifth of one- and two-year-old children consume soft drinks. Those toddlers drink an average of 7 ounces—nearly one cup—per day."[1] Some estimates are that nearly three-quarters of all children over the age of six months regularly use caffeine.[2] Caffeine, a methylated xanthine, is a stimulant drug. How do you feel about children using a drug? Did they get the habit from TV, their friends, or from watching Mom and Dad?

This is assuming caffeine-users are able to have any children in the first place, for women drinking caffeine have more difficulty conceiving than those who avoid caffeine.[3] Because of the risk of Reye's Syndrome, most parents avoid letting their kids take aspirin. But caffeine, as well as alcohol, is among recognized factors that can cause gastric ulcers. All these drugs, including caffeine, decrease the strength of the stomach lining. Caffeine also interferes with normal blood sugar levels.[4]

Miscarriage or low-birthweight babies, heart attack, elevated blood pressure, benign breast lumps, panic attacks, and lower academic performance may result from habitual, maintained caffeine use. With caffeine consumption at the equivalent of seven to ten cups of coffee a day, and for an extended period of time, there can be observable and even permanent damage to the rhythm of the heartbeat. Medical research and common sense alike indicate that staying off caffeine is well worth doing.

How do you stop caffeine intake without the withdrawal headaches? And then, how do you avoid the recurrent urge to raid your local Starbucks a few days later?

• Vitamin C reduces caffeine withdrawal symptoms, especially the headache. Studies have also shown that vitamin C reduces cravings for drugs, including nicotine and even narcotics such as heroin.[5] My suggestion: Take enough C to be symptom free, whatever the amount may be. Although it normally can take a couple of months to get over a caffeine habit, high antitoxic doses of vitamin C can greatly speed the process.

• Behavior modification: To work the psychological end of the street, substitute a nice cup of something else for your morning coffee.

Postum, herb-tea blends, hot water and lemon, or hot cider are all good choices. Enjoy the society, the ritual, and the cold-weather, creature comfort of pouring and holding a steaming mug of caffeine-free something-else in your hands. Even decaf is a good start.

• "What about tea?" you may be asking. Yes, there is caffeine in regular tea, roughly half that of coffee. Tea also contains some antioxidants, which are good for you. But then, fruits and vegetables contain a far greater variety of antioxidants and zero caffeine.

People often ask which is better, green tea or black tea? You may be somewhat surprised at the answer: their leaves are picked off of the very same plant, *Camellia sinensis.* The difference is that green tea is not aged (fermented), whereas black tea is. Uncrushed, unoxidized green tea leaves are healthier for you. But both naturally contain caffeine. A 5-ounce cup of brewed tea has roughly the same amount as a 12-ounce caffeine-containing soft drink.

• Because caffeine causes a "flushing out" of vitamin C and the B vitamins, I think vitamin supplements are especially important for the caffeine user and for the would-be quitter. Vast numbers of Americans are serious caffeine users. Caffeine is even found in diet aids and extra-strength pain relievers. For long-term caffeine afficionados, it is possible that a small homeopathic dose of unroasted coffee, *Coffea Cruda* 6X, might help you break away.

Remember, if you "have to have" your morning cup of coffee, that is a dependency. Any dependency that has physical symptoms, such as headache, as the consequence of quitting is a true addiction. This includes caffeine. Maybe it is time for us to wake up and not smell the coffee.

Cancer

People with cancer are fairly often cured for no known reason. Sometimes called "spontaneous remission," it happens every day. Somehow, the body has destroyed the cancer by itself. Anything we can do to encourage this is worthwhile. One way we may be able to assist the body is with vitamins and other nutrients.

There are several nutritional aspects to consider in cancer treatment. One of the most valuable is vitamin C, especially when given intravenously. A number of other nutrients and dietary approaches have shown effectiveness against cancer. Here is a case when you may need to fire your present doctor and hire a different one that will work with you. And there is much that can be done.

Vitamin C—"Treatment with high doses ascorbic acid either by mouth or intravenously or both carries no risk and does provide substantial advantages over chemotherapy and surgery used as the sole treatment," according to Abram Hoffer, M.D., Ph.D. In extremely high intravenous concentrations, vitamin C kills cancer cells without harming normal healthy cells.[1]

Vitamin C is essential to the formation of collagen, the protein "glue" that holds our cells together. Collagen binds your cells, just as mortar binds bricks together in a wall. If collagen is abundant and strong, your cells hold together well and tumors have a tough time spreading through them. Strong collagen can thereby slow or even arrest the spread of cancer. Cancer cells secrete a substance called hyaluronidase, which helps them eat away at collagen and break out into the rest of the body.[2] High vitamin C levels maximize collagen production. If cancer cells are going to try to spread by destroying a person's collagen, it just makes sense to make stronger collagen to keep them from doing it. To do this, a person fighting cancer probably needs enormous amounts of any substance that helps make collagen. Persons with cancer commonly have exceptionally low levels of vitamin C in their bodies, which might help explain why their collagen has not been able to prevent cancer from spreading. There is nothing to lose and everything to gain by trying regular high doses of vitamin C with every cancer patient.

Another reason to use vitamin C in cancer treatments is that vitamin C helps strengthen the immune system. Maximum immune function is vital if we want the body to kill cancer. Yet medical treatments such as radiation and chemotherapy can actually weaken the immune system a great deal. There are, then, really two reasons to bolster immunity with vitamin C. First, large quantities of the vitamin often enable a person to more easily tolerate large doses of radiation and chemotherapy, with far fewer side effects. Vitamin C does not interfere with chemotherapy.[3] Second, stronger immune function can only help the patient to fight the disease better in general.

In England, it once was not uncommon for terminally ill patients to receive narcotics to ease their pain. One side benefit of vitamin C studies at Vale of Leven Hospital in Scotland was profound pain relief. Patients given 10 grams (10,000mg) of intravenous vitamin C each day had greatly reduced pain even after the narcotic was discontinued.[4]

Administration: Vitamin C is most effective given intravenously. Vitamin C may also be taken by mouth, but this is not ideal. To approximate the constancy of an intravenous drip, it is necessary to have very frequent oral doses. An oral dose of the vitamin every half hour is not excessive. The amount of each dose is the maximum amount that a person can tolerate without diarrhea. This is called "titrating to bowel tolerance."[5] Loose stools indicate bodily saturation with the vitamin. Results may require truly large daily totals. Remember that oral doses are not as efficient as intravenous vitamin C, so it takes much more to do the job.

Vitamin C given orally has to be absorbed through the digestive tract, and a good bit of it isn't. Generally speaking, the sicker the patient, the more C she can hold. Most healthy people would experience bowel tolerance at a daily total of less than 20,000 milligrams (20g). This indicates a need for relatively little of the vitamin. A person with cancer may have a besieged immune system that would soak up as much as 100,000 milligrams (100g) per day or possibly even more. That is a lot of vitamin C, but then we are also asking a lot of it.

It is important to be consistent with large quantities of vitamin C. It needs to be taken every day and often. Taking too little of the vitamin sporadically is of little value. Taking too much at one time may result in a false saturation diarrhea. Most people taking 5,000 milligrams or more of vitamin C in a single dose will experience temporary loose stools. Yet, the cancer patient might really be able to hold twenty times that amount if taken in smaller, divided doses throughout the entire day. It must be emphasized that the just-barely sub-laxative level of vitamin C is the therapeutic level. This varies from person to person and must be established individually. All successful vitamin C studies for cancer have used high doses—the higher the dose, the better the outcome has been.

The Vitamin C Controversy: Physician reports from doctors such as Dr. Hoffer, who has worked with over 1,200 cancer patients, repeatedly indicate that those taking large quantities of vitamin C achieve significantly longer life and vastly improved quality of life.[6] I cannot imagine any more important and uplifting news for the family of a cancer patient.

Not everyone agrees with this. Certain politically powerful medical authorities have openly discouraged cancer patients from taking large doses of vitamin C. It is unethical for any doctor to deny therapy that might be of value to her patient. Still, the number of cancer patients who have ever had their doctor recommend a therapeutic trial of large quantities of vitamin C remains small.

The grounds for disparaging vitamin C usually center on three inaccurate claims: (1) vitamin C is ineffective against cancer; (2) vitamin C interferes with convitional cancer therapies; and (3) vitamin C is in itself harmful to the cancer patient. Let's set the record straight.

There are many controlled studies demonstrating that vitamin C is in itself effective against cancer.[7] Dose determines effectiveness. Some of the most successful early studies were done in Japan, using over 30,000 milligrams of vitamin C a day. More recently, clinical reports from orthomolecular (megavitamin) physicians, such as Hugh D. Riordan, M.D., indicate that even higher quantities of vitamin C work better. Dr. Riordan has found that 100,000 milligrams per day of vitamin C, given by intravenous infusion, actually kills cancer cells without harming healthy body cells.[8] Vitamin C at high concentrations is toxic to cancer cells in vitro.[9] Selective toxicity, the principle of conventional drug chemotherapy, can be also be accomplished effectively (and more safely) with I.V. vitamin C.[10]

Vitamin C administered orally in high doses reduces the side effects of chemotherapy, surgery, and radiation therapy. Patients on a strong nutritional program have far less nausea and often experience little or no hair loss during chemo. They experience reduced pain and swelling following radiation. They have faster, uncomplicated healing after surgery. Such vitamin-mediated benefits mean that oncologists can give vitamin-taking patients the full dose of conventional chemotherapy, rather than having to cut the dose to keep the patient from giving up entirely. Obviously, full-strength chemo is more likely to be effective against cancer than reduced-strength chemo. A similar benefit is at work with radiation therapy. Therefore, vitamin C, far from being detrimental, makes a most positive contribution to the conventional treatment of cancer.

Even at very high doses, vitamin C is an unusually safe substance; countless studies over a seventy-year period have repeatedly verified this. As an antioxidant, collagen-building coenzyme, and reinforcer of the immune system, vitamin C is vital to a cancer patient. Yet the blood work of cancer patients will invariably show that they have abnormally low levels of the vitamin. What is dangerous is vitamin deficiency.[11]

Vitamin A (as carotene)—High doses of vitamin A have proved effective against a number of forms of cancer. Acceptance of vitamin A therapy is probably slow due to the potential toxicity of the oil form of the vitamin when taken in enormous quantities for a long time. However, the vitamin A precursor, carotene or pro–vitamin A, is strictly nontoxic regardless of quantity or duration of therapy. A harmless carotenosis, or orange-colored skin, is the only side effect of even the most massive carotene intake. The body converts beta-carotene into vitamin A only as it needs to and the carotenes are probably more active against cancer than preformed oil vitamin A.

While the effective amount of carotene may exceed 500,000IU daily, that amount can be obtained from eight to ten glasses of fresh carrot juice. Such a natural source guarantees a mixture of many different forms of carotene. Adding some tomatoes into the mix provides lycopene, another anticancer carotenoid. Compared to fresh veggie juice, synthetic beta-carotene supplements are of little value.

"Most people have heard of beta-carotene, but this is only one of a large number of carotenoids which are present in colored vegetables and fruits such as carrots, beets, tomatoes and greens," states Dr. Hoffer. "The evidence is very powerful that these mixed carotenoids as found in these foods will decrease the incidence of cancer but there is a question about the efficacy of the pure beta-carotene. There is still a vigorous debate about this. I prefer carrot juice to the beta-carotene."

Vitamin E—Vitamin E is an antioxidant and free-radical scavenger that seems to help prevent cell damage related to cancer. It is a fat-soluble vitamin with no known toxicity. Doses of 800IU to 1,200IU are commonly employed. Dr. Hoffer prefers to use the water-soluble form of vitamin E, known as "d-alpha tocopherol succinate" for cancer patients. "This water soluble form has the greatest efficacy in controlling cancer cell growth in the test tube."[12]

Selenium—Regions of the United States with this trace mineral in their soil appear to have less cancer than those regions that don't. Research has indicated that selenium works with vitamin E both to protect body cells and to slow tumor growth. "I use selenium, 200mcg, three times per day (total 600mcg)," states Dr. Hoffer. "I think the toxicity of selenium has been greatly exaggerated. I had a patient who developed a severe lymphoma. He was operated on, but it came back. He had radiation and it recurred. He was given three months to live. I had started him on selenium, 600mcg per day. Like many patients, he thought if 600 is good, more is even better. He came back and said he was taking 2 milligrams per day, or 2,000mcg. I became a bit concerned about that and suggested he cut down to 1,000. In any event, he recovered and he has now been alive for seven years."[13]

For persons in good health, a normal supplementation dose for selenium is generally between 100 micrograms and 200 micrograms daily. Dr. Hoffer's higher amount is intended specifically for cancer patients with a doctor's supervision.

Niacin (vitamin B3)—"There have been seven international conferences on niacin and cancer," writes Dr. Hoffer. "This vitamin is an essential component of the enzyme systems that repair broken DNA molecules. The dose ranges from 100mg to 1,000mg three times daily (total 3,000mg per day). Several studies have found that the response rate of cancer of the head and neck was 10 percent on radiation alone but increased to 80 percent when patients were given large doses of niacinamide."[14]

Folic Acid (folate)—"Several studies have found this important vitamin has anticancer properties, for cancer of the cervix and of the lung," states Dr. Hoffer. "The dose range is from 1mg to 30mg daily. It can be taken (in such doses) only on prescription."[15]

Coenzyme Q10—"Dr. Karl Folkers discovered this substance, also called ubiquinone," says Dr. Hoffer. "Toward the end of his long and distinguished career, he regretted that he had not called it a vitamin. It is an odd vitamin, since young people are able to make enough from the lower numbered ubiquinones such as Q6 or Q8 whereas older people and anyone ill is not able to make enough. It thus becomes a vitamin later in life and when one becomes ill."[16] A few clinical studies have shown that large doses of coenzyme Q10 have anticancer properties, especially for breast cancer. CoQ10 is expensive, but nonprescription. Therapeutic doses range from 300 to 600 milligrams daily.

Calcium and Magnesium—These two minerals have been found helpful in cases of bowel cancer. Adults should receive 1,000–1,500 milligrams of calcium daily from their food and supplements, and half as much magnesium.[17]

"The sicker a person is, the more nutrients are needed in optimum doses to help the body's reparative mechanisms," states Dr. Hoffer. "Treatment must be started as soon as the diagnosis is suspected and made, and should be concurrent with any other treatment recommended by oncologists and cancer specialists." He predicts that eventually all cancer specialists will use these orthomolecular techniques. Supplements should be maintained while chemotherapy or radiation are being used, because patients do not suffer as much from the side effects and recover much more quickly.

Dr. Hoffer relates his experience working with cancer patients: "I did not interfere with the treatment done by the oncologists. What I tried to do was to improve their general health, to improve their immune system, to the point that they could cope more successfully with their tumors. The first thing I would do would be to create a bit of hope. I don't think many doctors in cancer clinics realize the absolute importance of hope.

"Then I advise my patients what kind of nutrition they ought to follow. The first thing I try to do is to cut their fat way down. I try to cut it down below 30 percent of calories, down to 20 or 10, if possible. I find that, in our culture, the easiest way to do that is to totally eliminate all dairy products. If you eliminate all dairy products and cut out all fatty meats, it's pretty hard to get too much fat in the diet. So, I put them all on a dairy-free program. I reduce, but I don't eliminate, meat and fish, and I ask them to increase their vegetables, especially raw, as much as they can. I think it's a good, reasonable diet, which most people can follow without too much difficulty. Having spent some time with them going over what they ought to eat, I begin to talk about the nutrients. The first one, of course, is vitamin C. I am convinced today that vitamin C is the most important single nutrient that one can give to any person with cancer.

"What are this program's advantages? Well, first of all, the increase in longevity. We have increased the longevity from 5.7 months to approximately 100 months, which is very substantial, and half of the patients are still alive. There has been a tremendous decrease in pain and anxiety, even amongst those who were dying. We do not have the final answer, but we have at least a partial answer. The use of nutrients, like vitamins C and B3 increase the efficacy of chemotherapy by increasing its killing effect on the tumor and decreasing its toxicity on normal tissues. The same has been shown to be true with radiation therapy.

"My conclusion is that the best treatment for cancer today is a combination of the best that modern medicine can offer, surgery, radiation, chemotherapy, combined with the best of what orthomolecular physicians can offer, which is nutrition, nutrients and hope."[18]

Gerson Cancer Therapy—The Gerson diet protocol, developed by the late Max Gerson, M.D., works toward the overall detoxification and nutritional restoration of the entire body, focusing on the liver. "Dr. Gerson found that the underlying problems of all cancer patients are toxicity and deficiency," states Dr. Gerson's daughter, Charlotte. "He found that one of the important features of his therapy had to be the hourly administration of fresh vegetable juices. These supply ample nutrients, as well as fluids to help flush out the kidneys. When the high levels of nutrients re-enter tissues, toxins accumulated over many years are forced into the bloodstream. The toxins are then filtered out by the liver. The liver is easily overburdened by the continuous release of toxins. Dr. Gerson found that he could provide help to the liver by the caffeine in coffee, absorbed from the colon. The caffeine stimulates the liver/bile ducts to open, releasing the poisons into the intestinal tract for excretion."[19]

Charlotte Gerson's entire life has been immersed in healing people, first learning while assisting her father, and later teaching his method to the world. I personally have seen what the Gerson program can do for the terminally ill cancer patient. I have been called upon to help in a couple of high-profile, but last minute, cases. One patient was a well-known sports figure. He was given some months to live and was not happy about it, as he was still in his fifties. He asked what his best shot would be for inoperable, untreatable metastasized cancer. I told him—the Gerson therapy. He did it, not in its entirety, but with enthusiasm. And, he lived considerably longer than he was expected to. But what really impressed me was the dramatic improvement in his energy level: from fatigue and weakness, he went instantly to a vibrant life. He maintained a more-than-full schedule for so long that even people who knew he had cancer forgot that he was sick.

I saw a similar level of success with a prominent New York businessman with untreatable liver cancer. He began to do much, but by no means all, of the Gerson program, and was subsequently able to extensively travel the world with his family. He lived years longer than expected, with a high quality of life confirmed by all who saw him. Looking only at these two patients, critics of Gerson's method might think that, without complete and unequivocal cure, there is little to crow about, but such a view is unproductive. Both these patients' families will tell you that added years and added quality of life are worth juicing the vegetables for.

For decades, cancer treatment and research has been almost entirely restricted to cut, zap and drug: surgery, radiation, and chemotherapy. Billions and billions of dollars have been expended investigating every cure but a nutritional one. Dr. Gerson guaranteed his own ostracism when he dedicated his life to find out why patients lived, and what could be done to be sure they did. It has been ridicule, not science, that has kept the Gerson therapy away from your local oncologist's office. The therapy's infamous coffee enema (don't worry: it's at body temperature) offers at least two vital benefits for a seriously ill patient: pain relief and detoxification. Gerson's extensive medical experience taught him that both are accomplished. Patients and physicians who follow Gerson's protocol have seen that he's right.

"I am familiar with the Gerson method and believe that it has a lot of merit," says Dr. Hoffer. "I have always been frustrated that it was not taken seriously and studied intensively as it should be. I think it has a very good track record."

If there is a down side to vegetable juices, I have yet to hear it. The worst reproach I've encountered is that, while harmless, vegetable juices have no special properties against cancer. But we now know that vegetables do help prevent and arrest cancer. Tomatoes are loaded with lycopene, proven effective against prostate cancer. Orange and green vegetables are tremendous sources of carotene. Broccoli, cauliflower, kale, Brussels sprouts, and cabbage (the cruciform vegetables) are all high in sulforaphane, a botanical heavyweight in the fight against cancer.[20] Juice consists of the entire cytoplasmic contents of a vegetable's cells, but without an unpalatable excess of indigestible fibrous cell wall. The two chief purposes of juicing are to increase the quantity of vegetables consumed, and to increase a patient's absorption of what is consumed. Juicing is good, and Gerson was right.

The Gerson therapy is labor intensive and takes a minimum of eighteen months to complete. Hospitalization is not a requirement. Dr. Gerson achieved remarkable results even from diagnosed terminally ill patients. You would think that it would be difficult to justify denying any patient the potential benefits of this proven nutritional program, but to most oncologists, it remains a "fringe" therapy to this day.

Prince Charles was soundly criticized by British doctors when he said in June 2004: "I know of one patient who turned to the Gerson therapy having been told she was suffering from terminal cancer and would not survive another course of chemotherapy. Happily, seven years later, she is alive and well. So it is vital that, rather than dismissing such experiences, we should further investigate the beneficial nature of these treatments."

Part of the Gerson program is the ever-controversial but crucial liver-detoxifying coffee enemas. But the heart of the program is nutritional, based on high-vegetable, low-salt diet, vegetable juices, and supplements of potassium, iodine, digestive enzymes, liver extract, niacin, and (by prescription) thyroid, and vitamin B12 injections. It is a lot of work to be sure. My experience in working with very sick patients and their families is that they are easily overwhelmed with instruction, no matter how vital that instruction may be. When done at home, the Gerson program requires a dedicated, involved, and cooperative family effort.

It needs to be said often that the Gerson therapy is not specifically a cancer treatment. Dr. Gerson saw it as a metabolic treatment, one that cleanses the human organism while strengthening the body's ability to heal itself. Not surprisingly, therefore, the Gerson therapy is effective against a wide variety of diseases, from migraines to lupus. The Gerson approach has been shown, for over six decades, to significantly improve both quality of life and length of life in the sickest, the most hopeless, of cancer patients. Many people have been completely cured on the Gerson therapy.[21]

Traditional medical treatments for cancer have focused on how to go in and kill cancer with chemicals or radiation. It is likely that this approach will evolve in favor of trying to get the patient's body to kill the cancer. A well-nourished body has the very best chance of doing this. During the crisis of cancer, the immune system needs to be boosted with a concentrated, plant-based diet and appropriately high doses of supplemental nutrients. In addition, extremely high intravenous doses of vitamin C, which kill cancer cells, may well be the chemotherapy of the future. And it can be done today.

Cardiovascular Disease

Cardiovascular disease (CVD) is by far the number-one killer of both men and women. And yet, most cardiovascular illness can be prevented. This makes it the perfect place to fire your doctor in a big way, because many heart and circulatory ailments can be halted and even reversed through nutritional therapy. While a detailed consideration of this topic is far too big for this book, I present here a working summation of natural cardiovascular therapies to get you started right now.

1. Eat less fat: This you already know; a near-vegetarian diet is the simplest, cheapest way to do it.

2. Don't smoke: This you know, too, but are you doing it? For ways to kick the tobacco habit, see the Tobacco Addiction section.

3. Lose excess weight. For practical, natural suggestions, please see the section labeled Weight, Excess.

4. Exercise more: Moderate exercise makes your ticker strong, your pipes clear, and your blood pressure healthfully low. Try walking or workout videos. If you can, exercise with a friend or a family member.

Just how good are the above four measures? The American Heart Association says heart disease deaths could be reduced by a third if people just ate better and exercised. Cigarettes kill over 400,000 Americans annually; stop smoking and CVD mortality will sink like a stone. Add supplements and take away meat, and the death rate would drop even farther. You could say that about most chronic illnesses, but with cardiovascular disease there is really no scientific controversy about it—it's smoking, failing to eat right, and refusal to exercise that is damaging our heart and its attendant plumbing.

There is far less agreement over the cure for CVD. There is money in arteries; as long as surgeons become millionaires from open-heart surgery, we can expect them to give short shrift to competitive, curative nutrition. After all, vitamins and a near-vegetarian diet are immeasurably cheaper and safer than by-pass surgery. I have often wondered how re-placing a few inches of coronary arteries is any kind of cure. Unless the patient changes his diet and lifestyle, won't the grafted blood vessels get all gummed up the way the first set did? And if you plan to change your diet to prevent that, why wait for surgery to force it? The fact that bypass grafts will sometimes be performed more than once on the same patient shows that some people are just not getting the message.

And the message is good news, indeed: "alternative" therapies work and are well proven. The stress-reduction and vegetarian-diet plan of Dean Ornish, M.D., has been demonstrated to reduce arterial blockages without surgery.[1] Lecithin and other supplements have been in use for decades and high doses of vitamin E for CVD disease spans an incredible seventy years.

Atherosclerosis

Atherosclerosis or "hardening of the arteries" is the underlying pathology behind most cardiovascular disease. Narrowed blood vessels prevent proper blood circulation, raise blood pressure, and catch wandering blood clots more easily. The result may be slow decline or instant death. The answer is neither surgical nor pharmaceutical, it is nutritional.

Lecithin—Take 2–4 tablespoons per day. Lecithin is a lipotrophic (fat-moving) agent that helps keep fatty deposits off the inside of your arteries. This both prevents and reverses atherosclerosis.[2] As too much fat is a problem for your body and its blood vessels, too little of the essential fatty acids (EFAs) is a problem for the ticker. Actually, your body does not need to eat any fat at all. Aside from taste and texture, the only role of dietary fat is to provide the EFAs, linolenic acid, and linoleic acid. Fatty acids are the preferred food source for the heart. Lecithin contains abundant linoleic acid and some linolenic as well. Heart-happy linolenic acid, found in fish oils, is also available in seeds, walnuts, and vegetables. This is why a near-vegetarian diet, which includes some fish, is best for health maintenance. Fish oils (for linolenic acid) and lecithin (for linoleic acid) are essential for a healthy circulatory system.

Each tablespoon (7.5g) of lecithin granules contains about 1,700 milligrams of phosphatidyl choline, 1,000 milligrams of phosphatidyl inositol, and about 2,200 milligrams of essential fatty acids. These valuable substances tend to be undersupplied by our daily diet.

Lecithin tastes crummy, which is why lecithin in capsules is so popular. These are admittedly convenient, but are also expensive. In order to get one tablespoon of lecithin, you have to take eight to twelve capsules. Since an effective supplemental dose is three or more tablespoons daily, that's a lot of capsules to swallow. Much less costly is liquid lecithin. A taste for liquid lecithin has to be acquired; it is easier to take if you first coat the spoon with milk or molasses. After taking liquid lecithin, have a "chaser" of any dairy product or molasses.

Lecithin is cheapest bought in bulk at a health food store as *granular* lecithin. Probably the best way to take a lot of lecithin easily is to stir the granules quickly into juice or milk. Personally, I think milk best covers the taste, but pineapple juice works well, too. Lecithin granules won't dissolve, but rather will drift about as you drink. They can also be used as a topping on any cold food. All supplemental forms of lecithin are made from soybeans. An alternate, but minimal, nonsoy source is egg yolk. Generally, maximum benefit is obtained when you eat the yolk lightly cooked (such as in a soft-boiled egg).

Diet—Eat less sugar. Even if you ate little or no cholesterol, your body will still make it. Sugar can cause your body to produce excess cholesterol. Sugar also raises your body's insulin levels and your triglycerides with it. Eat less meat as well. Even lean meat contains fat and cholesterol. High protein diets are not healthy in the long run.

Incorporate more fiber into your diet. While the scientists are figuring out why high-fiber diets reduce cardiovascular disease, just do it because it works. Eat, if you can, more wheat germ and brewer's (nutritional) yeast. Wheat germ is a much better than average source of magnesium and vitamin E, while nutritional yeast is a source of chromium and vitamin B12.

Additional Nutrients—Take more niacin (vitamin B3), between 1,000 milligrams and 3,000 milligrams per day. Abram Hoffer, M.D., one of the originators of niacin therapy to lower cholesterol, explains the difference between the common kinds of niacin: "Niacin lowers cholesterol, elevates high density lipoprotein (HDL) cholesterol, and reduces the ravages of heart disease, but causes flushing when it is first taken. The flushing reaction dissipates in time and in most cases is gone or very minor within a matter of weeks. Niacinamide has no effect on blood fats (lipids), but is not a vasodilator. A third form, inositol hexaniacinate, will lower cholesterol without the flushing side effect, although not quite as well as pure niacin will."

Take chromium, 200–400 micrograms per day; this mineral helps keep blood sugar (and therefore insulin) levels constant. Also add magnesium, 300–600 milligrams per day. This amount includes your diet, so if you eat a lot of vegetables and well-chewed nuts, you will need less in supplement form. Magnesium citrate is one of the best absorbed forms of magnesium; magnesium oxide, which is more common, is also acceptable.

Take coenzyme Q10, a vitaminlike substance that is absolute first aid for any cardiac case. It is not cheap, but 300–600 milligrams a day can save lives. Also take 400–800IU (and possibly more) of natural vitamin E (D-alpha tocopherol plus natural mixed tocopherols) daily.

Eat more lysine (2,000–6,000mg per day). The amino acid lysine is available as a supplement, but it is also found in fish, eggs, dairy products, and potatoes. The best source is legumes (beans, peas, lentils); use them as a main dish for two meals a day and you can easily eat enough lysine at no supplemental cost.

Take more vitamin C, several thousand milligrams per day. Vitamin C supplementation prevents atherosclerosis by stopping the buildup of artery-clogging lipoprotein A or Lp(a).[3] However, the use of vitamin C to prevent and reverse atherosclerosis does not really represent new knowledge. For decades it has been known that vitamin C deficiency raises cholesterol levels. What's more, vitamin C also prevents stroke. It does so by strengthening intercellular collagen, which prevents damage and bleeding (and subsequent clotting) on the inside wall of your blood vessels.

Stress Reduction—While most of the suggestions offered in this section are dietary, there is one other big way to help your heart: meditate. According to cardiologist John Zamarra, M.D., "There is more research on the benefits of the TM (Transcendental Meditation) program than any other medical procedure to improve health."[4]

Hospital admissions for cardiovascular disease were reduced by an astounding 87 percent among long-time meditators using the TM technique. The research was well controlled; these patients still had routine medical exams and physicals, so there was no confounding reason that they might have been merely avoiding medical care.[5] If there were a cardiovascular drug that even approached 87 percent effectiveness, it would be considered a miracle drug. Plus, meditation also lowers high blood pressure by 11mm Hg (systolic).[6] Imagine: Meditation beats medication!

Stroke and Heart Attack

A stroke is a loose blood clot lodged in the brain. There is a stroke every minute in America and over half a million annually. One-third are fatal, making strokes one of the leading causes of death in this country. A heart attack (myocardial infarction) is a blood clot caught in the heart's coronary arteries. Half of all heart attacks are fatal. In the United States, there are nearly three heart attacks per minute.

Their common cause is a blood clot. Clots are the result of bleeding. The source of such bleeding can be too little vitamin C: a vitamin C–deficient (scorbutic) artery can literally "bleed" into itself. William J. McCormick, M.D., reviewed the nutritional causes of heart disease and noted that four out of five coronary cases in hospitals show vitamin C deficiency.[7] As early as 1941, low vitamin C status was seen as the cause of coronary thrombosis cases. Supplementation with even a moderate quantity of vitamin C has been shown to prevent disease and save lives. Just 500 milligrams daily results in a 42 percent lower risk of death from heart disease and a 35 percent lower risk of death from any cause.[8] Vitamin B6 (pyridoxine) is also important to cardiovascular health. For thirty years, it has been known that laboratory animals receiving the human B6 dose equivalent of just 75 milligrams daily do not get strokes, even when fed a high-fat diet.[9] Since women on oral contraceptives are three times more likely at any age to have a stroke, B6 supplementation is vital. A B6 deficiency is serious and can also cause hardening of the arteries.[10] Furthermore, B6 is necessary for your body to produce its own lecithin, and lecithin has been used clinically to clear out fatty livers and even clogged arteries.

Vitamin D has been shown to have therapeutic as well as preventive use in cardiovascular disease. For example, hypertension appears to decline with vitamin D supplementation, whether or not the person is deficient. It is also thought that a shortage of vitamin D may contribute to abnormal mineral metabolism, leading to congestive heart failure.

Vitamin E—During the 1940s and 1950s, Drs. Wilfrid and Evan Shute gave their coronary thrombosis patients 450–1,600IU of natural vitamin E per day. In acute cases, they started with the high amount; in existing cases, they started with the lower amount and gradually worked up. Thrombophlebitis patients received 600–1,600IU daily; patients with angina symptoms received twice that amount.[11] My dad was one of them: on 1,600IU per day, he never had angina again.

One of vitamin E's many properties is that it helps strengthen and regulate the heartbeat. This is usually very desirable, but there are exceptions to every rule. Much cardiovascular disease is caused by, or accompanied by, hypertension (high blood pressure). The Shutes started hypertensive patients on around 75IU per day for a few weeks, increased to 150IU for a few weeks more, then gave 300IU, and then higher over time. The caution is due to the fact that in some hypertensives, a sudden blast of vitamin E can cause a temporary rise in blood pressure. Gradually increasing the dose eliminates this issue. And, over time, high doses of vitamin E have been shown to reduce high blood pressure.[12]

Persons taking drugs such as Coumadin (warfarin) commonly find that their prothrombin clotting time tests indicate a decreased need for "blood-thinning" drugs. The intelligent way to deal with this is to work with your doctor, who is responsible for your prescription. Commonsense caution: Since the effective dose of vitamin E varies with the individual condition, it is always a good idea to have medical supervision.

Vitamin E, according to the Shutes, can "melt" fresh clots like an antithrombic drug and prevent embolism. In high doses, the vitamin also improves collateral (small blood vessel) circulation, which is potentially more important than you might think: In just one square inch of your skin, there are 19 feet of blood vessels. The doctors also found that vitamin E mildly dilates blood vessels, keeps capillary walls healthy and flexible, raises low platelet counts, and prevents hemolysis of red blood cells.

The Shutes were among the very first medical doctors to clinically employ large doses of a vitamin in place of conventional drug therapy. Like many pioneers, they caught all the arrows. Almost all of the criticism seemed to come from the medical press, which seemed singularly resistant to even try the Shute's approach, let alone endorse it. One can only wonder what failed to get the medical profession's attention sooner, given the spectacular, wonder drug–style patient recoveries that the Shutes had already seen by mid-century:

1936: Vitamin E–rich wheat germ oil cures angina.

1940: Vitamin E suspected as preventive of fibroids and endometriosis, and curative of atherosclerosis.

1946: Vitamin E demonstrated effective in cases of claudication, thrombosis, cirrhosis, and phlebitis. Vitamin E strengthens and regulates heartbeat.

1947: Vitamin E successfully used as therapy for gangrene and inflammation of blood vessels.

1950: Vitamin E shown to be effective treatment for varicose veins.

It is not easy to see how such promise could be ignored for long. But it was. The American Medical Association even refused to let the Shute's present their findings at national medical conventions. Before the Shutes' viewpoint on vitamin E can be disregarded, we must consider that they successfully treated more than 30,000 cardiac patients over a period of more than thirty years.

Vitamin E is a fat-soluble vitamin with no known toxicity. Vitamin E is remarkably safe; the Shutes gave quantities as high as 3,200IU per day without causing harm. The natural form of vitamin E is called D-alpha tocopherol and is made from vegetable oil. The synthetic form is DL-alpha tocopherol. Not a big difference in name, but there is evidence that the natural "D" (dextro-) molecular form of vitamin E is much more useful to the body than is the synthetic form.

A person in good health may typically begin with a supplemental amount of 200IU of vitamin E per day and try it for a couple of weeks. Then, 400IU might be taken daily for another two weeks. For the next two weeks, 600IU daily, and for the next two weeks, 800IU per day, and so on. One ultimately takes the least amount that gives the best results.[13]

Chronic Fatigue and Immune Dysfunction Syndrome (CFIDS)

Many of us have been exhausted seemingly forever. In the early 1800s, it was called febricula or vapors; later, neurasthenia, chronic brucellosis, hypoglycemia, myalgic encephalomyelitis, total allergy syndrome, chronic mononucleosis, chronic candidiasis, and postviral fatigue syndrome.[1] Now known as Chronic Fatigue and Immune Dysfunction Syndrome (CFIDS), it's still an epidemic condition without a pharmaceutical solution. Let's consider nutrition research and see what real options are available for the CFIDS patient that has been told to "learn to live with it."

Vitamin A (as carotene)—Chronic fatigue syndrome encompasses depressed immune function. Your immune system is stronger when beta-carotene is adequately supplied by the diet and vitamin A deficiency weakens immune function.[2] It's estimated that fewer than 10 percent of people actually consume sufficient carotenes, so a lifestyle change is virtually essential.

Beta-carotene supplements have been shown to strengthen the immune system by helping the body to build more helper T cells. The amount used in one study was 180 milligrams of beta-carotene per day; this is, theoretically, the equivalent of 300,000IU of vitamin A per day.[3]

The body (ideally) can derive 10,000IU of vitamin A activity from each 6 milligrams of beta-carotene consumed. The actual yield is almost certainly lower, however. Studies using small amounts of beta-carotene (20 milligrams or so) are likely to show no benefit, even though the "theoretical" yield would be over 30,000IU of vitamin A activity. Either that isn't enough or it isn't converted nearly as efficiently as supposed.

As previously mentioned in this book, the safest way to give vitamin A is as carotene, in fresh raw carrot juice. The body will convert carotene into vitamin A as needed, and overdose is automatically avoided. Excessively large doses of preformed, fish-oil vitamin A may actually depress immune function, but huge doses of carotene do not appear to have such a negative effect. Too many carrots and your skin will get a bit orange, but that is harmless.

Vitamin B complex—The very discovery of the B vitamins is itself a story of fatigue.

The disease beri-beri (meaning "I cannot, I cannot") relates to severe weakness and exhaustion. This "incurable" condition was found to be simply a deficiency of thiamine (vitamin B1). Eating whole brown rice, instead of polished white rice, was enough to effect a remarkable cure from fatigue that no drug on Earth could obtain.

Pellagra is niacin (vitamin B3) deficiency, which results in (among other things) weakness and lassitude.[4] Why? In your body, food must be broken down into simple molecules like glucose, and in your cells, energy must be released from glucose. A major part of this complex process is called the citric acid cycle, or Krebs cycle. This elaborate, energy-releasing pathway grinds to a complete halt without the B-complex vitamins. Your body without enough B vitamins is like a huge, rusty ferris wheel without oil—it's there, but it's not moving.

The four B vitamins most involved with our cellular energy cycle are thiamine, niacin, pantothenic acid, and riboflavin. Scientific research indicates, over and over again, that B complex (and other) vitamin deficiencies weaken immunity.[5] Nutritionists, dietitians and physicians often discount these findings by maintaining that vitamin deficiencies are extinct in our modern civilization. Such opinion does not stand up to close examination of the scientific literature, which confirms widespread nutritional failings coast to coast. Nor does it explain the large number of CFIDS patients who have taken large quantities of vitamin supplements and noticed remarkable improvements.

It is common supplemental practice to include a B-complex vitamin with every meal. Even more frequent doses have been known to help more severe cases.

Vitamin C—Very large doses of vitamin C have been successfully used to boost the immune system for fifty years. Frederick R. Klenner, M.D., pioneered megavitamin-C therapeutics back in the 1940s, giving thousands of milligrams of vitamin C by injection for a wide variety of viral illnesses. When encountering viral pneumonia, Dr. Klenner noted that patients often reported "severe frontal headache along with a feeling of weakness in the lower extremities so marked that the patient complains of a dragging sensation when moving about in bed. This weakness persists for some days." Dr. Klenner found that in forty-two cases over a five-year period, he had excellent results from using vitamin C (ascorbic acid) in massive doses.[6] One cannot easily help but draw a significant parallel between pneumonia and CFIDS symptoms.

Viral pneumonia is a worthy foe, but the supreme test for vitamin C's immune-enhancing effect must surely be AIDS. Robert F. Cathcart, M.D., has published his successes with enormous doses of vitamin C against many viral illnesses. Even among his patients with fully developed AIDS, improved length of life and quality of life are the rule, not the exception.[7]

How much vitamin C does one need for treating CFIDS? Too little and you miss maximum benefits; too much is wasteful. Dr. Cathcart gives vitamin C to bowel tolerance, which is the maximum amount the body can take without having loose bowels. Any person can monitor this level at home, all by themselves. Dr. Cathcart says that the sicker you are, the more C you can (and will) hold. As you get better, you will not be able to hold as much, so down comes the dose. It is a self-adjusting process.[8] According to the many persons I have interviewed, the "take all the vitamin C you can possibly hold" plan really works. Still, it is the one principle most consistently overlooked, even by doctors and authors writing about nutritional therapies for CFIDS.

Magnesium and Calcium—Magnesium is a catalyst for hundreds of biochemical reactions in each of your body's cells. Calcium and magnesium are necessary for nerve function and muscular activity. Calcium deficiency is almost universal: Americans consume at least one-third less than the modest RDA. Magnesium deficiency may run as high as 99 percent among U.S. teenagers.[9] These are reasons why a calcium-magnesium supplement should be included as a first-line measure against chronic fatigue. I think 800 milligrams of calcium and 300–400 milligrams magnesium, in divided doses and taken with meals, should be taken in addition to whatever calcium and magnesium may be obtained from diet.

Chromium—Both stress and infection increase the amount of chromium required for good health. On top of that, the U.S. Department of Agriculture has estimated that 90 percent of us are eating chromium-deficient diets.[10] High sugar intake actually drains the body of chromium.[11] Organic chromium supplements increase immune function in animals.[12] Taking 200–400 micrograms of organic chromium daily is a safe and worthwhile measure to try. Chromium polynicotinate or chromium picolinate are the best forms to take as supplements.

Zinc—Zinc may be "tail-end Charlie" of the nutritional alphabet, but it is near the top in importance. Of all the trace minerals, only iron is found in the body in greater quantity. Oddly enough, excessive iron consumption can reduce your zinc absorption from food. Most Americans do not even get the RDA of zinc, which is a very low 8–14 milligrams per day.

Nationwide zinc deficiency almost surely has contributed to CFIDS. It is well known that zinc is needed by dozens of the body's enzyme systems. Reduced immune function follows zinc deficiency.[13] Zinc is absolutely essential for lymphocytes, T-helper cells, T-suppressor cells, and natural killer cells. Even if you have a blood test showing nearly normal plasma zinc levels, you may still have too little zinc in the cells themselves. This means your immune system may be seriously weakened and tests may not reflect it.[14] Does this sound somewhat familiar to chronic fatigue patients?

Zinc has been shown to shorten the duration of the common cold by over 50 percent.[15] Zinc also displays antiviral activity and has demonstrated improved immune response with about 400 milligrams per day.[16] At doses of 50–150 milligrams per day, zinc is completely safe to take. However, long-term doses of over 300–600 milligrams per day, especially of non-natural zinc sulfate, may cause copper- or iron-deficiency anemia. If such high doses were indicated, a few milligrams per day of copper and 10–15 milligrams per day of iron will counter the problem.

Chronic Pain

Pain is often our wake-up call to action, when our bodies need to get a message to, and an effective response from, our busy brain—the squeaky wheel demanding grease. Putting in earplugs—in this case, taking pain-relieving drugs—does not fix a squeaky wheel. The best pain relief will help cure the cause of pain. At the very least, we want the hurt to go away temporarily without harmful side effects. Here are two alternatives to pharmaceutical products:

Phenylalanine—D- or DL-phenylalanine, the "right-handed" form of this common amino acid, is not actually a nutrient but an amino acid analgesic. It is nonprescription but rather costly for an effective dose. Practitioners using DLPA (dextro-levo-phenyl-alanine) normally employ it for chronic pain that is unresponsive to other measures, such as arthritis or lower back pain. While no substitute for medical or chiropractic care, DLPA may well be a suitable companion.

Research has indicated that migraines, joint pains, neuralgia, and even postoperative pain respond to DLPA, and it has been reported to reduce inflammation. DLPA does not deaden normal sensation even when taken for a lengthy period. The most dramatic pain-relief case I have seen was when a friend of mine had a large number of old dental fillings replaced within a short period of time. As a result, he experienced ongoing and severe jaw pain that no pharmaceutical painkiller could touch, and the dentist tried them all. In desperation, my friend tried DLPA, about 3,000 milligrams per day. He reported truly profound relief.

Phenylalanine is converted by the body into phenylethylamine. Low levels of phenylethylamine are correlated with clinical depression; if DLPA raises these levels, there is a real biochemical benefit. As a painkiller, it seems to act by keeping enzymes from breaking down the body's own morphinelike natural painkillers, the enkephalins and the endorphins. This makes a lot of sense: If the body relieves its own pain, a safe mechanism is probably at work. DLPA appears to assist that mechanism.

The dose of DLPA needed varies from person to person, and is generally determined by starting with 1,000 milligrams daily for two weeks and then gradually increasing to a level that provides relief. If 3,000 milligrams per day does not work after a month's time, it probably will not work at all. About two-thirds of those using it will report real improvement in this time.

The good news is that persons reporting pain relief will generally be able to lower their dose gradually and will often be able to maintain pain-free status with less DLPA than before. DLPA has a long duration of action, yet the body does not seem to build up a tolerance to it. You will probably not find just "D-phenylalanine" for sale, hence the focus here on DLPA. It is the D-form that is active; you cannot substitute the levo- ("L") form that is so widely found, at lower cost, in foods and stores.

The safety of DLPA is very good indeed. It is nonaddictive and virtually nontoxic. Some estimates place its safety on a par with vitamin C or fructose. Still, it is not to be used during pregnancy. Persons with phenylketonuria (PKU) obviously should not take any extra phenylalanine. Persons with high blood pressure should take DLPA after meals. Prescribed medication usually may still be taken with DLPA without interference.[1]

Vitamin C (Ascorbic Acid)—At high intake levels, vitamin C reduces pain. In the 1970s, researchers in Scotland gave 10 grams (10,000mg) of vitamin C intravenously each day to terminally ill cancer patients. Yes, the study was about vitamin C and cancer, but the unexpected finding was in pain relief.

In Great Britain, at the time, it was policy to provide terminal patients with any and all painkillers available, including addictive narcotics such as heroin. The argument was simply that if one were dying anyway, a drug's analgesic value outweighs any drawbacks such as dependency. Five of the ascorbate-treated patients who had been receiving large doses of narcotics were taken off these drugs a few days after the vitamin C was begun, because the vitamin C reduced the pain to such an extent that the drug was not needed.[2]

Any vitamin that approaches the pain-relieving power of morphine or heroin must be considered an important analgesic. Because the study used intravenous vitamin C, you can expect that oral doses would have to be considerably greater. Given the results, this is a remarkably safe and simple therapy.

Colitis Ulcers and Other Gastrointestinal Problem

Your digestive tract is well over twenty feet long. If you were to flatten out just your small intestine, its total absorptive area would be half the size of a basketball court. This is an important bit of real estate.

Nature-cure advocates tend to annoy medical specialists by looking at gastrointestinal (GI) problems such as colitis, ulcers, spastic colon, irritable bowel syndrome, and even Crohn's disease as manifestations of the same two problems: systemic toxemia (a polluted body) and malnutrition. This means that one is taking in too much of the wrong things and not enough of the right ones.

Persons with GI troubles simply must stop doing things that hurt their guts. Smoking, alcohol, coffee, meat, food additives, and stress should be systematically eliminated. If a person is not willing to stop doing things that hurt, there is a greatly reduced chance of success with things that help. I need add nothing about why drinking and smoking harm your digestive system. Coffee drinking and meat eating, though, are often allowed by doctors unwilling to stop those habits themselves. But one has to confront even the popular vices, if doing so can reduce suffering. Persons who move toward vegetarianism and away from coffee will not be disappointed.

A near-vegetarian diet has important advantages: it is high in bulk, relatively high in vitamin C, and high in carotene (vitamin A). However, if you have a long-suffering, sensitive, sick digestive tract, you do not want to just leap in with a high-fiber vegetarian diet. Juicing vegetables is a smart transitional move. Persons with severe intestinal problems should see their doctor first. It will be difficult for any physician to object to vegetable juices for even the most irritated of intestines.

The lining of your entire digestive tract is made up of epithelial tissue. Epithelial cells are "skin" cells. So, in a way, your skin covers both the outside and the inside of your body. You might think of yourself as a sleeping bag: there is an outer waterproof covering and an inner, softer lining. Since epithelial tissue is dependent on vitamins A and C for its health and integrity, and since a diet high in fruits, sprouts, and veggies is quite high in these vitamins, you can see the vegetarian's advantage. The additional bulk of a veggie diet makes stools softer and easier to pass. Pressure is reduced inside the colon and straining to have a bowel movement is eliminated. Persons with very sensitive intestines should juice their vegetables and even put their salads through a blender if necessary. This tastes a lot better than it sounds, and is an extremely gentle and digestible way to instantly improve nutritional status. Fruits and especially vegetables are so high in carotenes that supplemental vitamin A is not needed if you are juicing.

One of the first naturopathic textbooks I read was *Everybody's Guide to Nature Cure* by Dr. Harry Benjamin.[1] At the time, I resisted his beginning practically every treatment the same way: with a fast. His advice has withstood the test of time. Persons with GI troubles often get the most relief by just shutting down the digestive system for a while. A few days of fasting gives the body a chance to rest and repair. Health nuts know, and anatomical evidence confirms, that given this chance the body will take advantage of it.

Earlier I mentioned that your intestinal tract is lined with epithelial cells. These cells, called enterocytes, are replaced by your body every three to five days.[2] This suggests that a fast of similar length would best enable this reconstruction. Fasting is simply a temporary and logical measure. While it is possible for some people to fast on water alone, I think this is unnecessary. Equally good results can be obtained (with greater comfort) by vegetable juice fasting. Juice fasts are ideal because they provide the healing vitamins A and C. The minimal carbohydrate content of vegetable juices promotes normal blood sugar levels, provides electrolyte minerals, and prevents ketosis.

To give you an idea of the therapeutic potential of vegetable juices, consider the work of Garnett Cheney, M.D. He had 100 peptic-ulcer patients drink a quart of raw cabbage juice daily. The patients reported dramatically less pain, and x-ray examination confirmed faster healing time. There was no other change in their diet, and they did not have drug therapy. Within one week, 81 percent of the patients were symptom free; over two-thirds were better in just four days. Average healing time for patients given standard hospital treatment was over a month.[3] Dr. Cheney also used cabbage juice to treat gastric ulcers and duodenal ulcers.[4] Today, the sulforaphane-rich cabbage family (cruclform) vegetables, including Brussels sprouts, kale, cauliflower, and broccoli, are recommended to help prevent diseases including cancer.[5]

I know of people who have utilized cabbage juice along with vegetarian diet and fasting to heal all forms of gastrointestinal diseases without drugs and without surgery. In *Doctor Yourself,* I reported the case of a person who cured her untreatable rectal bleeding with cabbage juice. The attending physician confirmed her excellent but unexplained progress, asking her what she was doing. She told the doctor of her diet and about cabbage juice. His response was, "No, that couldn't be it." Now you know how the book you are reading got its name.

Extra vitamin C is very valuable to help heal lesions and inflammation all along the GI tract. Thousands of milligrams in divided doses are necessary for best results. Enough vitamin C should be taken to improve the condition, but not so much as might cause excessively loose bowels. A nonacidic or buffered vitamin C is ideal, because it will not irritate the digestive tract; calcium ascorbate works well for this purpose.

Other nutritional options include vitamin D, which has been shown to relieve inflammatory bowel disease.[6] Barley or oatmeal water have traditionally been used as gastrointestinal healers,[7] as has fresh aloe vera juice.

Some form of stress reduction is essential for digestive system health and healing. Whether it is prayer, meditation, yoga, music, or another approach, what matters most is that you actually learn how to relax efficiently and take the time to do it every day. This will carry over into mealtime.

Constipation

My mother was a true believer in laxatives. More than any other reason, this was because she was medicated with phenobarbital for her epilepsy; depressants like that cause constipation. But in her zeal was overcompensation. On what seemed like a daily basis, my brothers and I were instructed to "go stand in Castoria Corner," over by the cereal cupboard in the kitchen, for a dose of Fletcher's Castoria. Since 1868 (and still sold to this day), Fletcher's Castoria is the trade name for a flavored herbal laxative that kids were supposed to enjoy taking. This label claim was not, I assure you, written by a child.

I hated Castoria. What came out of all this was ingrained apprehension with laxatives and a growing interest in alternatives. Even as a little boy I'd learned that chewing food well, eating raw vegetables, and raiding my mother's dresser for her stash of chocolate-flavored Ex-Lax were all better than choking down that Castoria. Eventually, Mom relented and Castoria went by the wayside. Maybe it is because we grew to eat better or maybe we ran and hid more effectively.

To spare your kids the culinary purgatory of even worse-tasting castor oil, here's a tip:

Apply castor oil externally, as an overall body rub. The castor oil is absorbed through the skin and works just fine. Castor oil is cheap, and used this way, easy to take. There is a slight smell but that's a small price to pay for bypassing your taste buds.

I do not recommend the routine use of laxatives, but constipation is such a problem in a population that stubbornly rejects a high-fiber, plant-based diet that we often need to, as W.C. Fields said, "Take the bull by the tail and face the situation." Natural healing advocates have always maintained that much, if not most, illness is due to systemic toxemia—a polluted body. Good elimination can be a wonderful start for chronically unhealthy people, and a castor oil rubdown will plant a person on the potty in a matter of hours. Another way to do the trick is to take a heaping teaspoon (or three) of vitamin C powder (6,000–15,000mg or thereabouts).

The real answer to regularity is, of course, a regular routine of high-fiber, raw-food-and-juice, near-vegetarian eating. A plant-based diet will also help you sidestep cancer, heart disease, diabetes, and many more constipation-related killers. Scientific studies have confirmed an increased incidence of diverticular diseases, heart disease, and cancer among constipated persons. It is common for arthritics to have a history of chronic constipation. Probably at least one-third of all insulin-dependent diabetics would require less of the drug if they simply had more fiber in their diet.

Throughout much of Africa and Asia, people eat a great deal of vegetables, grains, and legumes (beans, lentils, etc.). These people have a digestive transit time of eighteen hours or less, meaning that what's left of the food they eat will be excreted about eighteen hours later. In Westernized cultures, a transit time twice as long (thirty-six hours) is the rule, and forty-eight to seventy-two hours is not uncommon. This means the wastes stay in the body much longer, allowing greater opportunity for toxins to be reabsorbed.

Your colon (or bowel) is designed to collect and hold wastes, but only for a while. If the colon is not emptied regularly, it begins to resemble a backed-up sewer. Fecal matter packed into the bowel can stretch it out of shape, which reduces muscle tone, and poor elimination is the result. Wastes then become more and more compacted and concentrated, and harder still to eliminate. Stools become foul smelling as normally beneficial colon bacteria give way to a polluted, pathogenic bowel.

Constipation is one ailment that you need never have again. Certainly it is important to put the right kind of food into your body, but it is also essential to get wastes out. The naturopaths of the last century, such as Dr. Harvey Kellogg, frequently addressed illness bowel-first, and with good reason. Here are ways to end constipation:

1. Become a vegetarian; eating less meat and more plant-based food guarantees easier bowel movements.
2. Eat lots of fresh, uncooked fruits and vegetables; salads are the answer, not laxatives.
3. Drink a glass or two of water, preferably warm, right after you awaken in the morning; herbal teas are good, too. Then, be sure to drink plenty of water all day long.
4. Make a habit of sitting on the toilet for five minutes right after breakfast—given the opportunity, your body will get in the habit of an early morning bowel movement.
5. Add fiber to your diet by eating better snacks: popcorn, vegetable sticks, fruit, and nuts are excellent.
6. Molasses is a good natural laxative if you need one; about one-third of a cup will do it. Freshly made raw cabbage juice or juiced zucchini also works well: one or two 8-ounce glasses will probably be enough. A can of sauerkraut, juice and all, can also

be used as a laxative. And, yes, stewed fruits (such as prunes) still work well.

7. Take a few thousand milligrams of vitamin C in one dose to produce a laxative effect; adding a few tablets of a magnesium supplement is even better. Milk of magnesia is magnesium-based.

8. You can encourage a bowel movement with a gentle abdominal massage. Generally, you follow the bowel with the massage. Begin in your lower belly, below and to the right of your navel; move up and then across. Then, move down your left abdomen and finish just above the groin area. Repeat this a few times, and in a while you will likely notice an urge to have a bowel movement. This is especially helpful for children. Do not massage if there is a pregnancy or any medical or surgical reason why you shouldn't.

9. Walking, yoga, bicycling, and other light-to-moderate exercise is always helpful for regularity.

Coughing

It has happened to everybody: you, or somebody in your family, is coughing most of the night. This is especially troubling when it happens to a child. Is there something you can do between cough syrup and a hospital? You bet there is.

Coltsfoot—As an alternative to prescription cough medicines, herbal remedies deserve consideration. Coltsfoot *(Tussilago farfara)* leaves made into a tea make an effective cough medicine. You can buy dried coltsfoot at an herb store and at some health food stores. Use a tablespoon or two of herb in each mug of hot water. For an adult, several mugs of coltsfoot tea can even stop the cough of pneumonia. I know, because I had pneumonia and was sick as a dog. Prescription cough medicine with codeine did not touch it. Two or three mugs of coltsfoot tea would eliminate the coughing for hours. It is not expensive and has a low likelihood of side effects with occasional use. Coltsfoot is not for extended use, and not for use during pregnancy or nursing.

Vitamin C—Coughing is generally a symptom of some other problem in the body. It is wise to "pull the rug out from under" the cough by helping the rest of the body get well.

Healthy bodies do not cough. Whether it is a cold, flu, or pneumonia, strengthening the immune system with vitamin C can only help. My simple dosage plan: "Take enough C to be symptom free, whatever the amount might be." That is usually just under the amount that would result in loose bowels.

When my daughter was four years old, she had a very severe cough. We endured it for two nights while doing everything doctors suggest including strict bed rest and codeine cough syrup. Yet, she still was coughing after forty-eight hours. I was sufficiently sick of sickness to start my daughter on a teaspoon (about 4,000mg) of vitamin C crystals in juice every hour. After a few hours, the cough was gone. We continued to give her vitamin C for the rest of the day, and she remained quiet and comfortable. She had a total of 36,000 milligrams of vitamin C.

During the night the cough came back. We got up, gave her a teaspoon of vitamin C, and everyone was shortly asleep once again. The next morning, the cough was back again, and we met it and banished it with vitamin C every hour. We kept the cough down by keeping her C up. Those all-night battles for a sick child are really tough. Vitamin C and coltsfoot are tough, too. When you use them, everybody sleeps much better.

Down Syndrome

Early in 1980, the medical and educational establishments were shaken to their socks. Ruth F. Harrell and colleagues, in a study published in *Proceedings of the National Academy of Sciences,* showed that high doses of vitamins improved intelligence and educational performance in learning disabled children, including those with Down syndrome.[1] Though to many observers this seemingly came straight out of left field, Dr. Harrell, who had been investigating vitamin effects on learning for forty years, was not inventing the idea of megavitamin therapy. But she succeeded in focusing much-needed public attention on the role of nutrition in learning disabilities.

A number of well-publicized studies conducted to "replicate" Dr. Harrell's work seemingly could not do so. Would-be "replications" fail the moment they start when they refuse to use adequate dosages. Surely it is the most basic condition for any replication that one must exactly copy the original experiment. Yet Dr. Harrell's "replicators" failed to adhere to her protocol, and consequently, but not surprisingly, failed to get her results.[2] The Harrell study was successful because her team gave learning-disabled kids much larger doses of vitamins than other researchers are inclined to use: over 100 times the *adult* (not child's) RDA for riboflavin; 37 times the RDA for niacin (given as niacinamide); 40 times the RDA for vitamin E; and 150 times the RDA for thiamine. Supplemental minerals were also given, as was natural dessicated thyroid.

Dr. Harrell's critics embrace the assumption that medicine must ultimately prove to be the better approach, and if there are any megadoses to be given, they shall be megadoses of pharmaceutical products. Vitamin therapy is unattractive to pharmaceutical companies. There is no money in products that cannot be patented. A tragic example is modern medicine's approach to Down syndrome.

If there is orthodox resistance to using vitamins to enhance student learning, there is a fortified roadblock to the suggestion that vitamins can help children with Down syndrome. Nutritional intervention may help the body to biochemically compensate for a genetic handicap. Roger Williams, discoverer of the vitamin pantothenic acid, termed this the "genetotrophic concept." Genetotrophic diseases are "diseases in which the genetic pattern of the afflicted individual requires an augmented supply of one or more nutrients, such that when these nutrients are adequately supplied the disease is ameliorated."[3] Ruth

Harrell's decades of research showed that it is plausible.

Thiamine (Vitamin B1)—To see the physical incapacitation thiamine deficiency (beriberi) causes in impoverished countries is all too easy. To see the mental incapacitation in American classrooms is not difficult, either. Yet both may be caused by thiamine deficiency and both helped by thiamine supplementation. Dr. Harrell zeroed in on this topic sixty years ago, demonstrating that supplemental thiamine improves learning. In one of her experiments, which involved 104 children, nine to nineteen years old, half were given vitamin B1 each day and the other half received a placebo. After six weeks, the group that was given the vitamin gained 25 percent more in learning ability than the other group.[4]

Carbohydrates, including sugar, increase the body's need for thiamine. Children eat a lot of sugar. This may be part of the mechanism of attention deficit disorder and other children's learning and behavior disorders, as many so-called "food faddists" or "health nuts" have proclaimed for decades.

Though it is a stretch to say that all learning and behavioral disabilities are due to inadequate vitamin intake, it is certain that some are. Behavioral deficiency tends to show up before nutritional deficiency is recognized.

Arthur Winter, M.D. indicates that in thiamine deficiency, "symptoms such as lack of well-being, anxiety, hysteria, depression, and loss of appetite preceded any clinical evidence of beriberi." He adds that other research has shown that "adverse behavioral changes precede physical findings in thiamine deficiency."[5]

B-Complex Vitamins—As a group, the B vitamins are absolutely vital to the nervous system. Specifically, it is well established that thiamine deficiency causes not only loss of nerve function, and ultimately paralysis, but also memory loss, reduced attention span, irritability, confusion, and depression.[6] Riboflavin (vitamin B2) deficiency causes nerve tissue damage that may lead to depression and hysteria.[7] Niacin (vitamin B3) deficiency causes memory loss and emotional instability, while pyridoxine (B6) deficiency results in neurotransmitter imbalances and confusion.[8] A deficiency of folic acid may lead to irritability, apathy, forgetfulness, and hostility.[9] And a cobalamin (vitamin B12) deficiency causes degeneration of the spinal cord, fatigue, disorientation, and moodiness.[10] Though these symptoms generally appear after prolonged deficiency, a shortage of any one of the B vitamins can be seen to lead to neurological damage sufficient to contribute to learning and behavioral troubles.

Adherents of conventional dietetics presuppose that anyone who claims that there are widespread vitamin deficiencies among children must proceed from a false assumption. Those who advocate vitamin therapy would answer that Down syndrome creates a "functional deficiency" that must be met with appropriate supplementation. The very idea that doses sufficiently high to effectively do so should be 100 times the RDA is positively repellent to most investigators.

Another often-heard argument is that, even when you acknowledge that children eat poorly, there is insufficient evidence that Down syndrome is aggravated by poor nutrition, or helped by good nutrition. After all, it is a genetically determined disease. But surely the genes do not operate in a nutrient vacuum. For example, vitamin E has recently been demonstrated to preferentially protect genetic material in Down patients' cells.[11] This would also suggest that antioxidant vitamin supplements would be an especially good idea for individuals with Down syndrome.

Although the greater question may be, "Can optimum nutrition help compensate for a genetic defect?" the essential question must be this: Can nutrition help a child with Down syndrome? One special education teacher commented that IQ gains in Dr. Harrell's study were so great that not only did parents and teachers notice it, but the whole neighborhood did. "Three of four children with Down syndrome gained between 10 and 25 units in IQ and also showed physical changes toward normal."[12] Perhaps Dr. Harrell's dramatic IQ results were merely due to the placebo effect. If so, I want every school district on earth to lay in a stock of sugar pills, for gains like this in only eight months are astounding.

When Dr. Harrell died in 1991, she was far from being alone in reporting success with high-dose nutrition therapy. Physicians such as Dr. Henry Turkel, who treated hundreds of Down children, observed that children on megadoses of nutrients "lost the typical Down's syndrome facial appearance."[13] The Harrell team's results are sufficiently compelling justification for a therapeutic trial of orthomolecular supplementation for every learning-impaired child.

Earaches and Ear Infections

Many medicines for earache are ineffective even though still commonly prescribed. Back in 1983, the *New England Journal of Medicine* reported that a three-year study of decongestants and antihistamines, as prescribed by ear specialists, showed that they are no better than giving nothing at all. In fact, they are worse, as they are expensive and cause unpleasant side effects. Nine out of ten ear specialists used them anyway in spite of this finding: "Resolution of middle-ear effusion occurred at four weeks in 38 percent of those treated with placebo and 34 percent of those treated with drug."[1]You read that right—the placebo beat the medication.

The good news is that ear infections can be effectively stopped much sooner when treated by alternative means. Here's how:

1. Simple earache is likely to be a symptom of an ear infection. Almost anything you do to fight the infection will fight the earache as well. Very large doses of vitamin C are especially effective. At saturation (bowel tolerance) levels, vitamin C is a natural antibiotic and antihistamine. It will

also reduce inflammation and fever, and is safer than pharmaceuticals.

2. Check to see if the upper neck bones are misaligned. If one or more of these cervical vertebrae are "out," the resulting impinged nerve or straining muscle can lead to an earache. To check this out, find the place where the neck, skull, and jaw meet. This spot is just under the ear. If gentle pressure on this spot is painful, you may have an earache that a chiropractor will be able to help.

3. Warm, damp compresses are a traditional earache treatment. A washcloth moistened in warm tap water works fine, and feels good.

4. To help relieve pressure and encourage natural drainage, you can try a simple massage technique. Gently press under each ear. Then continue pressing, moving downward and forward along and just under the edge of the jawbone. You have just massaged the eustachian tubes, the internal passages connecting each inner ear to its opening inside the upper throat. Repeatedly massaging like this aids in relaxing, dilating, and clearing this tube. Before resorting to surgically inserting artificial tubes, let's try full use of the ones we were born with!

5. Drink more water. Liquids make mucus more liquid and easier to clear from the body. Lots of water is good advice to help clear the ears, but high-carotene vegetable juice is even better. You can also get an appreciable amount of water from eating quantities of fresh fruit, which most kids naturally love to do if you simply let them.

6. Natural healing advocates believe that earaches and infections are fundamentally due to improper diet. Many kids are overfed milk, meat, white bread, sugar, and chemically doctored foods daily. This must stop, or the earaches won't. A near-vegetarian diet with lots of fruit, vegetable salads, whole grains, and non-animal protein results in healthier children.

Eczema (Atopic Dermatitis)

Eczema is inflamed, sensitive, itching skin. There is currently no cure for eczema, according to conventional medicine. That does not stop doctors from trying to treat it, of course, with emollients, tars, antihistamines, topical or oral steroids, immunomodulators, or a bevy of other drugs. Atopic (inflammatory) eczema is the most common, dry, very itchy kind of eczema. There is also allergic contact dermatitis, irritant contact dermatitis, infantile seborrheic eczema (cradle cap), adult seborrheic eczema, varicose eczema, and discoid eczema. Incidence of eczema is on the increase throughout the world: according to the American Academy of Dermatology, currently one baby in ten has eczema.[1] Think about it: 10 percent of babies have an incurable condition. Does that make sense? If you are a parent, it should make you curious about natural alternatives.

One such curious mom was Yvonne. Her baby had a rash on his arms and legs, midriff, and back—he was red and sore, everywhere. Any kind of clothing made him squirm and he had trouble sleeping from all the itching. When the baby wriggled, you could see that the rash was worse where the diaper contacted the skin. At first, Yvonne thought it was just diaper rash. "But diaper rash doesn't go from the ankles to the shoulders, does it?" said Yvonne.

Her pediatrician said it was eczema; then he started talking about trying out some medicines. She hadn't yet decided if she wanted to use them and wondered if there were any natural remedies that might help.

"Some natural healing folks recommend a topical application of a solution of chamomile leaves or even onion juice," I told her. "I think your best bet might be to feed your baby some yogurt."

Her eyebrows went up at that suggestion. "Yogurt? But I breast-feed my baby," she said. "Why would he need yogurt?"

"You are right to nurse your baby. But breast-fed or not, babies given supplemental yogurt have eczema less often," I said. "In fact, studies have found that when pregnant women eat yogurt, or a supplement of the beneficial microorganisms naturally in it, their babies subsequently are much less likely to develop eczema."

It's thought that yogurt helps from the inside out. *Lactobacillus acidophilus* and *Bifidobacteria,* the beneficial bacteria commonly found in yogurt, may help reduce a child's allergic response, quieting down its super-sensitivity to everything.[2] We know that acidophilus and other good bacteria help strengthen the immune system and build resistance to colds. These bacteria create a healthier intestinal environment by keeping pathogenic bacteria in check, and they also improve digestion.

I asked if her baby had been given antibiotics. Yvonne thought for a moment. "Yes, he has. Two, actually three, rounds of antibiotics since birth. He's almost seven months old now."

"That might have something to do with it, too," I said. "Antibiotics kill off good bacteria at least as well as they kill bad bacteria. Yogurt helps restore the digestive tract's normal population of the little critters. Instead of killing bacteria, we actually help them along. The process of encouraging a healthy population of microflora is called probiotics."

Yvonne thought it made sense to try it. "Yogurt has to be a lot safer than the steroid cream his pediatrician wants to put him on," she said.

I suggested that she give her baby just a little yogurt with every feeding. Half a teaspoonful or so of good quality, plain yogurt is probably enough. I heard back from Yvonne in a few days. "The eczema is gone," she said, happily. "The yogurt really did the trick. I noticed the difference immediately, and by the look of things, so did my baby."

Vitamin C may be a useful cure for eczema as well. For decades, there has been a series of published but ignored Russian studies exploring this theory. A very promising University of Texas study was reported in 1989 specifying an effective eczema-reducing dose of 50–75 milligrams vitamin C per kilogram body weight per day (about 25–35mg per pound). This amounts to a few hundred milligrams a day for an infant, 1,000 or 2,000 milligrams per day for a child, or 5,000 to 6,000 milligrams per day for an adult.[3] The success may be due to vitamin C's antihistamine effect, to its anti-inflammatory effect, to its immune-enhancing effect, or perhaps to all of the above.

Good old-fashioned sunlight often improves eczema. While everyone knows that overexposure to UVB rays is to be avoided, we may be going too far in ducking from the sun. Both ultraviolet B and ultraviolet A have been demonstrated to reduce the symptoms of eczema.[4] In my neighborhood, we kids were always kicked out of the house to play on a sunny day. Maybe we should, with intelligent moderation, do likewise today.

Additional related and relevant skin-healing suggestions can be found in the section on psoriasis.

Emphysema and Chronic Respiratory Diseases

My aunt needed oxygen to put on her socks. A severe case of emphysema, which a lifetime of smoking had failed to cure, was the reason. She was just one of an estimated 16 million Americans suffering from chronic obstructive pulmonary disease (COPD), which is primarily caused by tobacco use. The fourth leading cause of death, COPD kills over 100,000 annually. That number is increasing, and medical research has contributed virtually nothing to stop it.[1]

But you can stop it—by stopping smoking, by stopping other people from smoking, and by stopping nonsmokers from "involuntary smoking," also known as breathing secondhand smoke.[2] According to the American Lung Association, smokers are ten times more likely to die from lung disease than are nonsmokers.

What can be done for the disease itself?

1. Vitamin E helps the body, especially the heart, to do more work on less oxygen. This has been known for over fifty years, ever since Drs. Wilfrid and Evan Shute first used high doses (800 to 2,400IU or even greater) of vitamin E in the 1940s.

2. Carotenes (in orange and green vegetables) and lycopene (in tomatoes) are powerful antioxidants. At least some of the damage of emphysema is caused by free radicals. While vitamin C is the body's predominant antioxidant (vitamin E is the runner-up), vegetable juices will provide a great variety of additional plant-based helpers, including lutein and sulforaphane.

3. Persons with emphysema should investigate vitamin A therapy. A derivative of vitamin A, retinoic acid, has been shown to reverse emphysema in animals, actually restoring and replacing damaged air sacs, thus "providing nonsurgical remediation of emphysema and suggesting the possibility of a similar effect in humans."[3] However, in pregnant mammals, retinoic acid can cause birth defects. It may be possible, and is certainly safer, to instead use non-prescription vitamin A, or retinol, from fish oil. Retinol can be converted into retinoic acid in the body. Better yet, your body is already capable of converting carotene into retinol. While few emphysema patients are pregnant, the fact that carotene is nontoxic even in enormous doses is a compelling reason to select vegetables over pharmaceutical designer drugs.

4. Pricey though it is, I would recommend coenzyme Q10 for COPD sufferers, at least 300 milligrams daily, divided into six 50-milligram doses. This is a hospital-friendly supplement, as there are no known negative side effects and therefore no rational basis to deny it to any patient.

5. Some emphysema is due to inflammation. Vitamin C at saturation doses fights chronic inflammation better and more safely than anything else. Saturation of vitamin C is easily reached through frequent, high oral doses. Very ill patients may need to take vitamin C intravenously.

6. Chiropractic adjustment, while certainly not a cure for emphysema, may help reduce some shortness of breath. A wood back-massaging spool (e.g., a "Ma Roller") can also be useful for some do-it-yourself adjustments.

Fever

Your body successfully fights many illnesses by creating a fever. Robert Mendelsohn, M.D. routinely told patients to throw away their thermometers. Ancient medical wisdom says, "Give me a fever and I can cure anything." At a hospital in Rochester, New York, I picked up a what-to-do-for-fever booklet. It said that the hospital does not even treat a fever until it is 103.5°F, and then only for the comfort of the patient. While opinions vary, some medical authorities maintain that fevers as high as 106°F are not dangerous, except in infants. Febrile seizures, which rarely occur, almost never harm the child. Brain damage, the parents' big worry, can not occur until an astounding 108°F.[1]

So what do you do for a fever? Well, first do nothing at all—if it runs its course in a day or two, let it be.[2] If a fever is very high for very long, though, there is genuine cause for concern and need for action. Many uninterrupted days of a fever in excess of 104°F might possibly result in heat seizures, kidney failure, or a variety of other complications.

Fevers are not the trouble; they are the indicator of trouble. We need to deal with the cause of the fever and the fever will take care of itself. It is good to know why the body has a fever. In our house, we will accept a daytime fever up to 103.5°F without medication. We like to see it under 102°F at night. This mostly comes from our worrisome nature as parents. To reliably lower the fever, we use vitamin C and plenty of it.

The biggest plus for vitamin C is that it is remarkably safe. Another advantage of high-dose vitamin C therapy is that, while it is an excellent antipyretic, vitamin C acts as an antibiotic and antiviral, and also strengthens the immune system. In other words, vitamin C lowers a fever by eliminating its cause. The vitamin must be given very frequently and in sufficient quantity to get results. When sick, I think one should take vitamin C as often as humanly possible, even every ten minutes if necessary. Either bowel tolerance and/or cessation of symptoms indicates that you took enough.

Bed rest and liquids have always been and still are very helpful for fever. In addition to water and instead of sugary "juice drinks," use freshly made vegetable juices. Carrot juice in particular is fairly tasty and loaded with carotene. Many fevers are accompanied by infection, which rapidly depletes the liver of its vitamin A reserves. Carotene is the cheapest and safest way to take in large amounts of provitamin A.

Of course, a sick body needs sleep. A niacin supplement will shorten the time it takes to fall asleep and actually act as a natural sedative. There may be an additional niacin benefit to someone with a fever: The superficial vasodilation resulting from a niacin flush, while it initially makes you feel warm, will in about ten or twenty minutes cause a loss of some heat from the body.

Homeopathy may be appropriate to try during a fever. Nonprescription homeopathic preparations have a nearly 200-year history of safety. They are so dilute that toxicity is next to impossible. One might wonder how something so safe can be so helpful to the body. It was during a major outbreak of scarlet fever that homeopathic medicine first received validation. Records showed that more patients survived with homeopathic treatment than did with conventional medicine. Two classic remedies that I've often used at home are *Belladonna and Ferrum Phosphate.*[3] Many a fever is relieved by chiropractic adjustment of the upper vertebrae of the neck. It is common to have a feverish child recover much more rapidly than usual after manipulative treatment.

There is a lot of unnecessary confusion over whether or not to "feed a fever." The actual saying, by the way, is "Starve a cold lest you feed a fever." Naturopathic theory holds that controlled, therapeutic juice fasting promotes recovery from many illnesses. We are not talking starvation, but rather a vacation from our usual pattern of over-eating. Juices, especially raw vegetable juices, actually provide above-average nourishment. One could easily show that vegetable juice fasting really isn't a "fast" at all—it is an especially healthful, inexpensive, natural, uncooked, modified liquid diet. I think that if you want results fast, then fast for results.

Fungus Problems

When I was a boy, there were two realities I had to accept. The first was that our backyard was too small for a pony. The second was that I was going to have athlete's foot forever. My brothers and I all had athlete's foot. We did everything right and still it persisted: We carefully dried between our toes, we doused our feet with antiseptics, we used foot powders, and we changed our socks constantly. Nothing worked.

My first real lesson in natural healing occurred the year summer camp began in rural Bergen, New York. The YMCA opened a camp with no place to swim. The bordering creek was stagnant and muddy and the camp's outdoor pool was still a dream. So, the counselors put us on a bus, dressed in swimsuits and sneakers, and took us to a nearby farm. Some arrangement had been made so we could swim in the farmer's cow pond.

When we were finished swimming, we were a lot dirtier than we ever got at the Y. We sat on the ground in the sun and quickly put on our socks, without time to dry our feet, before catching the bus back to camp. No disinfectant in sight. Immediately that summer, my athlete's foot went away.

Looking back, I think it was the sunlight that did it. Fungi in general, and athlete's foot fungi in particular, love darkness. When we swam outside and dressed outside, the sun got to our toes. Sunlight did what sanitation and drugs could not. Ringworm is not a worm at all, but another fungus. If you've ever had this on your tummy, under your arm, or behind a knee, you'll recall that these are generally places that are covered by clothes. Not to give you an excuse to become a nudist, but sunlight is an effective, natural treatment for skin fungus. When it is not sunny, camping weather, careful use of a sun lamp will work just as well. Caution: always wear heavily tinted eye protection when using a sun lamp and sensibly limit your exposure.

Another approach to "ringworm" fungus patches on the body is to apply tincture of iodine. This kills them as well or better than anything the doctor will tell the pharmacy to sell you. Iodine tincture is very cheap to buy. You will of course want to keep it out of the reach of children, for it is a poison if swallowed. I've found that it is only necessary to apply the iodine tincture every third day. The fungus is usually gone in a week or so. Iodine seems to irritate and dry the skin when applied too frequently, but you will probably only need a few applications to do the trick.

Fungal growths under the toenail are more stubborn, but a combination of sunlight and topical iodine will still generally be effective. It is an obvious point, but sandals really make a lot of sense. They allow light and dryness to intrude on the fungi's much preferred habitat of moist darkness. Try these tips and there will no longer be a fungus among us.

Gallstones

You need never suffer with a gallstone, ever. If you are overweight, diabetic, facing old age, pregnant, on estrogen therapy, or just plain eat wrong, this statement is especially important to you, as you are likely at greater risk for gallstones than most. Gallstones are largely made from cholesterol. You can stop eating cholesterol, stop making excess cholesterol, or dissolve existing cholesterol.

Vitamin C—Vitamin C in quantity stops gallstones before they start. "Ascorbic acid (vitamin C), which affects the catabolism of cholesterol to bile acids and, in turn, the development of gallbladder disease in experimental animals, may reduce the risk of clinical gallbladder disease in humans."[1],[2]

Vegetarian Diet—The bile you need to help you digest fats is concentrated in the gallbladder. During this digestive process, water is removed; the resulting concentrated cholesterol can be too much to remain in solution and cholesterol gallstones may precipitate out. In addition to hurting, gallstones obstruct the bile duct and thereby interfere with fat digestion. One indicator is light-colored stools. Bilirubin, the bile pigment, normally darkens them to brown-green.

High-fiber foods and low-fat meals help prevent gallbladder problems. Low-cholesterol diets help, too. Now, where can we find a high-fiber, low-fat, low-cholesterol diet? A vegetarian diet, of course. It needs to be stated and restated that cholesterol is only found in animal products. On top of that, your own body manufactures cholesterol for you. That's another big reason why you have the biological green light to become a vegetarian.

There are some people who make way too much cholesterol. Over the years, I have known quite a number of people whose cholesterol used to be through the roof for various reasons. They became vegetarian, focused on fiber, cut out sugar, started juicing vegetables, took their vitamin C and lecithin, and down came the cholesterol numbers.

Lecithin—Phospholipids in bile help emulsify, or dissolve, cholesterol. Lecithin (which is a phospholipid) is therefore well worth trying for gallstones. Three to five tablespoons of lecithin daily is more likely to be effective than a few capsules. Even a large 1,200-milligram capsule contains only about 1/8 tablespoon of lecithin. Lecithin is a very safe food substance, not expensive, nonprescription, and available at any health food store. One dose of this is not going to do it; plan on taking the lecithin as a part of your daily routine.

Additional Options—Drinking a mixture of 4 ounces of olive oil and 2 ounces of lemon juice is an old gallstone-flushing standby among traditional naturopaths. Many persons have reported successful use. One might want first to dissolve them (or at least make them smaller) with lecithin before flushing them out. Supplementing with the B vitamins supports proper liver function to help in the flushing process; the most effective way to take them is in a B-complex tablet several times daily. I also think a low-sugar diet, which cannot possibly hurt, is also worth incorporating.

Commonsense caution: If you are hurting, don't be a gallstone martyr. Get medical attention right away.

Headaches

Before you reach for a drug, it is worth your while to try natural ways to get rid of headache pain. Here are some methods that can bring real relief:

1. Are your neck bones (cervical vertebrae) misaligned? Many headaches can, and do, result from this. When vertebrae are turned or twisted, the muscles attached to them are tensed and pulled. In some cases, the nerves that emerge between each vertebra can be pressured or even pinched. This causes discomfort and pain that extends up into and over the head. In my experience, it is rare to see a case of a simple headache or migraine without the neck being out as well. What to do? You could start by seeing a chiropractor. Neither aspirin, acetaminophen, nor ibuprofen will realign your neck bones; pain relievers will not remove the source of a headache. A chiropractor often can.

2. For simple tension headaches, there are two homeopathic remedies that work: *Kali Phos* (potassium phosphate) and *Mag Phos* (magnesium phosphate). *Kali Phos* is the traditional natural remedy for headaches that are nervous or emotional in origin. If your headache goes away when you are doing something you enjoy, and comes back later when you're not, then try

Kali Phos. Stress, overwork, eyestrain, motion sickness, anxiety, and fretfulness are all indicators pointing to a need for *Kali Phos.* This remedy is especially good for children. *Mag Phos* is the remedy for pulling, cramping, spasmodic pain. *Mag phos* headaches tend to feel better when you are warm or when heat is applied.

Also known as "Schuessler cell salts," these mineral-based remedies are not drugs and neither has any side effects. Label directions are simple and homeopathic remedies are harmless. They have stood the test of time with nearly two centuries of worldwide use. Both are nonprescription and available at health food stores or from a homeopathic supplier.

3. Acupressure (acupuncture without needles) is often remarkably effective for headaches. You can try a series of pressure-point massages known as the Chinese Eye Exercises (see How to Do Six Chinese Eye Exercises).

4. What you eat or drink can make the difference in whether or not you have a headache. Chemical food additives, excess salt, dairy products (milk in particular), dehydration, or constipation may provoke a headache. If you consume any appreciable quantity of alcohol, don't bother crying about your headache. One old folk remedy is an ice pack for the head and

a mustard application under the nose. Yes, you use that inexpensive yellow prepared mustard right from the supermarket. Slather some under your snoot. Sure, it sounds funny. It looks even funnier.

All of the above approaches to headache relief are simple. Try them first—if a simple method cures it, then it was a simple headache. If the headache persists, you should consult a physician.

Migraines

Ironically, one of the most common of all prescription drug side effects is headache. Don't be bailing out a bottomless boat: Look up the side effects of any medication you take in the *Physicians' Desk Reference (PDR),* available at any library, pharmacy, or doctor's office. Start your headache program by first avoiding what is known to cause headaches.

Some migraines are hormonal in origin, as many women will be willing to verify. Natural health advocates have long maintained that the human body often suffers from internal toxic accumulations. They might be caused by poor elimination, eating too much of the wrong thing, or not getting enough of the right thing. Meat may contain unwanted hormones because cattle are fattened with them—yet another reason to become a vegetarian. Eating lots of fiber helps reduce hormonal buildup. It is well established that dietary fiber grabs hold of excess estrogen and eliminates it.

HOW TO DO SIX CHINESE EYE EXERCISES

These easy exercises to reduce eyestrain will help anyone, so take off those specs or take out those contacts, and let's begin.

EXERCISE 1: TEMPLE MASSAGE

With the pointer finger of each hand, massage your temples (the side of the head level with the eyes) in the depression that you will find there. If you wear glasses, the depressed location is right underneath each side of your glasses frame.

EXERCISE 2: NOSE-BRIDGE MASSAGE

Use the finger and thumb of one hand to gently pinch and massage the uppermost part of the nose. Again, if you wear glasses, this spot is under where the glasses sit upon your nose.

EXERCISE 3: FOREHEAD AND SCALP-LINE MASSAGE

This is a tricky one. Place the ball of your thumb along the underside of the upper margin of your eyesocket, find the supraorbital notch, and press. In other words, press up under the eyebrow with the ball of your thumb. Just under the top of each eye socket there is a little notch. No kidding—you can feel it. This tells you that you've got the right place. Press carefully upward.

At the same time, take your fingers and rest them along your front hairline (or where your front hairline used to be!). Draw the fingers down together, while drawing the thumb up, bringing it all together as you gently mush your forehead skin in the middle. I call this exercise the "Boris Karloff exercise" because you feel (if not look) like the Frankenstein monster in full forehead make-up.

EXERCISE 4: MID-FACE MASSAGE

Smile. An upper line formed by your grin curves up on each side toward your nose. One finger's distance out from each nostril, right on this smile line, is the location for this massage point. (The facial nerve emerges from the maxilla bone there.) After stimulating this point, try taking a deep breath through your nose. Many people find that this helps clear their sinuses, reduces sinus pressure, and relieves their sinus headaches.

So far, we have massaged, and relaxed, all four major muscle areas around the eye.

The eye can move in all directions because of the four attachments.

EXERCISE 5: CLOSED EYELID MASSAGE

This is one of my favorites and it is quite relaxing. Close your eyes and lightly and rapidly stroke the lids with your fingertips. Back and forth, top and bottom lids.

EXERCISE 6: ACUPRESSURE POINT ON THE HAND

Even though they're not close to the eye muscles, reflex or trigger points operate throughout the human organism. One such point, helpful for headaches, is in your hands, literally. With your palm open and your thumb up, you will notice a ridge of skin between your thumb and the base of your forefinger. Take the thumb of your opposite hand and invert it over this fold of skin bent like a little tent. Roll the thumb further over the side and you will locate a point about a thumb's distance in. Meet your thumb with the forefinger and press together.[1] Ooh! Feel that?

Helpful Hints: One may generally do the exercises several times a day, each one for a count of about fifteen. Always stimulate points bilaterally; that is, be sure to do the points with each eye, on both sides of the face and on each hand. Your fingernails should be short to avoid hurting yourself. Do not perform the exercises if you have a good reason not to. It is probably best to avoid using any pressure points while pregnant unless you have first checked with your doctor or midwife.

Although it sounds deceptively simple in principle, it may be possible to mitigate the toxin problem by diluting it. One medical doctor I know recommends that her patients drink a full glass of water every five or ten minutes for an hour until the headache goes away. I've tried it and it works. This technique costs nothing and may make all the difference in your day.

If you have not yet tried the Gerson therapy of vegetable juices and a salt-free diet, you are missing out on the most effective migraine therapy there is. Best known today as a nutritional approach to fighting cancer, the Gerson program is actually a systemic, holistic one that cleanses the human organism while strengthening the body's ability to heal itself. Properly feed the body and the body fixes what is wrong.

Dr. Max Gerson, a fully qualified medical doctor, suffered from incurable, blindingly debilitating migraine headaches. In desperation, Dr. Gerson had tried literally everything he could to relieve his pain. No medicine helped him. He then, as a last resort, began to wonder if diet might have anything to do with it. He noticed improvement for the first time when he ate an unprocessed, natural diet high in vegetables. But it was when he turned to drinking quantities of vegetable juices that his migraines were eradicated. He was as surprised as you would be, perhaps even more so because he was a doctor who had been taught nothing of natural healing, except perhaps professional contempt for it.

Word got around and people started to seek out this doctor who cured migraines when other doctors failed to. Dr. Gerson began to note that many of his migraine patients were also getting cures of assorted conditions that they hadn't initially told him about. He reasoned that juicing was a "metabolic therapy," nonspecific and broad spectrum in nature. The Gerson therapy has been in continual usage for eighty years, and its successes are documented and numerous.[2] And there is no down side to trying vegetable juices.

Doses of niacin high enough to cause a strong "flush" may profoundly relieve migraine pain. I attended a conference where a researcher presented this concept.[3] It caught my attention and, of course, I then mentioned it to a migraine sufferer. She took 500 milligrams of niacin (enough to immediately flush most people) every hour or so. While she had the migraine, she never flushed, even though she normally flushes very readily on far less niacin. She repeated the 500-milligram niacin dose over and over. When she finally flushed, the migraine pain was greatly diminished.

Herpes, Cold Sores, HPV (Human Papillma Virus), & Shingles (Herpes Zoster)

For persons told, "There is no cure for herpes," it is high time for a second opinion. There may be no pharmaceutical cure, nor medical cure, nor well-publicized cure. Before you resign yourself to accepting recurring, painful, and otherwise problematic herpes lesions as your lot in life, try the advice of Robert. F. Cathcart, M.D.: make a paste with vitamin C powder and a little water and apply it directly to external herpes lesions. Ascorbic acid works best, in my opinion, but may smart a bit. Calcium ascorbate is nonacidic and is "ouchless." It works so well, writes Dr. Cathcart, that "frequently, one application will suffice for herpes.... Applications to intact skin where the patient perceives an outbreak is about to occur will completely abort the attack. Several applications may be necessary to penetrate through the intact skin."[1]

You will likely find a significant reduction in both discomfort and in lesion size overnight. If the lesions were fluid filled (that liquid is loaded with viruses), you will notice that the lesions quickly become drier. If lesions have broken and the fluid has leaked out, apply the paste not only on, but liberally around the whole area. Repeat this process twice daily until the skin is completely healed.

Will doing so guarantee that every herpes virus on you is really and sincerely dead? No. Good antiviral though vitamin C is, there are survivors to almost any massacre. Be smart, and assume accordingly. Is herpes contagious? You bet it is. Use all necessary precautions to avoid spreading it.

For shingles, high oral doses (and possibly intravenous administration) of vitamin C appear to be most effective.[2] Megadoses of vitamin C sounds too simple to work, but the therapy has been used for decades. Remember, the strongest antiviral properties of vitamin C are to be found at the highest doses. Other troublesome skin virus problems can be effectively treated with high topical doses of vitamin C. HPV (human papilloma virus) responds amazingly well (and very quickly) to topical vitamin-C paste therapy, as does the common cold sore, herpes simplex.

There is no way to get a higher concentration than pure vitamin C powder applied directly to herpes lesions or HPV "warts." Remember: ascorbic acid powder, though most effective, can smart a bit if there is a break in the skin. If the skin is raw or tender, you can use buffered vitamin C powder, such as calcium ascorbate or sodium ascorbate. Or, for those who want the best results for the least cash, just mix in some sodium bicarbonate (baking soda) to make ascorbic acid pH neutral. I have knowledge of cases where not only has such treatment promptly gotten rid of lesions in a few days, but there has been no recurrence even over considerable lengths of time.

Another great natural enemy of the cold sore is the amino acid L-lysine. You can get lots of lysine by eating lots of beans. An effective dose is about 3–4 grams (3,000–4,000mg) of lysine daily. That is about a can and a half of beans a day.

BOOSTING YOUR IMMUNE SYSTEM

The essence of disease prevention is to strengthen an individual's immune system. It is futile to focus on the preemptive killing of every germ, every time, everywhere; it cannot be done. Rather than live inside a bubble, scramble for the latest and greatest antibiotic, or panic if your vaccination card is incomplete, why not concentrate on the many ways you can fortify the immune system yourself?

Ducks swim in water but do not get wet. This is because they have oiled their feathers to form a natural barrier impervious to moisture. We can do the same with our immune systems and germs. We live in a world full of germs. Most of them are harmless and many are actually beneficial. Cows, by the way, cannot really eat grass. But the digestive bacteria in the cow's rumen can. Helpful bacteria in your digestive tract make you healthy, too. Some bacteria actually make vitamins for you, notably B12 and vitamin K. Bacteria help break down your food and process wastes. And, yes, some bacteria are nasty. But if the body is healthy, bacteria, pathogenic or not, are largely irrelevant.

We live in a world full of antibiotic over-prescription, with a resultant rise in the number of drug-resistant bacteria. The importance of utilizing harmless natural modalities to boost the immune system is therefore more important than ever. A healthy immune system is built every day by your lifestyle choices, especially your nutrition choices.

- Immune Booster 1: Take lots of vitamin C to help defend yourself against viruses and bacteria. Strengthen your resolve with scientific studies on the antitoxic, antibiotic, and antiviral properties of megadoses of vitamin C.

- Immune Booster 2: Conquer chronic tiredness. Get to bed earlier. Set the video recorder and watch that TV show tomorrow! You can get a more satisfying night's sleep by darkening your room—the darker your sleeping environment, the more melatonin (your body's sleep hormone) you automatically make.

- Immune Booster 3: Take a good multivitamin twice each day. Research has shown that people who take supplements have higher numbers of immune T cells and natural killer cells, plus enhanced antibody response and immune cell activity.[1] Vitamin-takers are sick only half as many days per year as those who do not take supplements.[2]

- Immune Booster 4: Take supplemental vitamin E. A placebo-controlled, double-blind trial showed that 800IU of vitamin E per day improves immune responsiveness in the elderly. What is really interesting is that the response was seen in only thirty days.[3]

• Immune Booster 5: Drink lots of vegetable juices. Carotene in high doses specifically strengthens the immune system by helping the body to build more helper T cells. The amount used in one study was 180 milligrams of beta-carotene per day. The study produced positive results in only two weeks.[4]

• Immune Booster 6: Stop smoking. It is the greatest preventable danger to the greatest number of people. In the United States alone, tobacco kills 51 people an hour.

The bottom line—a naturally strong immune system effectively resists disease. If it didn't, we would be extinct. Take the steps above to heart and we can substantially strengthen our immune systems, right now, at low cost, and with no prescription.

384

Indigestion

A puzzle for you: you are an air traffic controller and your mission is to launch three different aircraft so that their flights do not conflict with each other. The three aircraft are a propeller-driven private plane, a commercial jumbo jet, and a hot-air balloon. To ensure that they are not in the same airspace at the same time, in which order will you launch them?

The answer is: jet first, private plane second, and hot-air balloon last. Why? Clear the fastest out first. Getting the 500-mile-per-hour jet out of the way first means the slower airplane won't encounter it. And launch the balloon last, for it will necessarily linger in the airspace the longest.

Nutritionally, this is analogous to the "layered eating" plan I learned over twenty years ago from Dr. Christopher Gian-Cursio, a famous New York naturopath. His view was that since complex, higher-protein foods take the longest to digest, they should have the stomach to themselves. To accomplish this, he directed patients to start their meal with quick-digesting fresh vegetable juices. Vegetable salad was next, and protein foods came last. This is one of the best no-cost ways to fight indigestion.

Other ways to improve your digestion:

1. If a food always bothers you, just eliminate it. There is no shortage of choices; eat something else instead. My Dad used to eat pastrami and he always had an upset stomach. So he stopped, and so did the symptoms.

2. Eat when you are really hungry. Digestion is strongest when you truly need to eat. Food tastes better then, too, for "hunger is the best mustard."

3 Chew your food thoroughly. We know it, we say it, but we do not do it. Mechanical digestion is nearly as important as chemical digestion. Your teeth are for cutting and grinding. Since you brush them, and fill them, and floss them, why not use them? One of the reasons people suffer indigestion is they eat too fast, which really means they swallow too soon. If food goes down in chunks, it will end up in your colon in chunks.

4. Eliminating meat from your diet is likely to eliminate distress from your belly. I know a person who cured his chronic indigestion just by giving up pork. For another fellow, it was quitting hot dogs that helped the most. Meat contains

zero fiber, clogs your pipes, and decays in your digestive tract. Ugh.

5. More fiber in general may help. Roughage helps keep everything moving and automatically stimulates the digestive process. Salads, raw vegetables and fruits, well-chewed nuts, whole grains, sprouts, and legumes (peas, beans, lentils) are all good choices.

6. Eat more rice. While bagels and pizza are particularly "gassy," rice is the opposite. Remember that rice cereal is recommended as a first solid food for babies because it is so easy to digest.

7. Yogurt and other cultured dairy products are an easy source of beneficial *L. acidophilus* bacteria (as well as protein and calcium). Such friendly bacteria digest much of your food for you. Every time you take antibiotics, it kills off these good bacteria; that is one reason for so much indigestion in America. If dairy products make you stuffy, dilute your yogurt with water. If you don't like less thick yogurt, just drink a glass or two of water before eating any dairy product. If you wish to completely do without milk products, you can buy *acidophilus* capsules at any health food store.

8. Try a multiple digestive enzyme supplement to improve digestion and absorption of

foods in general. Such a product will commonly contain pancrelipase, papain, hydrochloric acid, ox bile, bromelain, and amylase in one tablet. Totally vegetarian digestive supplements are also available. Begin with only half of the recommended amount and gradually increase as needed to get the most comfortable result. More will usually be needed for larger meals and higher-protein meals. The elderly will especially benefit from such supplementation.

9. To get bonus digestive enzymes from your food, eat more raw bean sprouts and fresh or dried papaya, figs, and pineapple. Pineapple contains the enzyme bromelain and papaya contains papain. Sprouts and figs contain a variety of beneficial enzymes. Cooking temperatures destroy enzymes, so try to eat these (and more of your foods in general) raw, whenever possible.

10 Raw vegetable juices are very easy to digest. People with really troubled tummies often make great improvements with the addition of carrot, cabbage, and other vegetable juices to their diet. Naturopathic authorities frequently recommend a short period of fasting on vegetable juices alone.

11. Get a medical opinion if indigestion persists. If you are told that you have an allergy, or are lactose intolerant, ask for

the basis of that diagnosis. Only about one in three "lactose intolerant" people actually tests out to have the condition. Even lactose intolerant people may be able to eat small quantities of cultured dairy products, such as aged cheeses and yogurt. Vegetarianism is always a sensible option. Many a so-called allergy goes away promptly with the addition of substantial amounts of vitamin C to each meal.

12. To improve your digestion, don't just sit there, do something! That something is exercise. Regular exercise, especially between meals and stretching before bed, will make a world of digestive difference.

Lupus

Lupus, which is considered an autoimmune disease, affects 1.5 million Americans and is much more common in women than men. Medical science does not know what causes it. To me, this immediately suggests that it may be related to nutrition. Many things can trigger lupus, such as trauma, puberty or menopause, childbirth, viral infection, and even medication. These events also take a nutritional toll on the human body, especially a body that has had only borderline nutrient intakes. Undernutrition has been known to set the body up for many chronic diseases, including other autoimmune conditions such as multiple sclerosis.

Max Gerson, M.D., was successfully treating lupus using diet as early as the 1930s.[1] We should not dismiss either the approach or the date out of hand. A time-honored unorthodox cure is still a cure, unfashionable as it may be among our pharmaphilic (drug-loving) medical specialists of today. The Gerson diet is very high in vegetables and their juices, and therefore very high in antioxidants. Antioxidants have been known to fight lupus for a long time. In 1948, Drs. Wilfrid and Evan Shute observed that vitamin E, another antioxidant, greatly helped cases of lupus. More recently, Robert F.

Cathcart, M.D., and Thomas Levy, M.D., have both reported that vitamin C in saturation doses is an effective treatment for lupus. Vitamin C, too, is an antioxidant. I think we may be onto something here.

Dr. Levy has commented that it might seem paradoxical that vitamin C, which is a well-known immune system booster, would be of value in treating an autoimmune disease. But the fact remains that huge vitamin C doses get clinical improvement.[2] Dr. Cathcart thinks that the antioxidant (electron-donating) property of vitamin C is the reason it works: "(M)assive doses of ascorbic acid—determined by bowel tolerance to ascorbic acid in the range of 30 to 100 to 200 grams a day (or use intravenous sodium ascorbate in the range of 60 to 120 grams a day)—will shut down inflammatory reactions mediated by free radicals."[3]

Because so little is known about lupus, the meganutritional approach remains intriguing. All of the doctors mentioned above deserve a listen, and their methods, a fair trial.

Macular Degeneration

If there ever was a clear example of an ounce of prevention beating a pound of cure, it would be macular degeneration. "Macula" means "spot," which in this case is on the retina. This is where visual images are focused on the inside of the back of the eye. A lack of antioxidants in the diet puts the retina at risk, causing premature aging and deterioration. Therefore, consuming generous amounts of the body's principal protective antioxidants, namely vitamins C and E, the carotenes, and small amounts of selenium and zinc, will help protect your sight. Start now, for macular degeneration is the primary cause of vision loss in the elderly.

If you have already been diagnosed with the condition, your doctor has probably told you that there is no medical treatment to rely on. If so, then there is no reason not to try nutrition. If antioxidants can prevent macular degeneration, larger amounts of them may help reverse it. The theory is easy enough to test and safe enough to try. Vitamins E and C and carotene are nontoxic. Too much vitamin C is indicated by very loose bowels. Excessive carotene, which is the orange color in carrots, is indicated by orange-colored skin.

Vitamin E is so safe that premature babies are specifically given it to prevent oxygen damage to their retinas. These infants require about 200IU a day for the treatment to be effective. That is the adult dose equivalent of about 7,000IU of vitamin E daily. Little clinical need has ever existed in adults for even half of that amount. However, the U.S. government recommendation of only 10–15IU per day is not even enough to stop macular degeneration in a hamster. Between 600 and 1,200IU daily is a common therapeutic level for a person. It is only possible to obtain such amounts by taking a supplement.

Selenium increases the effectiveness of vitamin E in the body. Only a little selenium is needed, say 100–200 micrograms daily. Too much selenium can be toxic, and extended use of amounts over 600 micrograms daily are to be avoided.

Zinc is another important mineral for the retina. Zinc deficiency in America is the rule, not the exception. Most of us don't even consume the small RDA of 15 milligrams per day. Zinc deficiency is especially prevalent in older persons. The signs of too little zinc in the diet are a weak immune system, poor wound healing, loss of taste and smell, psoriasis-like skin lesions, prostate problems, rheumatoid arthritis, and senility. Up to 660 milligrams of zinc a day has been used in some clinical studies, but there is an eventual risk of copper deficiency and anemia if such a high level is maintained. Just one-eighth of that amount, less than 100 milligrams per day, may be enough to slow or stop the process of macular degeneration. The amino acid chelate form of zinc is well absorbed. Pumpkin seeds are high in zinc. Or eat a lot of mollusks, oysters in particular.

Instead of beta-carotene supplements, try carrot juice. Yes, it contains a great deal of beta-carotene, but it also contains dozens of other beneficial carotenes, not just the "beta" form. Freshly made from your own juicer, raw carrot juice tastes good and provides many other valuable nutrients. Even a single carrot a day substantially reduces a person's risk of macular degeneration. We've all known since we were toddlers that "carrots are good for our eyes." But nearly one in four of us doesn't eat even a single serving a day of any vegetable.

In addition to carrots, consumption of fresh, raw foods may help much more. I know of a person whose degeneration of the retina was very severe and she had lost much of her sight. In desperation, she began a nearly 100 percent raw food diet. She ate mostly salads and a jar or two of home-grown sprouts a day. I won't say that she loved doing it, but she loved the results: Not only was she no longer losing her sight, she was actually gaining it back. Over a period of a year, her ophthalmologist confirmed improvement. Her recovery was remarkable and, medically speaking, highly improbable. She didn't care; she could see.

Motor Neuron Diseases

Motor neuron diseases (MND) involve the degeneration of the nerve cells (neurons) that control movement (motor function). They include amyotrophic lateral sclerosis (ALS), progressive bulbar palsy (PBP), primary lateral sclerosis (PLS) and progressive muscular atrophy (PMA). The conventional-therapy outlook is not at all good. According to the Motor Neuron Disease Association, most of those so diagnosed have a life expectancy averaging only two to five years, but a small number of people with MND have lived for ten years or more.[1]

I am intrigued that some people with motor neuron diseases live twice or even five times longer than others. Why? Could it have something to do with what they eat?

Frederick R. Klenner, M.D., successfully employed megavitamin therapy for multiple sclerosis and myasthenia gravis.[2] I am aware that these illnesses do not fit the strict description of motor neuron diseases, but they do, however, involve mobility and neurons. I speculate that the various stems might all spring from the same nutritionally deficient roots. There is an easy and obvious way to test this theory: begin a therapeutic trial and see.

Here is a summary of Dr. Klenner's intensive nutritional treatment for MS and MG, which may be applicable to MND:

- Vitamin B1 (thiamine): 1,500 to 4,000mg per day, orally and by injection
- Vitamin B2 (riboflavin): 250 to 1,000mg per day
- Vitamin B3 (niacin): 500mg up to many thousands of milligrams daily, enough to cause repeated, warm-feeling vasodilation ("flushing")
- Vitamin B6 (pyridoxine): 300–800mg per day
- Vitamin B12 (cobalamin): 1,000 micrograms three times a week by injection
- Vitamin C (ascorbic acid): 10,000–20,000mg or more per day
- Vitamin E (d-alpha tocopherol): 800 to 1,600IU per day

All the above doses need to be divided up throughout the day. Dr. Klenner also prescribed a number of other nutrients, including choline (1,000 to 2,000mg per day), magnesium (300–1,200mg per day in divided doses), and zinc (60mg per day). Calcium, lecithin, folic acid, linoleic and linolenic essential fatty acids, and a daily multivitamin/mineral supplement are also recommended.[3] I strongly support the addition of vitamin D, in a dose of 2,000IU per day, as people with MS typically are vitamin D deficient.[4]

Why such a large variety of nutrients? Because there is no such thing as monotherapy with nutrition. "One drug, one disease" is a failed legend of the drug doctor. All vitamins are important. Which wheel on your car can you do without? Which wing on an airplane can you afford to leave behind?

Why such large quantities of nutrients? Because that's what does the job. You don't take the amount that you think should work; you take the amount that gets results. A sick body has exaggeratedly high needs for many vitamins—you can either meet that need or fret about why you didn't. And what if someone has MS, MG, or any of the motor neuron diseases? Again, I am not suggesting that they are all the same illness, but they may all have a common basis: unacknowledged, untreated, long-term vitamin deficiency. Therefore, they all may benefit from Dr. Klenner's approach.[5]

Muscular Dystrophy

Everybody knows what muscles are, and when they don't work, the weakness, frailty, and incapacity of a child with muscular dystrophy (MD) makes for many a poignant poster and tearful telethon. According to the National Institutes of Health, "There is no specific treatment for any of the forms of MD."[1] Such despairing, autocratic, but research-friendly pronouncements must not be seen as the last word until we adequately factor in maternal and fetal malnutrition as a cause of this disease. For if nutrient deficiency can cause an illness, nutrient therapy may ameliorate, or even cure, that illness.

Malnutrition causes muscular dystrophy? Very possibly, because muscular dystrophy literally is malnutrition. The very word *dystrophy* is defined as "defective nutrition" or "any disorder caused by defective nutrition."[2] When we consider all that this means, we are poised to head down a steep slope. Nothing gets you into emotional hot water faster than being perceived as blaming a baby's problems on the mother's diet. It is very difficult to know for sure if a birth defect is the result of genetics or environmental factors. The mother represents half of a developing baby's heredity, but almost all of the developing baby's environment. Every single cell in a baby is the product of inherited DNA instruction. But every single cell is also the product of parental diet.

Ova (human eggs) are formed during the fetal stage of a female's life. In other words, all of a woman's eggs were formed while she was developing inside her mother, before she herself was born. This means that what your grandmother ate significantly contributed to your health. Think that over: what looks like a genetic problem may be a nutritional one. I call this "dinner table heredity." Just because a problem comes out of the womb does not mean that that problem is genetic only. Yet the National Institutes of Health unequivocally declares MD to be a genetic disease.

There is an important interrelationship between food and genes, called the genetotrophic concept, originated by Roger J. Williams, Ph.D. Dr. Williams, the discoverer of the B vitamin pantothenic acid, has explained in his books and papers how biochemical birth defects may be overcome with optimal nutrition.

In genetotrophic diseases, genetic abnormality leads to nutritional disability. To compensate, the body requires the availability of larger than normal quantities of one or more nutrients for the affected gene to successfully express itself. For that particular person, normal dietary vitamin intakes are quite inadequate for normal function. It is a bit like trying to take a hot bath with the drain open: it can be done, but you are going to need a lot more hot water.

I think that muscular dystrophy may constitute a good example of a genetotrophic disease. Furthermore, this also goes a long way to answering the perennial parents' question as to how one child can be healthy while the sibling is afflicted with MD ... when Mom ate pretty much the same diet during both pregnancies. There may be both a genetic component and a nutritional component. Rather than a nutrient deficiency, MD may more exactly be considered to be a genetically influenced nutrient dependency.

So, the real question is, "To what extent might individual nutrients enable the sufferer to overcome the existing condition?" There is considerable good news, and it is all nutritional.

Coenzyme Q10—By now, coenzyme Q10 (CoQ10 or ubiquinone) should probably be accepted as a vitamin. Many other vitamins are coenzymes. CoQ10 is found in small quantities in foods. Most young people make CoQ10 in their bodies, but a youngster with muscular dystrophy may either make too little or have a bigger requirement because of the illness.

It has been established that heart muscle greatly benefits from CoQ10 supplementation, resulting in improvement in cases of congestive heart failure and even cardiomyopathy. Striated cardiac muscle and striated voluntary (skeletal) muscle are not that dissimilar. Furthermore, researchers have found that cardiac disease is commonly associated with muscular dystrophy. Impaired heart muscle function in patients with muscular diseases is comparable to that of impaired skeletal muscle. Both may be helped by CoQ10.[3]

Because CoQ10 is so absolutely vital to muscle cells, involved with growth control, cellular energy production, and other essential life functions, it warrants special consideration for persons with muscular dystrophy. In two placebo-controlled, double-blind trials, using 100 milligrams per day of CoQ10 in persons of varying ages with muscular dystrophies, re-searchers reported that those receiving CoQ10 demonstrated "definitely improved physical performance."[4]

However, I submit that 300–600 milligrams of CoQ10 per day would be a more effective dose, especially for an older child with MD. For most families, the limiting factors will be cost or medical disapproval. As there are no harmful side effects with CoQ10, it is worth a serious therapeutic trial.

Vitamin E—Like CoQ10, vitamin E is an antioxidant. There is a long history of scientific suspicion, largely untested, that antioxidants are of unusual benefit to individuals with muscular dystrophy. Linus Pauling, Ph.D., wrote about MD in *How to Live Longer and Feel Better:* "It was recognized more than fifty years ago that a low intake of E leads to muscular dystrophy, a disorder of the skeletal muscles characterized by weakness similar to that caused by a deficiency of vitamin C.... The medical authorities do not mention the possible value of vitamins in controlling muscular dystrophies. The evidence about the involvement of vitamin E and vitamin C as well as B6 and other vitamins in the functioning of muscles suggests that the optimum intakes of these nutrients should be of value to the patients."[5]

Unfortunately, little research has been done in the last twenty years to establish the benefits of vitamins for MD. I found three studies, one with fifteen patients using vitamin E and selenium that reported "minimal" benefits[6] and a second with sixteen patients showing "slight" benefit.[7] I think they would have obtained far better results with larger doses of selenium, much larger doses of vitamin E, and using only the natural form of vitamin E.

The third study, using 600 milligrams of vitamin E and a relatively high amount of selenium got very good results in all five patients studied. "All improved their grip strength ... two normalized their gait, another two can now sit down on their heels and stand up, one patient can now walk on his toes, one can now get up from lying on the floor without using a chair, and two patients have improved their physical capacity.... No side effects were observed."[8]

Why no new, large-scale studies of high dose selenium–vitamin E therapy? Because drugless therapy is ignored by drug companies and consequently remains unpromoted and unknown to physicians. No investment is made and no research is done where there is no money to be recovered. Drug companies do not expect to find, nor do they want to find, a cure that does not involve a drug. A tragic example is modern medicine's approach to muscular dystrophy. There is no drug that corrects malnutrition, and never will be.

Agricultural scientists know this. You will have little trouble finding numerous research studies on the role of selenium or vitamin E in preventing muscular dystrophies in chickens, cattle, or lambs. Yet, in spite of the long, expensive history of research on MD, only a very small portion has involved vitamins, and much of it was quite some time ago. In 1953, one medical textbook made the following statement: "The peculiar muscular degeneration of muscular dystrophy produced in animals is caused and is only caused by lack of vitamin E. Human muscular dystrophy shows identically the same peculiar degeneration. The key to the cure of muscular dystrophy is vitamin E."[9]

Low doses of synthetic vitamin E will not work. It has to be the natural "D-alpha" form, and plenty of it, preferably from or with wheat germ or wheat germ oil.

Lecithin—Lecithin has been shown to improve therapeutic response when included along with vitamin E supplementation. This is probably due to the fact that lecithin contains a great deal of both inositol and phosphatidyl choline, which appear to reduce creatinuria in those with muscular dystrophy. Daily dosage used is about 20 grams, about three tablespoons, a day.[10]

Selenium—Blood levels of the trace mineral selenium are reduced in muscular dystrophy. "Myotonic dystrophy and all its major symptoms (including muscle dystrophy) can be cured or prevented in animals by selenium supplementation."[11] This includes rabbits, calves, and, in my opinion, people.

Selenium works closely with vitamin E and helps the body more efficiently utilize the vitamin. This important biochemical synergy only works if both nutrients are present. Normally, it takes very little selenium, about 100–200 micrograms a day, to protect your cells and membranes from harmful oxidation via a protective selenium-containing enzyme, glutathione peroxidase, found in all body cells. A muscular dystrophy patient probably needs more.

Foods containing selenium include nutritional (or brewer's) yeast, seafood, legumes, whole grains, animal products, and vegetables. However, food is an unreliable source of selenium, as selenium content of soils varies around the nation. For normally healthy individuals, overdose of selenium is possible with chronic excessive dietary intake. But bear in mind that in one of the MD studies, muscular dystrophy patients showed improvement with a daily dose of up to 1,400 micrograms of elemental selenium over a period of nearly two years. Toxicity is clearly not an issue.

A Medline search at the National Library of Medicine, in Washington, D.C., will locate over 18,300 studies that relate to muscular dystrophy. Yet I have seen no evidence whatsoever that current MD research includes megavitamin/mineral therapy. It has already been shown that selenium, vitamin E, and CoQ10 levels are decreased in people with muscular dystrophy.[12] What is it taking so long to apply that knowledge to those suffering today?

Osteoporosis

You either have to prevent calcium loss from bones or put calcium back into them if you want to avoid osteoporosis. While estrogen therapy slows calcium loss, it does not fundamentally stop, prevent, or reverse it. Nutritional therapy can, without estrogen's accompanying risks.

Calcium—Osteoporosis is much more common in women than men. In the diets of most women, a calcium deficiency begins at about age thirty-five and will become twice as bad by menopause. To prevent osteoporosis, young and middle-aged women should be encouraged to consume calcium. Pretty obvious advice, since prevention beats cure any day.

But can bones be remineralized in old age? The test is simply to give more calcium and the vitamin D necessary for its absorption and uptake into bone. In June 1984, the *American Journal of Clinical Nutrition* reported that 1,800 milligrams of calcium given daily to post-menopausal women produced significant results. This research, conducted in Australia, was verified by both x-ray and measurement of urinary hydroxyproline. How long did it take to achieve the results? Eight days.

Estrogen does not make bones stronger. As a matter of fact, estrogen administration may cause a reduction in bone remodeling rates and may actually increase the risk of fracture.[1] Since estrogen therapy carries an increased risk of endometrial cancer, calcium therapy makes a lot of sense. If you wonder why it is not promoted more enthusiastically, I suggest that it may make a lot of sense but does not make a lot of dollars. The medical and pharmaceutical industries stand to profit rather little from such a cheap cure as calcium.

Because of its calcium content, dairy food is better than meat. As a former dairyman, I am probably more kind to milk products than some. However, I advocate cultured milk products (cheese, yogurt) but not fluid milk, to get calcium.

Vitamin D—For strengthening bones, vitamin D is actually even more important than calcium. For decades, a milk-fed public has had its attention focused on calcium and largely diverted from the "other" important osteoporosis-preventing factor, vitamin D. Not only is vitamin D necessary for calcium deposition in the body, it is necessary for absorbing calcium into the body in the first place.[2]

Most persons with osteoporosis have low vitamin D levels. Along with calcium, 800IU of vitamin D daily (about twice the RDA) has been shown to increase bone density and to reduce hip fractures by an astounding 43 percent.[3]

There are over 250,000 hip fractures annually among persons over age sixty-five. Fractures and their complications are a major cause of death in the elderly. Up to 27 percent of hip fracture victims die within six months of their fall, usually of complications from surgery or infections,[4] so vitamin D therapy can save lives as well as bones. That the recommended dietary intake of vitamin D has been tripled for the elderly is an indication that this fact is not unknown, but even 600IU of vitamin D is probably too little.

Interestingly, vitamin D may offer another benefit for osteoporosis: Studies have found that "when older individuals take vitamin D supplements, they have less of a tendency to sway while standing or walking, and may therefore be less likely to fall."[5]

Current RDAs/DRIs for vitamin D are 200IU (5mcg) for all persons up to age fifty, 400IU (10mcg) for ages fifty-one to seventy, and for those seventy-one years and older, 600IU (15mcg). The present recommendations are an improvement; however, there is evidence that even three times the DRI for an adult is still not enough if a person is not receiving much sunlight.[6] These government recommendations are probably inadequate for disease prevention. Since sun exposure can provide the equivalent of 250 micrograms (10,000IU) of vitamin D per day, a significant increase may be in order, perhaps to several thousand IU per day.[7]

Vitamin D deficiency is widespread and is especially common in the elderly, who all too commonly eat the worst diet, take the most medication, and get the least sunlight. Furthermore, the normal aging process decreases the body's ability to make vitamin D from what sunlight may be received. Supplementation is essential, and I think 1,000 to 2,000IU per day is appropriate for every adult not living in the Sun Belt.

Ways to Avoid Osteoporosis

1. Drink less alcohol. "High intakes of alcohol, caffeine and protein cause significant negative calcium balance."[8] Outside of inadequate diet, alcohol is the most likely silent partner there is in osteoporosis and resulting fractures.
2. Use less caffeine. Caffeine is found in many soft drinks and diet aids as well as in extra-strength pain relievers. There is certainly little food value in coffee and soda.
3. Eat less protein. Americans consume about 100 to 120 grams of protein daily, three times the world average, and at least twice as much as we need. As for the high-protein, low-carbohydrate, weight-loss diets

that some people enter into, that's just heading further in the wrong direction. Eat less meat, or none at all, and the risk of osteoporosis declines. Avoiding meat and especially cola "soft drinks," which are both sources of dietary phosphorus, are important steps. Chronic excess phosphorus intake causes a calcium washout in the body. Vegetables and dairy products are good sources of calcium, and near-vegetarians naturally eat more of them.

4. Get more magnesium. Vegetables and especially nuts provide the mineral magnesium, which works in concert with calcium and is involved in hundreds of biochemical reactions in your body. Deficiency is common at all ages and is a certainty in the elderly. Taking 300–600 milligrams per day of magnesium is a good supplemental policy.

5. Move the bones or lose the bones. Ask any astronaut: Exercise helps build bone. Walking is ideal, but whatever exercise program you will actually do regularly is the best one for you.

6. Get more boron. Boron, a trace mineral, helps strengthen bone. Urinary excretion of calcium and magnesium is higher when you are boron deficient. Researchers have found that calcium-deficient animals have

"vertebrae that contained higher calcium content and required more force to break" than did the vertebrae of animals fed a low-boron diet.[9] Take about 3 milligrams daily to help prevent osteoporosis.

7. Eat natural, whole foods. A diet of organically grown, mineral-rich food makes stronger bones and speeds the healing of broken ones. Look to the soil. Years ago, research showed the average age for a broken hip in supermarket-fed Dallas County, Texas, to be sixty-three years. In rural, mineral-rich Deaf Smith County, Texas, it was eighty-one years of age. The average time for the fracture to heal in Dallas County was six to nine months; in Deaf Smith County, it was only eight weeks![10]

8. No tobacco. Cigarette smoking is a known risk factor in osteoporosis as well as for practically everything else.

9. Avoid fluoride. Not only does fluoridation fail to protect bones from fracture, it actually contributes to *increased* fractures.[11] Plus, the National Cancer Institute found a fluoride-related increase in osteosarcoma (a bone cancer) in young males.[12]

Prostate Problems

Let's briefly consider three common problems associated with the prostate: infection (prostatitis), enlargement (benign prostatic hypertrophy), and malignancy.

Prostatitis: Bacterial infection of the prostate may be acute or chronic; nonbacterial prostatitis is actually more common. Saturation doses of vitamin C are at least as effective as antibiotics in these conditions. We know this through the work of Frederick R. Klenner, M.D., Robert Cathcart, M.D., and other physicians who have for decades used very large doses of vitamin C to cure infections. Vitamin C is admittedly nonspecific, but no more so than the pharmaceutical antibiotics that are given for infection. Vitamin C has the advantage of being cheaper and considerably safer than drugs. Saturation of vitamin C is indicated by diarrhea, so take just under the amount that would produce loose stools. It will be a lot, measured in grams, not milligrams. The need for vitamin C will diminish as the infection subsides. A maintenance dose effectively helps to prevent a recurrence.

Infection or other stress results in lower blood zinc levels in general and lower prostate levels in particular. In prostatitis, zinc levels are only one-tenth of those in a normal prostate.[1] One time-tested prostate remedy is eating pumpkin seeds, which are a good source of zinc, as are shellfish (especially oysters) and nutritional yeast. A daily zinc supplement totaling 50–100 milligrams is frequently recommended in the natural healing literature, and that amount cannot be faulted by medical literature. Since men lose zinc in every seminal emission, their need for the mineral is higher than women's. Research at the Center for the Study of Prostatic Diseases, in Chicago, employed 50–100 milligrams of zinc per day for two weeks up to four months. There was prompt improvement in 70 percent of the cases.[2]

Benign Prostatic Hypertrophy (BPH) or Hyperplasia: Conventional medicine has historically indicated surgery as "definitive" therapy for this condition. Medication such as terazosin HCl or doxazosin mesylate is now commonly prescribed first, one of the more popular being finasteride. These drugs are actually more dangerous substitutes for an herbal remedy (as at least half of all pharmaceuticals are). The classic herb pirated in this case is the saw palmetto berry.

Saw palmetto is a shrub that grows in Georgia and Florida. The leaves are palmlike and the stems are saw-toothed, hence the name. According to *The Herb Book* by Dr. John Lust, a teaspoon of the dark-colored berries is steeped in one cup of water, and that is taken once or twice daily. There are no side effects or contraindications listed. European studies have confirmed that saw palmetto berries are a statistically significant therapy for enlarged prostate. They are clearly a safer treatment, and cheaper as well.

Zinc deficiency results in prostate enlargement, and zinc supplementation can shrink enlarged prostate glands. Very few men obtain even the low RDA of 15 milligrams of zinc a day. Larger supplemental doses, commonly between 50 and 100 milligrams daily, may help shrink a swollen prostate. Toxicity of zinc is very low and side effects begin at about 500 milligrams daily, vastly more than any guy would ever need to take. (Even at that level, supplemental iron and copper alleviate the side effects.) How effective is zinc therapy? Researchers from Cook County Hospital studied over 5,000 patients and have confirmed that zinc prevents prostate enlargement.[3]

Vitamin C would almost certainly be of benefit to a person with an enlarged prostate as well. Infection would be avoided, and many men report that vitamin C makes urination easier.

Prostate Cancer: There is much that can be done to prevent prostate cancer, the second leading cancer killer of American men. Adequate zinc and abundant vitamin C both help to strengthen the body's immune system and prevent cancer. As mentioned above, optimum prostate health requires these nutrients in particular. Abram Hoffer, M.D., reports on a patient who had a prostate tumor that had spread to his pelvic bones. A cancer clinic had declared him untreatable. "He responded to the (meganutrient) regimen and died nine years later, at age 80 clear of cancer."[4]

There is no doubt whatsoever that diet has a major role in allowing—or inhibiting—prostate cancer. A study at the Harvard University School of Public Health indicated that you are 250 percent more likely to suffer from advanced prostate cancer if you eat red meat every day than if you eat red meat only once a week. The message is clear and generally ignored: Move your diet in the direction of vegetarianism.[5]

Prostate cancer is very slow growing. 146 Because of this, radical measures such as radiation or surgery are often reasonably postponed. This "watchful waiting," to see if surgery is truly needed, is advocated by an increasing number of doctors. Obviously, regular medical examination and follow-up is important. Although there is some question as to whether or not it actually saves lives, the prostate-specific antigen (PSA) blood test is one way to monitor the prostate's condition. The actual benefits of surgery and radiation therapy are statistically quite small. After ten years, only slightly more of the treated patients are still alive than those that did nothing at all.[6]

An especially good diet and appropriately generous use of supplements may positively influence the situation. It certainly cannot hurt to have lots of raw salad foods, sprouts, and fresh vegetable juices every day. Natural health research has continually emphasized these measures to help fight cancer. A particularly good example is the work of Max Gerson, M.D., whose diet I previously discussed. Dr. Gerson used a mostly raw food and fresh vegetable juice diet for cancer patients with remarkably good results. He also used substantial quantities of vitamin supplements.[7] More recently, eating a lot of lycopene-rich, fresh tomatoes has been shown to greatly reduce prostate cancer risk.[8] Even peanuts can help, as they contain phytosterols, particularly beta-sitosterol, which is protective against colon, breast, and prostate cancer.[9]

Soy products may yield a special benefit. Japanese men have especially low death rates from prostate cancer. Even though they get the disease as often as American men, Japanese men are only about one-fifth as likely to die from it. The Japanese eat a lot of tofu, tempeh, miso, soy milk, and other soy foods. Even animals fed a lot of soybeans have far less prostate cancer. There are at least two specific substances in soybeans that seem to help fight cancer: genistein and daidzein. These natural chemicals, called isoflavones, are especially effective against some hormone-dependent cancers, which includes prostate cancer.[10]

Psoriasis

Conventional medical thinking says that psoriasis has an unknown cause and no real cure. If the medical doctor's black bag is empty, that does not mean that there's nothing else to do. It means that it is now necessary to open Nature's nutritional knapsack. With psoriasis, there definitely are clues worth tracking down. The therapeutic use of fish oils, vegetable juice fasting, zinc, and vitamins do indeed offer hope for psoriasis.

Omega-3 Fish Oils—Psoriasis may be partly due to a difficulty in the way the body handles oils or to a lack of oils in the diet itself. Studies have shown that consuming an omega-3 fatty acid found in fish called EPA (eicosapentaenoic acid) may provide symptom relief. Most vegetable oils that you eat are omega-6 fatty acids. The two most common omega-3 fatty acids in fish oil are EPA and DHA (docosahexaenoic acid). People who don't eat fish need to know that there is a third, vegetarian omega-3 called linolenic acid (not omega-6 linoleic acid). Linolenic acid is found in some vegetable oils, lecithin, nuts, and leafy green vegetables.

Linolenic acid is slowly converted into both DHA and EPA in the body. Could this be the problem that psoriasis patients have, namely, that they are slow to make this conversion? If so, the psoriasis patient probably needs fish in the diet to provide EPA ready-made. It is a sensible thing to do anyway. The Japanese have among the longest life expectancies of all the "Western-ized" cultures, and they eat a lot of fish. They also eat very little red meat. A way the omega-3 fatty acids might work is by actually getting into each cell membrane, making them more bendable, adaptable, and durable. Improved immune response is another benefit of fish oil consumption.

Oily fish (trout, mackerel, salmon) are the best sources and a little dab will do you. Nonoily fish (cod, flounder, haddock) are also worth having, but you would need to eat a bit more of them. Tuna packed in (omega-6 vegetable) oil does not count. Alternatively, you could eat a lot of leafy green vegetables, eat nuts more often, and take an EPA supplement. Around 300 to 1,000 milligrams of EPA daily is frequently recommended.

Vegetable Juice Fasting—Since vegetables, especially green ones, provide omega-3 linolenic acid, a diet fortified with quantities of fresh vegetable juice makes more sense than ever. You also avoid any worries about fish and water pollution. Grow your own veggies and you can avoid pesticides and other agricultural chemicals as well.

A diet of juiced vegetables may provide such an abundance of linolenic acid that it overcomes any bodily reluctance to metabolize it properly. I know of two people who tested this theory by going on periodic one-week juice fasts. Both individuals had been properly diagnosed with psoriasis by medical specialists. Over a period of weeks, both fully recovered. Since psoriasis often comes and goes anyway, the real significance is that each person has remained symptom free for many years now.

Vegetable juice fasting is not starvation. It is just a temporary diet of lots of liquefied salad. A lot of veggies go into the daily quart or two of juice that a person commonly drinks while fasting. That is not too much liquid; doctors often recommend four to eight glasses of water daily. And do not let anyone tell you that "it is too much vegetable" in the diet; you simply cannot hurt yourself with produce. The juices provide carbohydrates, minerals, vitamins, and more protein than you might think. It is certainly a low-fat diet; adding fish oil addresses that.

Zinc—Your skin contains one-fifth of your body's zinc supply. Rats and mice that are deficient in zinc develop a skin condition called keratogenesis that is very similar to human psoriasis.[1] Zinc deficiency in humans is the rule, not the exception. In spite of this, it is uncommon to find either dietitians or doctors recommending a supplement of this mineral.

Research has shown that supplements of zinc are safe up to about 600 milligrams daily. At that huge dose, over a period of weeks or months, a copper deficiency may develop. A more sensible daily dose of 50–100 milligrams may be maintained for as long as desired. A good multivitamin taken along with the zinc will provide some balancing copper. The "amino acid chelated" form of zinc is more easily tolerated and better absorbed than zinc sulfate or other inorganic forms of the mineral.

Vitamin Supplementation—The skin is your largest and most visible organ. It is therefore a good indicator of health in general and vitamin shortages are often indicated by skin problems. Clinical deficiencies of riboflavin (B2), niacin (B3), vitamin A, and vitamin C all result in skin problems that no drug will fix. At the very least, psoriasis patients should be urged to take a good multivitamin twice daily. Everyone knows that it can't hurt, but not everyone appreciates just how much it might help. Additional vitamin A is best taken as nontoxic carotene, which is in vegetable juices.

A B-complex supplement provides a balance of all B vitamins, thus ensuring safety. Vitamin C is also nontoxic, even in very large doses. Supplemental vitamin D also helps heal psoriasis.[2]

Respiratory Infections

Now here is a well-traveled highway: snif-fle—> slight cold—> bad cold—> pneumonia. Vitamin C can help stop this trip before it starts. The further you've gone down the path of sickness, the more vitamin C it will take to heal. The faster a locomotive is going, the more braking power it takes to stop it. Dr. Linus Pauling says to start taking multigram doses of vitamin C at the very first sniffle. I do; it works.

It is common for people to raise their eye-brows when many therapeutic claims are made for a single vitamin. "Vitamin C for colds, maybe. But pneumonia? C'mon!" The central thesis of megavitamin therapy may help explain it: *the reason one vitamin can heal so many conditions is that a deficiency of one vitamin can cause many conditions.* Disease is often the aggravated result of vitamin deficiency. If this seems to be too much emphasis on nutri-tion and not enough on microbes, remember that we live with viruses and bacteria all about us, all the time. Yet everyone is not sick all of the time. Differing nutritional status is at least as important a consideration as any other.

Vitamin C, for example, is good for so many illnesses that to the medical profession it seems too good to be true. What a nice problem to have: this substance is too useful. Of course, doctors use the same drug for any number of viral diseases. Their argument, and mine too, is that there is a virus that must be stopped. Antiviral drugs try to kill viruses like an A-bomb; vitamin C works through the body's immune system like the French Resistance. You can fight the war either way you choose, but I'd rather avoid the fallout side effects from the drugs.

Colds and Flu

Vitamin C works exceptionally well as an antiviral, but only if you take enough. Enough is called "saturation" and is indicated by loose stools. Try taking vitamin C until saturation is reached. While symptoms persist, 20,000IU of vitamin A daily and a few grams of bioflavonoids (from fruits and vegetables, or supplements) will also help. When sick, I drink lots of carrot juice and don't need to take extra vitamin A. During illness, if you eat almost entirely fruits and vegetables, you won't need the bioflavonoid supplement either. The biggest difference you will find in treating influenza is that your saturation level of vitamin C will be higher (perhaps much higher) than with the common cold.

There is a trick to almost everything, and the trick to really sensational results with vitamin C is to use enough, and use it immediately. Dr. Pauling's advice still stands: At the very first sniffle, cough, or sneeze, take a big dose of vitamin C powder in water or juice. This is called a "loading dose." The intention is to promptly ingest as much vitamin C as you can without having loose bowels. Everyone, even kids, can learn what their particular level is.

Here is another technique to try, and it is also Dr. Pauling's: To help control a cold, try a topical application of sodium ascorbate (a buffered, nonacidic form of vitamin C) dissolved in water (3,000 milligrams of sodium ascorbate in about 2 ounces of water). Try introducing 20 drops of the solution into each nostril with an eyedropper. This might be more helpful because the local concentration of vitamin C is much more than is possible with oral administration.[1]

Bronchitis and Pneumonia

In May 2002, the journal Lancet published a study showing that azithromycin, an antibiotic commonly used against bronchitis, is no more effective than low-dose vitamin C in treating the condition.[2] Antibiotics in general seem ineffective against acute bronchitis. The medical supposition is that perhaps this is because bronchitis is a viral disease, not a bacterial one. To a megadose vitamin C user, such a distinction is academic. Orthomolecular physician Robert F. Cathcart, M.D., once said that disease names can be a waste of time. He prefers to classify illness by how much vitamin C it takes to cure them. Bronchitis, for example, might be a "60-gram (per day) cold"; pneumonia might then be a "120-gram cold."

Preventing is obviously easier than treating severe illness. Immediate use of large doses of vitamin C (2,000–3,000mg every half hour) up to saturation will usually stop a cold from escalating to pneumonia. But if it has become pneumonia, treat serious illness seriously: in the very young or the very old, pneumonia can kill; do not hesitate to seek medical attention.

And while you do, here is a second opinion. Dr. Cathcart advocates treating pneumonia with up to 200,000 milligrams of vitamin C daily, often intravenously (I.V.). You and I can simulate a 24-hour I.V. of vitamin C by taking it by mouth very, very often. When I had pneumonia, it took 2,000 milligrams of vitamin C every six minutes to get me to saturation. My oral daily dose was over 100,000 milligrams. Fever, cough, and other symptoms were reduced in hours; complete recovery took just a few days. Bronchitis clears up even faster. That is performance at least as good as any pharmaceutical, and the vitamin is both safer and cheaper.

Treating respiratory infections with massive amounts of vitamin C is not a new idea. Frederick R. Klenner, M.D., and William J. McCormick, M.D., used this approach successfully for decades beginning in the 1940s. People who think that vitamin C generally has merit, but that massive doses are ineffective or somehow harmful, would do well to read the original papers for themselves (see the Bibliography). Clinical evidence confirms the powerful antibiotic/antiviral effect of vitamin C when used in sufficient quantity.[3]

Vitamin C can be used alone or along with medicines if one chooses. Clearly prescription drugs are not up to the job; some 75,000 Americans die from pneumonia each year. There is no question that aggressive use of vitamin C would lower that figure a great deal. This applies to SARS (severe acute respiratory syndrome) as well.

Sinus Congestion

Before taking a decongestant for your stuffed-up sinuses, try the following natural alternatives.

- Watch your food intake. Stuffy, low-fiber foods like meat, white bread, and candy at least indirectly contribute to sinus congestion. Choral directors the world over know that dairy products are notoriously mucus-producing. The simple way to test this is to drop these items from your diet and see if you feel better and breathe easier.

- Added chemicals in food may cause stuffiness in some people. This means that avoiding artificial colors, artificial flavors, and preservatives might help you. Chemicals have no nutritive value anyway, so why not?

- Ayurvedic medicine (the traditional health care of India) recommends particular foods to ease your breathing, based on your Ayurvedic body type. Stuffy sinuses are likely a sign of a *kapha* imbalance, caused by eating too many heavy, pasty foods. The appropriate Ayurvedic response would be to drink more water and eat hot, spicy foods.

- My grandfather used to relieve congestion by breathing in the vapors from a jar of freshly opened horseradish. He also sprinkled cayenne pepper all over his soup. My daughter literally sips cayenne pepper sauce straight from the bottle if she gets stuffy. These instant remedies are found right in your own kitchen.

- Drink water and plenty of it. Liquids change mucus from a troublesome solid that makes breathing difficult into an easy-to-cough-up liquid.[1] Lots of water is good advice, but vegetable juice is even better. You can also get an appreciable amount of water from eating quantities of fresh fruit.

- Gentle facial massage may bring sinus relief, as may a hot, steamy shower.

- If you had to choose a conventional, over-the-counter decongestant, it would be "Vicks Vaporub" (or its generic equivalent). Think of it as an herbal remedy, because it is: a mixture of various plant extracts, including nutmeg, camphor, and eucalyptus oils. Most folks massage a bit into their neck or chest, but, as kids, my brothers and I used to put a dab in each nostril. The label directions do not recommend this, but we seem to have suffered no harm.

- The best natural health philosophy is one that treats causes rather than just symp-toms. For this reason, I maintain that peri-odic vegetable juice fasting is the overall best approach to clear sinuses. Sinus congestion is virtually nonexistent when you juice a lot and eat right.

Sore Muscles

An alcohol extract of two common flowers makes one of the best topical first-aid treatments for bumps, bruises, and muscle strains. Calendula *(Calendula officinalis)* is an annual, like a marigold, with a dense orange or yellow flower about the size and shape of a mum. Hypericum *(Hypericum perforatum)* is also called St. John's wort. It is a wild "weed" that may appear in your garden whether or not you expected it. The flowers are small, yellow, and star-shaped, attached to a leggy branching plant about one or two feet tall. You can grow or purchase these herbs. I pick mine when I walk paths in the country.

The only additional ingredient you require is alcohol as a solvent. Since you are making a liniment to put on the skin, it might be possible to use rubbing alcohol, but I do not recommend it. Isopropyl alcohol is poisonous. I suggest using brandy instead, just in case someone accidentally thought the tincture was to be taken internally. Brandy is around 40 percent alcohol, strong enough to extract the goodness of the flowers and to act as a preservative as well. (Gin and rum work, too.) Take perhaps half a cup of flowers, toss them into a small glass jar, add enough brandy to float them, and cover tightly. After about a week, strain off the flowers and pour the solution into dropper bottles. It keeps for years.

Whenever we pull a muscle, stub a toe, bump a corner, have a fall, or suffer any sports-type injury, out comes the "Hyper-Cal" mixture. (Serious injury, of course, requires more than just herbs; get all appropriate health care necessary.) You can also purchase these tinctures and health food stores, but it is hard to beat natural medicine from your own garden!

Sugar Craving

In some ways, sugar cravings resemble alcohol cravings: both are simple carbohydrates and both can be addressed nutritionally. A number of "sugar addicts" have people in their family that are addicted to other things. Perhaps they all have addictive personalities. Perhaps not. I assert that there is a nutritional way that, as one person put it, "might help me in my ongoing white-knuckled struggle as I hurry past the baked goods and candy."

Probably the most reliable and most powerful help for the sugar junkie is to diligently follow Dr. Roger J. William's nutritional program for alcoholism.[1] Large quantities of the B-complex vitamins are a cornerstone of such treatment. I suggest taking the entire B complex at least six times daily. Chromium, vitamin C, lecithin, the amino acid L-glutamine, and a vegetable-rich,high-fiber,complex-carbohydrate diet are also very important. Over the last decades, I have seen the following approach help many people:

- Vitamin C in quantity (10,000–20,000mg per day or more). High doses of vitamin C increase your body's production of mood-boosting epinephrine (adrenaline) and serotonin.

- Vitamin B complex, consisting of about 50 milligrams of each of the major B vitamins, six times daily. The B-complex vitamins work best in concert with each other. Frequent divided doses are the key to effective use of the B complex.
- L-Glutamine, 2,000–3,000 milligrams per day. This amino acid helps decrease physiological cravings for alcohol and may help some people with sugar cravings. It works best taken on an empty stomach.
- Lecithin, 2–4 tablespoons daily. This nutrient provides inositol and choline, which are related to the B-complex vitamins. Lecithin also helps improve glucose tolerance.
- Chromium, at least 200 micrograms to perhaps 400 micrograms of chromium polynicotinate daily. Chromium greatly improves carbohydrate metabolism and helps control blood sugar levels.
- A good high-potency multivitamin/mineral supplement, containing magnesium (400mg) and the antioxidants carotene and vitamin E (d-alpha-tocopherol).

Tobacco Addiction

Many people are familiar with this prayer: "Give me strength to change the things I can, the serenity to accept the things I can't, and the wisdom to know the difference." Well, smoking is something we can take personal control over. Stop smoking now. Nag someone you love to stop smoking. Do whatever it takes to save their life, or yours. Besides, nine out of ten smokers say they'd like to quit, and nine out of ten who do quit used no special technique at all: they just stopped doing it.

While the "cold turkey" method can and does work, quitting is much easier if vitamin C is sprayed onto the back of the throat each time you want a cigarette. You can make your own vitamin C spray, fresh, every day. Using plain ascorbic acid crystals or powder (available from any health food store), dissolve as much as you can in an ounce or two of water. There is no specific measurement to make; just mix as much of the powdered vitamin C as will dissolve. It's just that simple. Buy a spray bottle at your local discount store.

Be sure to spray the back of your throat any time you crave a smoke. This not only helps you stop smoking, it also helps control hunger cravings and reduce nicotine-withdrawal weight gain. This technique was demonstrated effective in a randomized, controlled scientific study.[1]

Stress reduction also helps you kick the cigarette habit. Studies have demonstrated that meditation can be particularly helpful in overcoming addictions.[2]

Years ago, a national advice columnist published a reader's letter claiming that eating a pinch of tobacco before smoking a cigarette reduced the amount of smoking a person did. Maybe it was the yucky taste. Or perhaps it was the principle of homeopathy, which may be colloquially explained as "the hair of the dog that bit you." *Tobaccum* 6X, a harmless microdilution of tobacco, might be a more gum-friendly way to explore this idea.[3]

Remember: tobacco is the world's most dangerous weapon of mass destruction. The greatest cause of disease and death in every developed country is tobacco addiction. "The World Health Organization estimates that tobacco addiction kills 5 million people worldwide each year, including more than 400,000 Americans."[4] Diabetes is nearly twice as likely to develop in men and women who smoke.[5] And everyone knows that smoking causes cancer.

So, stop smoking—advice that can save over 400,000 lives a year is good advice indeed. Please take it.

Tooth Care

Here are a number of natural ways to keep smiling:

• Eat less sugar. All nutritionists and dentists agree that sugar promotes tooth decay, yet Americans consume over 120 pounds of sugar per person annually. Sugar contains no vitamins, no minerals, and no fiber. Decay-promoting bacteria love sugar, so starve them.

• Clean between your teeth. Use dental floss or those easy-to-use, plaque-removing, inter-dental cleaning sticks.

• Take extra vitamin C. Tooth health is dependent on gum health, and gum health is more closely related to vitamin C than to any other nutrient. The first symptom of scurvy is easily bleeding gums.

• Finish meals the way people did in past centuries—with cheese. Cheese inhibits bacterial growth in the mouth. Mozzarella, Monterey Jack, Swiss, and aged cheddar cheeses are all good for this purpose.

• Eat organically grown foods, preferably from your own garden. Hereford, Texas, became famous during the 1940s as "The Town Without a Toothache." Why was there practically no dental disease in this town? Because there were lots of organic minerals in the soil and the foods grown in it. So, any teeth grown there were also better fed and stronger. The local dentist practically went broke.[1]

- Pregnant women especially need calcium and multiple-mineral supplements to enable their developing baby to form strong teeth before birth. These same mineral supplements help her to make milk for the baby's continued tooth and bone development after delivery.

- A baby's tooth enamel is constructed in the womb. Ameloblasts adequately form the enamel in the fetus only if mom gets enough vitamin A. Carotene is best because too much fish oil vitamin A can be potentially harmful during pregnancy. All green and orange vegetables, and of course, carrot juice are ideal. It is pretty difficult to harm mother or child with produce!

- A multivitamin is a good idea for everyone. Prenatal for mom, liquid for baby, chewable for little kids, and don't forget teenagers and grownups in general. Research continues to show, decade after decade, that Americans continue to eat meals that are deficient in several vitamins, not just one.

- Rethink fluoride. Fluoride is so toxic that only one milligram constitutes a prescription dose. In spite of this, the Environmental Protection Agency (EPA) allows up to this amount in a single glass of drinking water.

Virtually every country in Europe has stopped fluoridation. Studies have shown that fluoride confers little, if any, real benefit. Persons who have grown up with fluoridated water have, on the average, only half a filling less than people who did not drink fluoridated water.[2]

• It is true that fluoride naturally and properly occurs mostly in bones and teeth. In extremely small amounts, it contributes to their hardness. Excess fluoride may be excreted in the urine or retained in the body. Overdose is both well known and widespread. Fluoride overdose (fluorosis) is characterized by mottling of the tooth enamel. This overdose condition is so common in India and many other countries that they must operate fluoride-removal facilities for their drinking water. Artificial fluoridation of water has also caused fluorosis in the United States. Curiously, fluoridation of public water supplies is rarely seen as the rather imprecise mass medication program that it in fact is.[3]

The alleged decay-preventing properties of fluoride are not as clearly established by scientific means as fluoridationists would have you believe. And the *Physicians' Desk Reference* has listed adverse reactions to fluoride as low as one-quarter part per million. Numerous studies have demonstrated adverse effects to bone caused by fluoride at levels equivalent to that found in public water supplies.[4] In an age of fluoride toothpastes, fluoride mouthwashes, and even fluoridated children's vitamins, it is very difficult to justify the significant hazard of mandating still more fluoride in everyone's drinking water.

Urinary Tract Infection (UTI)

"What the hell is Cipro?" Larry asked. He had been asking me questions about the chronic urinary tract infections he'd had, off and on, since he returned from duty overseas.

"It's a particularly strong antibiotic," I answered. "Why?"

"My doctor has been treating me for this urinary tract infection for months now. He started with sulfa, then erythromycin, then another antibiotic or three."

Each time he took the medicines, he noticed less burning and the blood flecks went away, but only for a while. The symptoms kept coming back, so his doctor was going to put him on Cipro.

"What would you do if you had this kind of UTI?" he asked.

I told him I'd try bowel tolerance saturation of vitamin C along with vegetable juice fasting. Vitamin C and the nutrients in vegetables help strengthen the immune system. Both provide antioxidant and antitoxic activity. Carotenes in vegetables specifically help the cells lining the urinary tract to resist infection. Vegetable juices are easily absorbed, so the carotenes get where they will do the most good. Vitamin C strengthens the collagen that holds cells together, which also resists infection. And, at bowel tolerance levels, vitamin C has a strong antibiotic effect. Plus, excess vitamin C is excreted in the urine. That means a whole lot of vitamin C will be washing over the insides of the urethra where the infection is.

Larry stared back at me. He had his typically tolerant look on his face. We often agreed to disagree. I surmised that this was going to be one of those times. "I think I'm going to try the Cipro," Larry said, finally. "I've had it with this infection."

He called me up a couple of weeks later. The Cipro worked, he said. Then, less than two weeks after that, he stopped by again. "It's back, damn it," said Larry. "And what's worse, the doctor said that the next antibiotics he wants to try are so rough that they require hospitalization. There is no way I want to go into a hospital for this."

He was quiet for a moment. "Juicing, eh?" Larry said abruptly. "How much?"

"All you want and all you can hold." I told him the idea was to eat nothing except veggie juice, perhaps with some fruit to relieve the routine when it gets too monotonous. He had a juicer, so he was ready to give it a try. And I recommended vitamin C to bowel tolerance.

"You take enough to be symptom free, no matter what the amount might be. And the amount is likely to be pretty high. But you do not take so much as to cause loose bowels."

So, Larry went and juiced up a storm, drinking 20 ounces at a sitting, and he took his vitamin C too. He was on the phone again in no time. "Man, did that work!" he said. "No burning, no sign of blood, no discomfort, no nothing. And this, without an antibiotic, after all the other ones had tried and failed. That's pretty neat." I've talked to him many a time since, and he's still juicing, still taking some vitamin C every day, and still completely free of any urinary tract infection.

Weight, Excess

We tend to overeat and still be undernourished. One possible explanation is that we overeat because we *are* undernourished. Overeating is perhaps a natural craving that attempts to increase our vitamin intake. The problem is, the more we eat, the more vitamins we need to metabolize the food, specifically more of the B vitamins and more lipid-protective vitamin E. And the more we eat to try to get these nutrients, the more calories we take in, and the more we weigh.

The way out is to just get off that train. Dieters, take your vitamins. You need plenty of them every day and that means supplements. Obtaining vitamins helps you eat right. Underweight people who eat right will gain weight; heavy people who eat right will lose weight. Vitamin pills contain no calories. The foods most people eat contain calories and no vitamins. I think a lot of people overeat because their bodies are understandably craving vitamins and also craving the good fats, the essential fatty acids (linolenic and linoleic acids). You can meet both cravings without blimping out.

Eat a tablespoon of lecithin (granulated, in milk or juice) about an hour before every meal.

Lecithin in quantity is a very good diet aid: It kills your appetite while giving your body the two essential fatty acids it is really looking for. Also, take a good multivitamin twice daily.

I'll let you in on a secret: The real trick to successful dieting is to never be hungry. If you are hungry, you are doing it wrong. I think far too many dieters are either down and dehydrated, crazy carnivores, or angry martyrs.

Diet Mistake Number 1: Down & Dehydrated —Drink lots of water, the colder the better. Your body has to burn calories in order to raise cold water to body temperature. Plus, drinking more water means you will eat less food. It will help fill your tummy with zero calories, cut your appetite, and it costs nothing.

And while you have that glass of water in your hand, take some vitamin C. One big reason people eat is to improve their mood. Vitamin C, a natural antidepressant, helps do this too. High doses of vitamin C promote the formation of epinephrine, or adrenaline. In fact, the body's primary reserves of vitamin C are found in the adrenal glands, and vitamin C is a specific treatment for adrenal exhaustion. You take more C and you feel peppier. Just you try it: take substantial vitamin C doses regularly throughout the day and see how well it works as an appetite suppressant. In four weeks, I lost nearly 20 pounds this way.

Diet Mistake Number 2: Crazy Carnivorism—Most meats contain a big slug of fat. Even lean meat is made up of 10 percent to 20 percent fat, and it has no fiber. You need protein, but you do not necessarily need to kill a critter to get it. Eat nuts instead. You will hear people say the opposite, but the truth is that nuts are a very good diet food. They are satisfying, crunchy, and have excellent mouth feel. Nuts are also incredibly filling if you eat them slowly and chew them well. Buy the good ones at the health food store: nothing stale, no salt, no oil, no tooth-rotting "honey roasting." Eating nuts will help you have the willpower to leave the meats and many other "fat-foods" alone. Nuts are high in the amino acid tryptophan, which your body makes into mood-elevating serotonin with a little help from vitamins C and B6. For people who "eat for the wrong reasons," who eat out of loneliness, despondency, or despair, nuts are a perfect answer. Peanuts and cashews are especially rich in tryptophan.

Diet Mistake Number 3: Angry Martyrdom—It's not what you eat, but what you eat a lot of that matters in trying to lose excess weight. So, don't have a tasteless diet! Eat all the salads and all the fruit you want. Raw-food vegetarians eat themselves slim. Want to cook the vegetables? Go ahead: cooking does not increase the calories in a food, but it does compact the food and you may eat more of it. A really big bowl of greens will cook down into a very small portion. Still, it's far better for you than the meat-mad, fat-frenzied, carbo-crazy way most people eat. Raw vegetarian foods are low calorie and delicious, and you can eat until you are full, really truly full, at every single meal.

If you do not want to go for the "full monty" of a raw food, vegetarian diet, then just do a regular no-junk-food, meatless diet and load up on foods that really do need cooking: the legumes. Peas, beans, and lentils are high in fiber, cheap, and filling. They are also high in the dieter's friend, tryptophan, the feel-good amino acid.

Be sure to eat squash, too. People who complain that vegetarian eating does not satisfy their hunger are doing it wrong. Follow the ways of the Native Americans and always invite all of the "Three Sisters" to your dinner table: grains, legumes, and squash. If you eat a lot of just one or two parts of this triad, you will likely still have the after-dinner munchies. When you have roughly equal servings of grains, beans, and squash at each meal, you prepare yourself for entry into a whole different between-meal world: a world in which you are happy and the cravings are gone. And I mean *gone!*

Other Ways to Help You Lose Weight

- Try fasting. Unless you have a limiting medical condition, you do not need food every day. If you are overweight, you do not even need food every week. Fat is stored food, so use it up! Make your body go to your fat reserves and burn 'em, by simply not eating. Drink lots of vegetable juices for fluids and electrolytes (minerals) and for some carbohydrates. The carbohydrates prevent ketosis and spare protein. You will gain energy, and you will lose fat, but not muscle. While fasting, take lots of vitamin C (buffered with calcium as needed), drink lots of water alternating with veggie juice or watered-down fruit juice, and take a multivitamin several times daily.
- Chemical energy is stored in chemical bonds, and there are a lot of chemical bonds in fat. So, if you are overweight, you contain a lot of stored-up energy. So go and expend it! The only way to lose weight is to burn more calories than you take in. This means either eat fewer calories or exercise more. Preferably both.

- Remember: You cannot get fat on a mostly raw food diet. This means you can eat all of the raw veggies, sprouts, salads, and fruits that you want. An easy way to lose weight even if you don't want to become a raw food vegetarian is to become a regular vegetarian. Drop meat and you drop weight.

- Another easy way to slim down: simply skip desserts. Instead, end your meal with fruit, especially dried fruits. Yes, they do contain sugar, but no fat. Just try eating two handfuls of raisins or dates—it is hard to do, because the natural mix of sugars, minerals, and fiber in fruit has a self-limiting effect on the appetite.

- Sweeten with dates, raisins, honey, or molasses. Again, these are sugar sources but you simply cannot eat a lot of them.

- Want to control your appetite without even giving up dessert? Adopt the motto of a perky eighty-four-year-old friend of ours: "Life is short: eat dessert first." Seriously, if you eat a bit of sweet food about fifteen minutes before your meal, you will eat less at the meal. This is at least partly because appetite is linked to blood sugar levels. Do you remember what your mother said? "Don't eat that candy now; it will spoil your appetite." Exactly!

- Yoga stretches are one of the best forms of exercise. The basic postures of yoga are described in many good books available on the subject. Yoga classes are inexpensive; check your local school or community center for a beginner's course. I learned yoga on board ship in the middle of the Pacific Ocean. That was over thirty years ago. I still remember the voyage, and I still do the yoga.

- Walking is probably the greatest exercise of all. Did you know that a mile of walking burns just about as many calories as a mile of running? And walking is easier on your knees and ankles. I love to walk. Get yourself a cool pair of sneakers and a dog, and you will too.

- Good weight loss need only be 1, perhaps 2, pounds per week. Crash diets often crash right back, with weight gained almost as quickly as it was shed. Take your time. Even allowing for a two-week vacation, a pound lost each week is 50 pounds a year.

- You've seen those weight-loss powders and liquid meals. How would you like to make your own? Combine 2 tablespoons of lecithin granules (a fat-transporting substance), 1/2 teaspoon of vitamin C powder, and 1 teaspoon of calcium-magnesium powder with your favorite sweet fruit juice.

Stir it well and drink. I usually follow it with a "chaser" of some more fruit juice. To improve the value, you can add 1 teaspoon of nutritional yeast for the B vitamins. Alternatively, you could take a B-complex supplement. I always take a multivitamin and 800IU of natural vitamin E along with the mixture.

Commonsense caution: Weight loss is not for anyone who is pregnant or nursing, nor is it for growing children, unless you are advised by a doctor to do so.

Yeast Infections

Some people think that to avoid yeast infections, you should avoid yeast. This sounds almost plausible until you think about it. Many yeast infections are caused by one particular species, *Candida albicans.* These fungal critters, which are found in any healthy body, are normally kept in balance by your resident flora of "good" bacteria and other microorganisms. But a depleted immune system, stress, poor nutrition, and especially antibiotic use, can bring on a *Candida* overgrowth.

You do not cook with *Candida* when you bake bread and you do not eat *Candida* when you eat cheese. And your body is quite happy digesting brewer's and nutritional yeasts, which are loaded with B vitamins and trace minerals. The problem isn't yeast from the diet but an unbalanced overgrowth of a microorganism that is already in you.

Therefore, an internal ecological approach makes sense. For the various forms of yeast infection, I first recommend vegetable juicing and a near-vegetarian diet, including plenty of unsweetened yogurt. This helps get the body's entire microbe population back into balance. Eliminating sugar is an absolute must. *Candida* love sugar, so starve them. In addition, to help bring prompt symptomatic relief, I suggest mega-doses of vitamin C to bowel tolerance (saturation). Used in sufficient quantity, I think it is superior to nystatin, imidazoles, or any other pharmaceutical you may be offered.

Oral Thrush (Candidiasis or Moniliasis)

Direct application of vitamin C is an effective antifungal treatment. Due to where thrush is commonly found, and to the fact that ascorbic acid is acidic, it is recommended that for topical use you select calcium ascorbate, sodium ascorbate, or any other nonacidic form of vitamin C. Adding a few drops of water to 1/2 teaspoon of buffered vitamin C powder makes a paste that will adhere to the skin when applied with a cotton swab. Another method is to make a vitamin C spray, using additional water and a sprayer bottle from your local discount store.

Homeopaths frequently recommend *Borax,* 3X or 6X, for thrush.

Vaginal Thrush (Candidiasis or Moniliasis)

Some women have effectively employed ascorbic acid vitamin C tablets (250mg) twice daily as vaginal inserts. Acidophilus, found in supplements or yogurt, is also very helpful. Getting a medical opinion before you self-treat makes common sense.

Fire Your Doctor! Health Truths

Of all the recommendations I've made to people in the past thirty years, it is these three axioms that have helped the most. If you have any health condition and have not yet tried these options, you may be suffering unnecessarily.

1. If you are not already familiar with "saturation" (bowel tolerance) of vitamin C, this is a good time to learn. Remember what Frederick R. Klenner, M.D., said: "I have never seen a patient that vitamin C would not benefit."

2. If you smoke, drink alcohol, crave caffeine, pig out on sugar, or eat meat or junk food, stop.

3. A near-vegetarian diet and juice fasting are tried-and-true therapies that heal and energize all parts of the body. If you have not tried them, you are volunteering to be sick.

Remember: If you are not a health nut, then what kind of a nut are you?

Quick Reference Guide to Additional Health Conditions

I am neither smart enough, nor are your arms strong enough, to pack all health knowledge of all topics into one volume. I know that when you, like me, peruse a self-care book, you are likely to be on special lookout for the ailments closest to home. So, in this section there are some very brief therapeutic options for an encore assortment of health problems.

While there is no such thing as a simple "magic bullet," the following "too simple to work" natural approaches can make a big difference and are worth a full and fair trial. Common-sense caution: Bear in mind that I am not a physician, and that these are opinions to weigh and alternatives to consider. There is rarely a short answer to any illness, and no one should think that what follows is anything close to the whole story. But perhaps it will motivate your further inquiry.

ADRENAL EXHAUSTION

Saturation of vitamin C is specific for this condition. Along with the eyes and spinal fluid, the adrenal glands are the major storehouse of vitamin C in your body. Megadose vitamin C may be worth an adjunctive therapeutic trial for those with Addison's disease.

ALOPECIA

Genetic factors aside, zinc deficiency is known to cause alopecia (hair loss) in animals. I think vitamin E and the essential fatty acids linoleic and linolenic acid are also important. Years ago, I stopped my own hair from thinning by taking lecithin, high doses of B complex, and zinc. It is still so thick that it pulls back at me when I comb it.

ANOREXIA NERVOSA

Much has been said on this subject, but rarely this: Zinc deficiency is known to depress appetite. Even more important: Intravenous multivitamins in quantity will do much to keep a hospitalized anorexic alive, buying time and improving recovery. I think niacin therapy is worth trying to help the psychological aspects of this illness.

BLOODY NOSE

It's too little vitamin C that's the problem. A bloody nose is an early sign of juvenile scurvy. Vitamin C deficiency causes spontaneous blood vessel leakage. Give your child lots of vitamin C and you will use up fewer tissues and wash fewer pillowcases. A daily dose of 500 milligrams of vitamin C per year of age is a good "rule of nose." Divide the dosage all through the day, amid meals and snacks.

BURNS

First aid for burns is immediate application of cold. Topical vitamin E, right from the capsule, and aloe gel squeezed directly from the plant's leaves also work very well.

First Degree Burns (redness, no blisters): At bedtime and again in the morning, gently rub in liberal amounts of vitamin E mixed with a teaspoonful of olive oil to help it spread.

Second Degree Burns (blisters): For this type of burn, forget the olive oil and apply concentrated vitamin E directly, gently, and frequently.

Third Degree Burns (damaged skin; skin missing): Drip vitamin E on the wound straight from the capsules and you do not have to touch the burned area at all. Risk of infection and need for skin grafting will be dramatically reduced. Be smart and get medical attention for any serious burn.

CONJUNCTIVITIS ("PINKEYE")

A twenty-two-year-old, contact-lens-wearing young woman with a history of occasional conjunctivitis had a recent flare-up, most noticeable by evening. There was considerable redness, discharge, swelling, and itching. She decided to try an alternative to her usual doctor-prescribed antibiotic eyedrops. The alternative was high-dose oral vitamin C therapy, beginning with a whopping 8,000 milligrams at 10p.m. The next morning, she took an initial dose of 4,000 milligrams at about 7a.m.; another 4,000 milligrams at 9a.m.; then 2,000 milligrams about every fifteen minutes until she reached bowel tolerance or "saturation." At this point, that took only about two more hours. She then cut back on the vitamin C but kept taking as much as she could hold, without actually having diarrhea, and her symptoms were gone by 4p.m. Total elapsed time to cure: eighteen hours, and she was asleep for half of that.

DANDRUFF

Here's a very common complaint with a very direct solution: Eat right, eat less, and try reducing your dairy intake. Persons with dandruff have found that if they reduce their consumption of milk products, their dandruff goes away. No medications, no special shampoos. I have seen this on my own scalp. More interestingly, I saw this with my dog.

Cobber (Australian for "buddy") was a scrawny, fourteen-week-old black-and-tan when he adopted me. He looked so skinny and pitiful that I simply had to come to his rescue. I fed him all the dog food he could eat, presoaked in raw milk and covered with raw cream from the farm. I topped this already mighty mixture with skim milk powder. The dog grew, in all directions, and he developed dandruff. I cut his feed in half, eliminated the dairy, and the dandruff went away. When I reintroduced the dairy foods, the dandruff came back. Once again, I stopped all milk products, and the dandruff went away again. The same works for people.

DIAPER RASH

Try topical vitamin E and dietary yogurt. Use less soap on your baby, and try the chemical free ones when you do use soap.

DRUG ADDICTION

Stress reduction substantially helps stop drug abuse.[1] Also, researchers have reported that patients previously receiving large doses of morphine or heroin exhibited virtually no withdrawal symptoms when also given high doses of vitamin C (10,000mg per day intravenously).[2]

EAR WAX

Trickle some vitamin E (squeezed from a capsule) into the ear canal. It works even better than the old home remedy, warm oil.

EPILEPSY (in Children)

Children using anti-epileptic medication demonstrate reduced blood levels of vitamin E, a sign of vitamin E deficiency. So, doctors at the University of Toronto gave epileptic children 400IU of natural vitamin E per day for several months, along with their medication. This combined treatment reduced the frequency of seizures in most of the children by over 60 percent; half of them "had a 90 to 100 percent reduction in seizures."[1]

ESOPHAGITIS

Drink cabbage juice, four glasses daily. Also helpful are aloe vera juice and nonacidic ("buffered") vitamin C.

EYE TWITCHES

A quartet of offbeat suggestions: Some people find that taking lecithin helps stop their twitches. Lecithin is rich in choline, which the body makes into the neurotransmitter acetylcholine. Or try the homeopathic remedy *Kali*

Phos 6X, available in health food stores. Also, regularly practice some form of stress reduction. Finally, knock off the caffeine.

FINGERNAIL SPOTS

What do those little white spots in the fingernails mean? Carl Pfeiffer, M.D., Ph.D., said that they commonly indicate zinc deficiency. I think he's right. As a young man I had those fingernail spots myself. Ever since I started taking 30–60 milligrams of zinc a day, they have vanished.

FOOD POISONING

Saturation (bowel tolerance) doses with vitamin C. An initial loading dose of one or two teaspoons (4,000–8,000mg), followed by 2,000 milligrams every half hour, is the right way to do it. Severe food poisoning, especially in children or the elderly, requires medical attention.

GLAUCOMA

Bowel tolerance (saturation) doses of vitamin C are absolutely mandatory for a therapeutic trial. Since the late 1960s, there have been a considerable number of scientific papers published on reducing intraocular pressure with high oral doses of vitamin C (over 30,000mg per day).[1]

GUMS, RECEDING

Calcium ascorbate, a nonacidic form of vitamin C, can be made into a paste with a little water and applied directly to the gums. I know a considerable number of people who have had receding gums greatly improve by using this trick. In at least one instance, scheduled gum surgery was canceled as a result.

HEPATITIS

George had chronic hepatitis B for seven years, and drugs weren't helping. "I haven't had many serious symptoms over the years except fatigue," he recounted. "My liver function tests and bilirubin counts remained elevated. Worse, the disease caused cirrhosis of my liver."

He had been treated on two occasions with prednisone, a steroid drug. Although this did improve his liver test results, the side effects were terrible and the tests elevated after he discontinued the drug. Then, when his tests again rose to an alarming level, his doctors told him there wasn't anything else they could do.

"It was at this time I became a health nut," says George. "I have been taking megadoses of vitamins faithfully and have concentrated on eating more fresh fruits and vegetables. I now take 25,000–30,000 milligrams of vitamin C a day; large amounts of B complex with B12; a mega-multivitamin; chelated magnesium; and vitamin E."

On his latest tests, George achieved the lowest level of bilirubin and the lowest liver function scores in over a year. And this without any prednisone. "My doctor is surprised and still skeptical about megavitamins," he says. "She says she can't condone what I'm doing—there's not enough "medical" research on it—but she does say I had better keep doing it."

George got these results in just nine weeks. I met him again more than ten years later. He was still taking "all those vitamins" and he was entirely symptom free.

LOSS OF TASTE AND SMELL

Try a zinc supplement, 25–50 milligrams daily, taken with a meal. Better yet, break the tablet in three pieces and take some with every meal. You'll get better absorption, and better results that way.

LYME DISEASE

If there were a one-word synonym for Lyme disease, it would be inflammation. Ascorbic acid (vitamin C) in quantity is the most powerful natural anti-inflammatory agent there is. At saturation (bowel tolerance) levels, ascorbate is therapeutically equivalent to, but is much safer than, antibiotics or corticosteroid drugs. Additionally, I have physician reports that the homeopathic remedy *Ledum,* in the 1M potency, greatly benefits persons with Lyme disease.

MEMORY LOSS

Take lecithin. Now write that down before you forget it.

MENSTRUAL CYCLE IRREGULARITY

This may sound like an offbeat idea, but here's what many of my adult students have reported help normalize periods: Try eating a few tablespoons of wheat germ daily. Put it on breakfast cereal or ice cream. Make sure the wheat germ is fresh or vacuum packed. I am not saying that this is the sure answer, but it surely is harmless to try. See a doctor if the problem persists.

MOLLUSCUM CONTAGIOSUM

I once saw a ten-year-old boy whose arms were seriously affected by this ailment. His parents then gave him saturation oral doses of vitamin C and applied vitamin C powder all over the pox-like, warty growths. The condition vanished in a matter of days. Now it is admittedly true that *Molluscum contagiosum* will go away on its own, but this typically takes months or years. The American Academy of Dermatology says that the illness, which is viral, is "more persistent in people with a weakened immune system." Exactly. Concentrated vitamin C is an antiviral without equal, and it is also the ticket to a strengthened immune system.

MONONUCLEOSIS

Mononucleosis is another one of those diseases that is generally believed to be hard to cure, but in fact is strikingly easy to cure. Saturation (bowel tolerance) levels of ascorbic acid (vitamin C) will obliterate the symptoms of mono in less than forty-eight hours. To a public that has been taught to view mono as a serious disease lasting six weeks to six months, this statement is the apex of medical heresy. It is too bad that so many physicians hold such strong opinions without ever having tried intensive vitamin C therapy. It works, and if you take enough, it works astonishingly fast.

MOTION SICKNESS (AIRSICKNESS)

For airsickness, try some in-flight *Kali Phos,* a homeopathic mineral preparation also known as a Schuessler cell salt. It is the greatest anti-nausea remedy on or off the Earth. When I learned to fly, I "decorated" many an aircraft: for you nonpilots, that means I puked during practically every flight lesson. When you vomit in a two-place trainer with a cabin about 36 inches wide, there is no room for decorum. So you push open the window, lean out, and let it go. It does not go far: a hundred-knot slipstream coupled with a cold aluminum fuselage ensures that your lunch instantly becomes a frozen mural on the airplane's side. This is somewhat humiliating to say the least. Ever since I've taken *Kali Phos* before (and perhaps during) a flight, I have not repeated the spectacle. *Kali Phos* is also great for kids and has no side effects. It is available at most health food stores. Try a 6X potency and see how well it works next time you take off.

NAUSEA

I'd suggest getting your neck checked by a chiropractor, as nausea may be caused by misaligned cervical vertebrae. Homeopathic remedies also help: for morning sickness, the homeopathic remedy *Natrum Phos* 6X is the first choice. For nausea from indigestion, stop eating what you have been eating, and juice fast instead. For nausea from nervous tension, you can't beat a regular practice of stress reduction.

NIGHTMARES

I think bad diet can equal bad dreams. Your brain gets the same nutrients, or garbage, as your stomach does. When in doubt, do not eat within three hours of bedtime. Regular exercise helps, too. I find that a mug of chamomile tea and 250 milligrams of niacin give me sweet dreams every time.

OBSESSIVE-COMPULSIVE DISORDER (OCD)

Take frequent oral doses of niacin in large quantity, plus vitamin C and the B-complex vitamins. Also important is adopting a caffeine-free, sugar-free, vegetarian diet. More heresy?

I take that as a compliment. Just try that niacin before you judge.

POSTPARTUM DEPRESSION

Try niacin, cashew nuts (for their tryptophan), and get a good babysitter.

POSTSURGICAL SWELLING

Swelling around an incision can be treated by topical vitamin E dropped onto the suture line. Physicians and hospitals cannot rationally object to this as long as you wait about five to seven days before application. This helps ensure that the wound has sufficiently closed. I recently saw this work rather dramatically in a case where there was a profound swelling (more like a large, hard, egglike lump) beneath a "dissolvable" sutured incision. The two-inch lump was greatly reduced overnight and gone in another day. Topical vitamin E also alleviates inflammation, itching, and that dry "pulling" feeling of a healing wound. Plus, it greatly reduces scarring.

ROSACEA

Doctors usually give antibiotics for roseacea. Saturation levels of vitamin C have a powerful antibiotic effect and it merits a therapeutic trial.

SCIATICA

Use saturation levels of vitamin C to reduce inflammation. Gentle stretching exercises, chiropractic care, and weight loss are extraordinarily helpful for sciatica relief. And if you haven't already done so, stop smoking.

SCLERODERMA

Scleroderma has responded favorably to long-term oral vitamin D (1,25-dihydroxychole-calciferol) therapy.[1] I also think changing to a high-vegetable and vegetable-juice diet would be worth trying. Good stuff from the garden might be more of an answer than you'd expect, and there is no down side to putting it to the test with scleroderma.

SLEEP DISORDERS

Instead of taking melatonin (a sleep hormone), make your own. Go to bed early and keep your bedroom dark, and your body will make plenty for you. Consider lining or doubling your curtains or drapes, adding blinds or a dark-colored window shade, and getting rid of brightly-lit digital clocks. Keep a nightlight on in your hallway for nighttime trips to the bathroom, but keep your bedroom door closed. These steps will keep your sleeping environment darker and your melatonin production will go up.

The "go to bed early" comment may be discounting some readers, who might say, "I can't go to bed early. There is too much to do." But if you are too busy to sleep, you are just too busy. Many people are sacrificing sleep for family time, TV, or work. In an age of cheap video recorders, the TV excuse can be easily dismissed without delay. Work pressures may be more difficult to deal with. I can hardly object to family time, but kids should not be up late either. An eight-grader needs ten to twelve hours of sleep a night, and even college students are supposed to get eight to ten hours a night. Well-rested kid(s) plus well-rested parent(s) has got to equal better quality time at home, and better school performance.

Afterword

Some day, health care without megavitamin therapy will be seen as we today see childbirth without sanitation or surgery without anesthetic. The natural healing alternatives to ever more medication may initially sound farfetched, but they all have one common characteristic: they work.

Unorthodox medicine, unpopular research, drugless healing, and especially megavitamin therapy have always been targets for criticism by allopathic, or drug-and-surgery, doctors. There's nothing wrong with disagreement in the health professions, because this keeps practitioners abreast of varied approaches to wellness. The problem starts when one school of treatment gains political power and creates biases, even in the laws of the land, against alternative modes of treatment. The American Medical Association has had this very opportunity. Although the A.M.A. now represents fewer than half of the physicians in the United States, it remains the strongest professional lobby in Washington and is a highly influential "union."

Leading-edge scientists, explorers, and "health nuts" have all had to struggle to demonstrate the truth of their theories.

Fortunately, they have done so with great success, and history bears them out. The laws are sometimes the last aspect of a country's rising consciousness to reflect change. For this reason, we must all "lobby" and call for health freedom.

If you read your state's Medical Practice Act (available at your public library), you may be amazed at the strong restrictions on "nonmedical" approaches to healing. Whether or not natural methods work typically is not considered relevant. Why? Because the issue is not health, but business. Medical practice laws protect the exclusiveness of the allopathic medical doctor from competition by rendering an outsider's practice illegal. Public health has precious little to do with it.

But alternatives work. They work so well that every year more than half of all Americans see nonmedical practitioners. But you have to make up your mind about that yourself, rather than having it made up by the medical politicians. Deciding, choosing, and verifying in your own life which health methods are truly life-supporting should be restricted by no law, doctor, or popular belief system.

THE AMERICAN HEALTH, UH, DISEASE CARE SYSTEM

There are fundamental problems with America's disease care system (we can call it this because it certainly is not a healthcare system). The quality of emergency care is superb, but what about chronic disease care, preventive medicine, nutrition, and wellness education? Delivery of these services is so pathetic that we are often better off without them. Here are some reasons:

1. **Financial Conflicts of Interest**—Doctors, hospitals, and pharmacies make the real money only when you are sick. The end result is obvious. Also, there is virtually no funding from pharmaceutical companies to support vitamin research. Why is that? Because there is no money for them in a cheap, nonprescription cure that already exists and cannot be patented.

2. **Government Out of Touch with the People**—Government may change the way it funds our failing "health" system, but the system itself continues on, fundamentally unchanged, with its drug-and-surgery orientation. Only voters can stop this.

3. **Avoidance of Individual Responsibility**—The elderly are the main users of the health system and are by far the chief

taxpayer-supported users. This age group is often strikingly resistant to diet and lifestyle change. What preventive health education the elderly are offered is as bland as a nursing home diet and just as useless. In addition, the poor are treated for diseases but not educated for health. Thus they stay dependent on dispensary-style medical "care." Real health demands long-term lifestyle changes for almost all Americans. Young or old, rich or poor, everyone has to move toward a nutrient-rich, low-sugar, near-vegetarian, chemical additive–free diet.

4. **Complacency and Misinformation from Health Professionals**—For decades, nutritionists and dietitians have preached that vitamin and mineral supplements are not needed if you just eat a balanced diet. It is a nice story, but it is only a story. Daily supplements are the only way that Americans can possibly get 800IU of vitamin E per day, the amount that prevents most cardiovascular disease. Daily supplements are the only way to get several thousand milligrams of vitamin C per day, the amount that is protective against many forms of cancer. Nutritional deficiency is the rule, not the exception, in the United States. It's simply not enough to keep

cholesterol and saturated fat *out* of your diet—you have to put something good *in.*

THE WAY OUT

Nobody likes a naysayer or prophet of doom, especially when the subject hits as close to home as health care. So, here's the way out:

1. Health care for every person requires that everyone take responsibility for their own health.
2. A country that manages to get tax forms to everyone can get a good daily multiple vitamin to everyone. Cost? Ten cents a day per person times 300 million Americans equals $30 million a day. Multiply that by 365 days in a year for a total of $11 billion annually. That is less than 1 percent of what we currently spend on health care each year in this country.
3. The government-promoted nutrient standards (RDAs and DRIs) must be raised significantly to truly be effective in preventing disease. Vitamin C should be increased by at least twenty times (from 60mg to 1,200mg daily); vitamin E should be increased by at least forty times (from a ridiculous 10–15IU to 400–600IU). This means supplements, so let's take them.
4. If you want to improve our nation's health, increase the tax on alcohol and cigarettes.

Two-thirds of all elderly hospital admissions are alcohol related. The single greatest cause of death is the cigarette. You may well object to paying for these habits with your taxes, but users are paying with their lives.

TAKE ACTION

When change is needed, the American people typically rise to the occasion, get out their pens, and write to their elected officials and to the press, and straighten them out. Here are some simple communication tactics that work well.

• **Writing to Congress:** When writing directly to your U.S. representative or senator, remember the "KISS" rule: Keep It Simple and Short. Important issues cannot wait, so please start writing today. Your library and the Internet have the local and Washington, D.C., addresses of all elected officials.

When writing, use regular postal mail and neatly handwrite your letter with a pen. Avoid form letters, e-mail, or petitions. They lack the impact of the personal, individual letter. Your letter does not have to be long, just to the point. Be sure to include your return address. Essentially, you could write as little as three sentences:

a) Identify what issue you are writing about.

b)   Briefly state your opinion.

c)   Ask for a written response.

Politeness always helps, but still press for a clear statement of their stand. Remember, you want a written answer. That creates a nice, quotable, permanent paper trail. That is why it is possible, even likely, that the elected official will not write back at all. If you don't receive a response within a couple of weeks or so, write again. Mention that you have already written once, and you want a reply! If you don't get a response this time, write to your local newspaper and tell them that your representative or senator does not seem to care about the public or about this issue. That will get you an impressively prompt response from virtually any elected official.

• **Writing to a Newspaper:** Make the issue hit home to move readers to action. For example, everyone is concerned about high taxes, their health, and their children. Show how their action, now, will help them, their families, and their pocketbook. What action? Have them do what you did: write! And be sure to say to whom they should write. Strengthen your letter with facts whenever you can. Provide testimony—how have you been affected by this issue? Remember that every letter, even if published by a small hometown advertiser or local paper, will be read by hundreds, or thousands, of people. Smaller newspapers especially are very willing to print your letters.

It has been said that no king with his scepter wields more power than an informed citizen holding a pen, and using it.

Select Bibliography

Balch, James F., and Phyllis A. Balch. *Prescription for Nutritional Healing,* 3rd ed. Garden City Park, NY: Avery, 2000. A fine presentation of specific therapeutic natural, nutritional procedures (protocols) for many illnesses, and it's authored by a nutritionist-physician team.

Cameron, Ewan, and Linus Pauling. *Cancer and Vitamin C* (revised ed.). Philadelphia: Camino Books, 1993. Cancer patients receiving intravenous vitamin C live on average five times longer than those who don't.

Carper, Jean. *Food: Your Miracle Medicine.* NewYork: HarperCollins, 1993. An easy-to-read, not-the-four-food-groups book that collects and summarizes recent nutritional research.

Chapman, J.B. *Dr Schuessler's Biochemistry.* London: New Era, 1973. The best short introduction to the subject of mineral homeopathy: Practical and cross-indexed for quick reference.

Cheraskin, E., and W.M. Ringsdorf. *Psychodietetics.* New York: Bantam, 1974. A classic book showing not only that we are what we eat, but that our behavior is strongly influenced by diet.

Cheraskin, E., W.M. Ringsdorf, and E.L. Sisley. *The Vitamin C Connection: Getting Well and Staying Well with Vitamin C.* New York: Harper and Row, 1983. Emanuel Cheraskin, M.D., and his coauthors have written an excellent guide to vitamin C therapy that thoroughly debunks many misconceptions about this enormously versatile, safe, and effective vitamin.

Chopra, Deepak. *Perfect Health.* New York: Harmony, 1991. A fine introduction to Ayurvedic medicine, written by a bestselling endocrinologist.

Clarke, John H. *The Prescriber* (9th Edition). Essex, England: C.W. Daniel, 1972. In this book, you can quickly look up any illness and obtain the homeopathic remedy for it, and its dose as well. Written by an M.D.

Cleave, T.L. *The Saccharine Disease.* New Canaan, CT: Keats, 1975. The first, and best, book showing that sugar causes chronic illness. Often criticized but never refuted. Written by a medical doctor.

Ford, M.W., S. Hillyard, and M.F. Koock. *The Deaf Smith Country Cookbook.* Lakewood, CO: Collier, 1973. My favorite, easy vegetarian cookbook.

Garrison, Robert H., Jr., and Elizabeth Somer. *The Nutrition Desk Reference* (2nd ed.). New Canaan, CT: Keats, 1990. A good single-volume summary of vitamins, minerals, and other nutrients. I used this as a textbook when I taught clinical nutrition to graduate students.

Gerson, Max. *A Cancer Therapy: Results of Fifty Cases* (3rd ed.). Del Mar, CA: Totality Books, 1977. First published in 1958; Gerson's successful case histories, and exhaustive details about the nutritional cancer protocol that cured his patients, is required reading for any family fighting cancer.

Gregory, Dick. *Dick Gregory's Natural Diet for Folks Who Eat: Cookin' With Mother Nature.* New York: Harper and Row, 1973. The best short introduction to nature-cure I've ever read, and it's funny, too. In 1970, I heard Dick Gregory speak, watched him juice, and was challenged by his raw foods message.

Hawkins, David, and Linus Pauling. *Orthomolecular Psychiatry.* San Francisco: W.H. Freeman, 1973. This textbook is a collection of technical papers, written by physicians for physicians, describing the science behind megavitamin therapy for schizophrenia and other mental illnesses.

Hoffer, Abram, and Morton Walker. *Orthomolecular Nutrition.* New Canaan, CT: Keats, 1978. One of the best introductions to vitamin therapy, expertly written and easy to understand.

485

Hoffer, Abram. *Vitamin B-3 and Schizophrenia: Discovery, Recovery, Controversy.* Kingston, Ontario, Canada: Quarry Press, 1998. Dr. Hoffer has successfully treated thousands of schizophrenic and psychotic patients for nearly half a century and he's seen that very sick people get well with megadoses of niacin.

Hoffer, Abram. *Dr. Hoffer's ABC of Natural Nutrition for Children.* Kingston, Ontario, Canada: Quarry Press, 1999. "Battered parents" of ADHD children need to know what to do, and *now.* Saying "no" to drugs also requires saying "yes" to something else. That something else is nutrition, properly employed, as Dr. Hoffer presents it.

Hoffer, Abram. *Vitamin C and Cancer: Discovery, Recovery, Controversy.* With Linus Pauling. Kingston, Ontario, Canada: Quarry Press, 1999. Dr. Hoffer offers well-researched, clinically tested, practical nutritional advice, plus dozens of documented case histories of vitamin-taking cancer patients who achieved significantly longer life, and vastly improved quality of life. I cannot imagine a more important and uplifting book for the family of a cancer patient.

Howell, Edward. *(Food) Enzymes for Health and Longevity.* Woodstock Valley, CT: Omangod Press, 1980. You'll have trouble finding this book, even with an interlibrary loan, but it is worth the effort. An amazing presentation of the value of raw food enzymes in the diet.

Illich, Ivan. *Medical Nemesis: The Expropriation of Health.* New York: Bantam, 1976. The first major criticism of the medical industry, heavily referenced and relentless.

Kulvinskas, Viktoras. *Survival into the 21st Century.* Wethersfield, CT: Omangod Press, 1975. This manual of sprouting is backed with a large number of medical references. Easily the most unusually illustrated book on sproutarianism ever written. You might pick it up for the Peter Max cover, but you stay for the information.

Levy, Thomas. E. *Vitamin C, Infectious Diseases, and Toxins: Curing the Incurable.* Philadelphia, PA: Xlibris Corporation, 2002. Vitamin C is the best broad-spectrum antibiotic, antihistamine, antitoxic, and antiviral substance there is. Over 1,200 scientific references are provided. Authored by a board-certified cardiologist.

Lilliston, Lynn. *Megavitamins.* New York: Fawcett, 1975. A short, handy, popular introduction.

Natural Hygiene Society (of America). *The Greatest Health Discovery.* Chicago: Natural Hygiene Press, 1972. Rare and very interesting book that tells the history of the whole foods, raw foods lifestyle in the United States. Yes, there were health nuts in the 1800s, and this is their story.

Passwater, Richard A. *Supernutrition.* New York: Pocket Books, 1975. A fine presentation on how and why to use vitamins and other nutritional supplements effectively. Practical and direct.

Pauling, Linus. *Vitamin C, the Common Cold, and the Flu.* New York: Freeman, 1976. Possibly the most influential popular health book ever written. Dr. Pauling rocked the medical boat with his scientifically substantiated thesis that megadoses of vitamin C prevent and cure colds and flu.

Pauling, Linus. *How to Live Longer and Feel Better.* New York: Freeman, 1986. Dr. Pauling presents a thorough case for megadoses of the various vitamins. He also answers his critics with facts from peer-reviewed scientific journals.

Price, Weston A. *Nutrition and Physical Degeneration.* La Mesa, CA: Price-Pottenger Foundation, 1945. A masterwork by a dentist who traveled the world studying the dentition of "primitive" peoples. His discovery? People who eat natural foods have beautiful choppers. Illustrated with photographs.

Shadman, Alonso J. *Who Is Your Doctor and Why?* New Canaan, CT: Keats, 1958. The story of a surgeon who, because he practiced homeopathy, hardly had to do any surgery. And when he did operate, Dr. Shadman never gave blood transfusions on the operating table.

Shames, Richard L., and Karilee H. Shames. *Thyroid Power.* New York: Harper Collins, 2001. A physician-authored guide with many specific, natural, useful, patient-friendly suggestions for hypothyroidism. The details of thyroid testing are explained better than in any other book I've seen.

Shute, Wilfrid E. *Vitamin E for Ailing and Healthy Hearts.* New York: Pyramid Books, 1969. Dr. Wilfrid Shute and his brother, Evan, were arguably the world's most experienced cardiologists, having treated tens of thousands of patients with vitamin E. As the risk of heart disease in America is double that of cancer, everyone would benefit greatly from this easy-to-understand and valuable book.

Shute, Wilfrid E. *Health Preserver: Defining the Versatility of Vitamin E.* Emmaus, PA: Rodale Press, 1977. Vitamin E is "too useful" for too many disease conditions? That's not what this physician says, showing how and why megadoses of the vitamin are so effective.

Shute, Wilfrid E. *Your Child and Vitamin E.* New Canaan, CT: Keats, 1979. Short and parent-friendly.

Sinclair, Upton. *The Jungle.* New York: New American Library, 1960. Classic work of social fiction based on a true and otherwise ignored story of filth in Chicago's meatpacking plants. The Pulitzer-Prize–winning author was a vegetarian, so you know it's going to be good.

Smith, Lendon H. *Clinical Guide to the Use of Vitamin C: The Clinical Experiences of Frederick R. Klenner, M.D.* Tacoma, WA: Life Sciences Press, 1991. Frederick Klenner spent nearly forty years successfully treating patients by administering enormous doses of vitamin C. "Vitamin C should be given to the patient while the doctors ponder the diagnosis," wrote Dr. Klenner. "I have never seen a patient that vitamin C would not benefit." [Also published as: *Vitamin C As a Fundamental Medicine: Abstracts of Dr. Frederick R. Klenner, M.D.'s Published and Unpublished Work* (1988).]

Stoll, Walt. *Saving Yourself from the Disease-Care Crisis.* Published by the author: 415 South Bonita Avenue, Second Floor, Panama City, FL324013963; www.askwaltstollmd.com. Physicians who used to teach at medical schools and then went full-time into natural healing are rare. But here's one, and his book is well written and right to the point.

Stone, Irwin. *The Healing Factor: Vitamin C against Disease.* New York: Grosset & Dunlap, 1972. Humans have inherited a genetic trait to need but not manufacture vitamin C. This book contains over fifty pages of scientific references, making it required reading for you and especially for your doctor. Topics covered include infections (bacterial and viral), allergies, asthma, eye diseases, ulcers, cancer, heart disease, diabetes, fractures, wounds, pregnancy complications, and glaucoma.

Straus, Howard. *Dr. Max Gerson: Healing the Hopeless.* Kingston, Ontario, Canada: Quarry Press, 2002. The hard-to-believe, but true, biography of Max Gerson, M.D., written by his grandson. The famous (some say infamous) originator of the vegetable juicing anticancer protocol may have been murdered.

Walford, Roy L. *Maximum Life Span.* New York: W.W. Norton, 1983. Can systematic underfeeding, plus nutritional supplements, increase longevity? A very entertaining and educational book, written by a physician specializing in gerontology.

Werbach, Melvyn, M.D., with Jeffrey Moss, D.D.S. *Textbook of Nutritional Medicine.* Tarzana, CA: Third Line Press, 1999. This book is a rarity among health books: at 750 pages, it is still remarkably concise. It takes only seconds to look up any of over eighty diseases that are known to respond to nutritional therapy. More than 5,600 references are provided. (Previously published as *Nutritional Influences on Illness.*)

Westlake, Aubrey T. *The Pattern of Health.* Berkeley, CA: Shambala/Random House, 1973. Here is the book that started my interest in natural healing. Long out of print, it is the wonderful, personal story of an English physician's search for medical truth.

Wigmore, Ann. *Recipes for Longer Life.* New York: Avery, 1980. "Raw foods cookbook" sounds a bit oxymoronic, but that's exactly what this is. You have never seen so many novel raw foods, salads, and salad dressing recipes in your life.

Williams, Roger J., and Dwight K. Kalita. *A Physician's Handbook on Orthomolecular Medicine.* New Canaan, CT: Keats, 1979. A veritable who's who of nutrition therapy, this excellent collection of papers on how high doses of vitamins cure disease has never gone out of date. Most highly recommended.

Internet Resources

What the printing press was to the sixteenth century, the Internet is to the twenty-first century: a free, open, mass exchange of information for every person. And that it truly is—a one-second Google search for "health" yields over 200,000,000 responses! So if the electronic "information highway" sometimes looms like an information landfill, well, just relax. Here are some of my favorite Internet sites for you to more easily begin your own personal search for wellness.

Orthomolecular (Nutritional) Medicine

The worldwide center for orthomolecular information, presented by Hugh D. Riordan, M.D., and colleagues: http://www.orthomolecular.org

Dr. Abram Hoffer's personal website discussing cancer is www.islandnet.com/~hoffer/

Dr. Hoffer's website discussing mental illness is www.islandnet.com/~hoffer/hofferhp.htm

The nutrition papers of vitamin discoverer Roger J. Williams, Ph.D., are available free of charge from www.cm.utexas.edu/williams

The authoritative source of megavitamin research papers, the *Journal of Orthomolecular Medicine:* www.orthomed.org

Read many articles from the *Journal of Orthomolecular Medicine* at: www.orthomed.org/jom/jom.htm or www.healthy.net/library/journals/ortho/index.html

A large and very fine noncommercial website focusing on preventing and reversing heart disease nutritionally: www.health-heart.org

The Townsend Letter for Doctors and Patients has many articles online at www.tldp.com

Dr. Harold Foster's website provides free downloads of his books on the nutritional control of AIDS, Alzheimer's disease, and on nutrition and schizophrenia: www.hdfoster.com

Jack Challem's *Nutrition Reporter,* an excellent therapeutic nutrition resource: www.thenutritionreporter.com/

Vitamin C

Read Linus Pauling's complete 1968 paper on megavitamin therapy atwww.orthomed.org/pauling2.htm

A 1974 Linus Pauling paper on the same subject is posted at www.orthomed.org/pauling.htm

Why and how Linus Pauling and colleagues believed that vitamin C and the amino acid lysine may prevent and cure atherosclerosis: www.internetwks.com/pauling/

Oregon State University's Linus Pauling Institute, a source of scholarly information on the safety and effectiveness of vitamin C and other nutrients: osu.orst.edu/dept/lpi/index.html

Dr. Robert F. Cathcart's papers on vitamin C as an antibiotic, antiviral, antihistamine, and more: www.orthomed.com

The Vitamin C Foundation is a great source of megavitamin information: www.vitamincfoundation.org/

C For Yourself is the type of site you search all over for; easy to use and very informative: www.cforyourself.com

Scott Roberts' very interesting site with a positive view on vitamins, especially vitamin C: heelspurs.com/cure.html

A large number of full-text papers on curing illness with vitamin C are posted at www.seanet.com/~alexs/ascorbate   This website contains classic papers by Drs. William J. McCormick, Frederick R. Klenner, Irwin Stone, Hugh D. Riordan, and other very important megavitamin researchers.

Nutrition, Foods and Food Additives

How being a "health nut" all started: www.bernarrmacfadden.com

A free, online library of organic gardening, natural farming, and nutrition: www.soilandhealth.org

Over five hundred natural hygiene links can be found at www.rawfoods.com

Paul Mason's references and full-text papers on magnesium can be found at www.mgwater.com

The pro-vegetarian Physicians' Committee for Responsible Medicine: www.pcrm.org

Improve your health and save cows from further abuse with a look at the exceptionally thorough www.notmilk.com

If you have the slightest concern about aspartame ("Nutrasweet") safety, see Dave Reitz's non-commercial information supersite: www.dorway.com

The nutrition research of Weston Price, D.D.S., and Francis Pottenger, M.D., can be found at www.health-and-healing.org/articles.html

More good articles on natural nutrition are at www.westonaprice.org

Alternative Medicine

A huge website of alternative health information: www.pnc.com.au/~cafmr/

Jonathan Chamberlain, author of *Fighting Cancer: A Survival Guide,* has posted his entire book for free public reading at www.fightingcancer.com/index.html

The Dr. Edward Bach flower remedies are a variant of both herbology and homeopathic medicine: www.bachcentre.com/

Fluoridation

If you have an interest in the medication added to your drinking water without your consent, you will want to see the following:

www.orgsites.com/ny/nyscof

www.fluoridenews.blogspot.com

www.fluoridealert.org

www.rvi.net/~fluoride/index.htm

www.inter-view.net/~sherrell/site_index.htm

www.garynull.com/issues/Fluoride/FluorideActionFile.htm

www.sonic.net/~kryptox/fluoride.htm

www.fluoride-journal.com/

www.fluoridation.com/

Current Issues in Natural Healing

John Hammell's clearinghouse for information about supplement restriction, alternative health regulation, and much more: www.iahf.com/index1.html

All concerned about the mercury in dental amalgam "silver" fillings should be sure to read vest.gu.se/~bosse/Mercury/Listings/mercburden.html

For articles on the downside of vaccination and genetic engineering, I recommend going to www.trufax.org/menu/bio.html

Well-written,well-referencedanti-vaccination websites include

www.909shot.com/ (National Vaccination Information Center)

www.vaccines.bizland.com/

www.vaccination.inoz.com/about.html

www.avn.org.au/

www.whale.to/vaccines.html

Endnotes

Preface

[1] Abram Hoffer, M.D., Ph.D., notes: "Occasionally niacin will increase darkening of the skin. This is due to the deposition of melaninlike pigments. With continuing niacin treatment, the darkening stops and leaves behind clean, normal skin. It is not dangerous at all, but has been confused with *Acanthosis nigricans,* which it is not."

[2] Abram Hoffer, M.D., Ph.D. notes: "Niacin is probably not quite as safe as water, but pretty close to it. Patients ask me, 'How dangerous is niacin therapy?' I answer them, 'You are going to live a lot longer. Is that a problem for you?' There have been no deaths ever from niacin. The LD 50 (the dosage that would kill half of those taking it) for dogs is 5,000 milligrams per kilogram body weight. That is equivalent to over half a pound of niacin per day for a 60kg human. No human takes 300,000 milligrams of niacin a day: they would be nauseous long before reaching a harmful dose. The top niacin dose ever was in a 16-year-old schizophrenic girl, who took 120 tablets (500mg each) in one day. That is 60,000mg of niacin. The 'voices' she had been

hearing were gone immediately. She then took 3,000mg a day to maintain wellness."

A Pep Talk to Get Started

[1] Saul, A.W. "Can Supplements Take the Place of a Bad Diet?" *Journal of Orthomolecular Medicine* 18:3-4(2003), 213-216; Saul, A.W. "Vitamin D: Deficiency, Diversity and Dosage." *Journal of Orthomolecular Medicine* 18:3–4(2003), 194–204.

[2] Classen, D.C., S.L. Pestotnik, R.S. Evans, et al. "Adverse Drug Events in Hospitalized Patients. Excess Length of Stay, Extra Costs, and Attributable Mortality." *JAMA* 277:4(1997), 301–306.

[3] If you wish to explore actual physician errors in prescribing, look at these important papers: Leape, L.L. "Error in Medicine." *JAMA* 272:23(1994), 1851–1857; Wears, R., and L.L. Leape. "Human Error in Emergency Medicine." *Ann Emerg Med* 34:3(1999), 370–372. (Comment on: *Ann Emerg Med* 34:3(1999), 373–383.) Leape, L.L. "Institute of Medicine Medical Error Figures Are Not Exaggerated." *JAMA* 284:1(2000), 95–97.

[4] Bates, D.W., N. Spell, D.J. Cullen, et al. "The Costs of Adverse Drug Events in Hospitalized Patients. Adverse Drug Events Prevention Study Group." *JAMA* 277:4(1997), 307–311.

[5] Cheraskin, E. "Healthcare: the fastest growing failing business." *Optimum Nutrition* 8:No2, 36–40. Autumn. Also see: Cheraskin, E. *Human Health and Homeostasis* (Birmingham, AL: Natural Reader Press, 1999).

[6] *The Truth About the Drug Companies* by Marcia Angell, M.D. (NY Random House, 2004)

[7] *Death By Modern Medicine* (The All About Book Series) by Dr. Carolyn Dean, M.D., with Trueman Tuck. 2005: Matrix Vérité. http://deathbymodernmedicine.com/

[8] Personal communication, reprinted in *Doctor Yourself Newsletter* 3:22-A (September 26, 2003) and posted at www.doctoryourself.com.

Educating Yourself

[1] From the Pittsburgh Health Club Newsletter (July 31, 1931).

[2] A very enjoyable and well-written book on this subject is *Detox Your World,* by Sharon "Shazzie" Holdstock (Cottenham, Cambridge, England: Rawcreation, 2003); web-site: www.rawcreation.com.

A Quick Start to Better Health

[1] Aubrey Sheiman. "Sugar and Dental Caries." *The Lancet* 8319 (1983), 282–284.

[2] "Aging Western Kidney" in: Williams, S.R. *Nutrition and Diet Therapy,* 7th ed. (St. Louis: Mosby, 1993), p.668. Reviews the following studies showing kidney damage from high-protein diets: Brenner, B.M., et al. "Dietary Protein Intake and the Progressive Nature of Kidney Disease." *NEJM* 307:11(1982), 652; Klahr, S., et al. "The Progression of Renal Disease." *NEJM* 318:25(1988), 657; Mitch, W.E., et al. *The Progressive Nature of Renal Disease* (New York: Churchill Livingston, 1986).

[3] Available on the Internet: www.nutrition.cornell.edu/ChinaProject/results.html. See also: Campbell, T.C., and J. Chen. "Diet and Chronic Degenerative Diseases: A Summary of Results from an Ecologic Study in Rural China." In: N.J. Temple, and D.P. Burkitt (eds.), *Western Diseases: Their Dietary Prevention and Reversibility* (Totowa, NJ: Humana Press, 1994), pp.67–118; Campbell, T.C., and J. Chen. "Diet and Chronic Degenerative Diseases: Perspectives from China." *Am J Clin Nutr* 59(1994), 1153S–1161S.

[4] Mathers, J.C. "Pulses and Carcinogenesis: Potential for the Prevention of Colon, Breast and Other Cancers." Br J Nutr 88:Suppl 3(2002), S273–S279.

[5] Orme-Johnson, D. "Medical Care Utilization and the Transcendental Meditation Program." *Psychosomatic Medicine* 49(1987),

502

493–507. Also: Heron, R.E., Hills, S.L., Mandarino, J.V., Orme-Johnson, D.W. Walton, K.G. "Reducing medical costs: the impact of Transcendental Meditation on government payments to physicians in Quebec." *American Journal of Health Promotion.* 1996;10:208–216.

[6] Padayatty, S.J., H. Sun, Y. Wang, et al. "Vitamin C Pharmacokinetics: Implications for Oral and Intravenous Use." *Ann Intern Med* 140:7(2004), 533–537; Gonzalez M.J., J.R. Miranda-Massari, E.M. Mora, et al. "Orthomolecular Oncology: A Mechanistic View of Intravenous Ascorbate's Chemotherapeutic Activity." *P R Health Sci J* 21:1(2002), 39–41. Riordan, N.H., H.D. Riordan, X. Meng, et al. "Intravenous Ascorbate as a Tumor Cytotoxic Chemotherapeutic Agent." *Med Hypotheses* 44:3(1995), 207–213.

[7] Levy, Thomas E., M.D., J.D. *Vitamin C, Infectious Diseases, and Toxins: Curing the Incurable* (Philadelphia: Xlibris Corporation, 2002), p. 36.

[8] Cathcart, R.F. "Vitamin C in the Treatment of Acquired Immune Deficiency Syndrome (AIDS)." *Med Hypotheses* 14(1984), 423–433. Also see: Cathcart, R.F. "Clinical Trial of Vitamin C." [Letter to the editor] *Med Tribune* (June 25, 1975); Cathcart, R.F. "The Method of Determining Proper Doses of Vitamin C for the Treatment of Disease by Titrating to Bowel Tolerance." *J*

Orthomolecular Psychiat 10 (1981), 125–132; Cathcart, R.F. "Titration to Bowel Tolerance, Anascorbemia, and Acute Induced Scurvy." *Med Hypotheses* 7(1981), 1359–1376; Cathcart, R.F. "Vitamin C, the Nontoxic, Nonrate-limited Antioxidant Free Radical Scavenger." *Med Hypotheses* 18(1985), 61–77; Cathcart, R.F. "The Vitamin C Treatment of Allergy and the Normally Unprimed State of Antibodies." *Med Hypotheses* 21(1986), 307–321; Cathcart, R.F. "A Unique Function for Ascorbate." *Med Hypotheses* 35 (1991), 32–37; Cathcart, R.F. "The Third Face of Vitamin C." *J Orthomolecular Med* 7(1993), 197–200.

Three Steps to Health

[1] Airola, P. *Health Secrets from Europe* (New York: Arco, 1972).

Go Meatless

[1] Sarasua, S., and D.A. Savitz. "Cured and Broiled Meat Consumption in Relation to Childhood Cancer: Denver, Colorado (United States)." *Cancer Causes Control* 5:2(1994), 141–148.

[2] Peters, J.M., S. Preston-Martin, S.J. London, et al. "Processed Meats and Risk of Childhood Leukemia (California, USA)." *Cancer Causes Control* 5:2(1994), 195–202.

[3] From Jean Carper's syndicated column in the Lancaster, PA, *Intelligencer-Journal* (June 22, 1994).

[4] Farrell, Warren, Ph.D. *The Myth of Male Power* (New York: Simon and Schuster, 1993), p.109.

[5] JAMA 176:9 (June 3, 1961), 806.

[6] See the Physicians Committee for Responsible Medicine website: www.pcrm.org/health/veginfo/vegetarian_foods.html.

[7] TBS Network program Earth (February 4, 1996).

[8] Price, Weston. *Nutrition and Physical Degeneration,* 15th ed. (New Canaan, CT: Keats, 2003), p.44.

[9] Ibid.

[10] www.fda.gov/fdac/features/895_vegdiet.html.

[11] Chen, J., T.C. Campbell, J. Li, et al. *Diet, Life-style and Mortality in China: A Study of the Characteristics of 65 Chinese Counties* (Oxford: Oxford University Press, 1991).

[12] Lappe, F.M., Joseph Collins, and Peter Rosset. Institute for Food and Development Policy. *World Hunger: Twelve Myths* (Berkeley, CA: Grove/Atlantic, 1998).

[13] Lyman, Howard F., with Glen Merzer. *Mad Cowboy: Plain Truth from the Cattle Rancher Who Won't Eat Meat* (New York: Scribner, 1998).

[14] Hussain, M., M. Banerjee, F.H. Sarkar, et al. "Soy Isoflavones in the Treatment of Prostate Cancer." *Nutr Cancer* 47:2(2003), 111–117; Harris, R.M., D.M. Wood, L. Bottomley, et al. "Phytoestrogens are Potent Inhibitors of Estrogen Sulfation: Implications for Breast Cancer Risk and Treatment." *J Clin Endocrinol Metab* 89:4(2004), 1779–1787; Yamamoto, S., T. Sobue, M. Kobayashi, et al. "Japan Public Health Center-Based Prospective Study on Cancer Cardiovascular Diseases Group. Soy, Isoflavones, and Breast Cancer Risk in Japan." *J Natl Cancer Inst* 95:12(2003), 906–913.

[15] Meyerowitz, S., M. Parman, and B. Robbins. *Sprouts The Miracle Food: The Complete Guide to Sprouting,* rev. ed. (Great Barrington, MA: Sproutman Publications, 1998); Wigmore, A. *The Sprouting Book* (New York: Avery Publishing, 1986).

[16] Hoffer, Abram, M.D., Ph.D. *Dr. Hoffer's ABC of Natural Nutrition for Children* (Kingston, Ontario: Quarry Press, 1999), p.91.

Tips for Healthier Eating

[1] Bansal, Sunita Pant. "Spirit of the Gandhian Diet." www.lifepositive.com/Body/holistic-recipes/recipes/gandhiandiet.asp.

[2] www.all-creatures.org/articles/ar-anag2003.html.

[3] *Dr. Julian Whitaker's Health & Healing* 8:10 (October 1998).

Juice Fasting

[1] Newman, C. "Why Are We So Fat?" *National Geographic* (August 2004), 46–61.

[2] There are over 106,000 deaths from pharmaceutical drugs each year in the United States, even when prescribed correctly and taken as prescribed. Leape, Lucian. "Error in Medicine." *JAMA* 272:23(1994), 1851. In addition, there are an estimated 150,000 more people killed by other aspects of medical care, including botched and unnecessary surgeries (12,000); hospital-caused infections (80,000); medication errors (7,000); and other medical mistakes (20,000). That makes a total of a staggering quarter-million deaths caused by the medical profession per year. This makes medical care one of the chief causes of death in the country. Starfield, B. *JAMA* 284(2000), 4. See also: Lazarou, J., B.H. Pomeranz, and P.N. Corey. "Incidence of Adverse Drug Reactions in Hospitalized Patients: A Meta-analysis of Prospective Studies." *JAMA* 279:15(1998), 1200–1205. "We estimated that in 1994 overall 2,216,000 (1,721,000–2,711,000) hospitalized patients had serious Adverse Drug Reactions and 106,000 (76,000–137,000) had fatal ADRs, making these reactions between the fourth and

sixth leading cause of death. The incidence of serious and fatal ADRs in U.S. hospitals was found to be extremely high."

[3] Cheney, G. "Vitamin U Therapy of Peptic Ulcer." *California Medicine* 77:4(1952), 248–252.; Cheney, G. "The Medical Management of Gastric Ulcers with Vitamin U Therapy." *Stanford Med Bull* 13:2(1955), 204–214; Cheney, G. "Vitamin U Concentrate Therapy of Peptic Ulcer." *Am J Gastroenterol* 21:3(1954), 230–250. Cheney, G. "The Nature of the Anti-peptic-ulcer Dietary Factor." *Stanford Med Bull* 8:3(1950), 144–161.

[4] Hara, M., et al. "Cruciferous Vegetables, Mushrooms, and Gastrointestinal Cancer Risks in a Multicenter, Hospital-based Case-control Study in Japan." *Nutr Cancer* 46:2(2003), 138–147.

[5] Jackson, S.J.T., and K.W. Singletary. "Sulforaphane Inhibits Human MCF-7 Mammary Cancer Cell Mitotic Progression and Tubulin Polymerization 1,2." *Nutr* 134(2004), 2229–2236.

Supplements and How to Use Them

[1] Lazarou, J., B.H. Pomeranz, and P.N. Corey. "Incidence of Adverse Drug Reactions in Hospitalized Patients: A Meta-analysis of

508

Prospective Studies." *JAMA* 279:15(1998), 1200–1205.

[2] Starfield, B. "Deficiencies in US Medical Care." *JAMA* 284:17(2000), 2184–2185. Starfield, B. "Is U.S. Health Really the Best in the World?" *JAMA* 284:4(2000), 483–485; See also: Leape, Lucian. "Error in Medicine." *JAMA* 272:23(1994), 1851; Leape, L.L. "Institute of Medicine Medical Error Figures Are Not Exaggerated." *JAMA* 284:1(2000), 95–97.

[3] American Association of Poison Control Centers' Toxic Exposure Surveillance System, 1998.

[4] Meyers, D.G., P.A. Maloley, and D. Weeks. "Safety of Antioxidant Vitamins." *Arch Intern Med* 156:9(1996), 925–935.

[5] Basu, S., B. Sengupta, and P.K. Paladhi. "Single Mega-dose Vitamin A Supplementation of Indian Mothers and Morbidity in Breastfed Young Infants." *Postgrad Med J* 79:933(2003), 397–402; Rahmathullah, L., J.M. Tielsch, R.D. Thulasiraj, et al. "Impact of Supplementing Newborn Infants with Vitamin A on Early Infant Mortality: Community Based Randomised Trial in Southern India." *BMJ* 327:7409(2003), 254.

[6] www.emedicine.com/emerg/topic638.htm.

[7] For more information on niacin, see: Hawkins, D., and L. Pauling. *Orthomolecular Psychiatry* (New York: Freeman, 1973). Here,

in one big volume, is more information than most doctors ever want to admit exists on using niacin, especially in treating schizophrenia and psychoses. Also: Hoffer, Abram. *Niacin Therapy in Psychiatry* (Springfield, IL: Charles Thomas, 1962); Hoffer, A., and H. Osmond. *The Chemical Basis of Clinical Psychiatry* (Springfield, IL: Charles Thomas, 1960). These books are what started it all; note the publishing dates.

[8] Brown, B.G., et al. "Simvastatin and Niacin, Antioxidant Vitamins, or the Combination for the Prevention of Coronary Disease." *NEJM* 345:22(2001), 1583–1592.

[9] Wynn, V. "Vitamins and Oral Contraceptive Use." *The Lancet* 1:7906(1975), 561–564.

[10] If you want to learn more about the therapeutic uses of vitamin C, try the following books: Linus Pauling, Ph.D. *How To Live Longer and Feel Better* (New York: Freeman, 1986); Stone, Irwin. *The Healing Factor: Vitamin C against Disease* (New York: Putnam, 1972); Cheraskin, Emanuel, M.D., et al. *The Vitamin C Connection* (New York: Harper and Row, 1983); Smith, Lendon H., M.D. *Clinical Guide to the Use of Vitamin C* (Tacoma, WA: Life Sciences Press, 1991); Levy, Thomas E., M.D., J.D. *Vitamin C, Infectious Diseases, and Toxins: Curing the Incurable* (Philadelphia: Xlibris Corporation, 2002); Hickey, Steven, and Hilary

510

Roberts. *Ascorbate: The Science of Vitamin C.* Available on the Internet: www.lulu.com.

[11] Murata, A., F. Morishige, and H. Yamaguchi. "Prolongation of Survival Times of Terminal Cancer Patients by Administration of Large Doses of Ascorbate." *Intl J Vitamin Nutr Res* 23: Suppl. (1982), 103–113; Also in: Hanck, A., ed., *Vitamin C: New Clinical Applications* (Bern: Huber, 1982), pp.103–113; Null, G., H. Robins, M. Tanenbaum, et al. "Vitamin C and the Treatment of Cancer: Abstracts and Commentary from the Scientific Literature." *Townsend Letter for Doctors and Patients* April/May (1997); Riordan, N.H., et al. "Intravenous Ascorbate as a Tumor Cytotoxic Chemotherapeutic Agent." *Med Hypotheses* 44:3(1995), 207–213.

[12] Enstrom, J.E., L.E. Kanim, and M.A. Klein. "Vitamin C Intake and Mortality among a Sample of the United States Population." *Epidemiology* 3:3(1992), 194–202.

[13] "In the large-scale Harvard Prospective Health Professional Follow-Up Study, those groups in the highest quintile of vitamin C intake (>1,500mg/day) had a lower risk of kidney stones than the groups in the lowest quintiles." Gerster, H. "No Contribution of Ascorbic Acid to Renal Calcium Oxalate Stones." *Ann Nutr Metab* 41:5(1997), 269–282;.

[14] Additional vitamin C safety references: O'Brien, J.E. *Vitamin C Really Does Slow Aging and Prevent Disease* (Boca Raton, FL: Globe Communications, 1993), p.13; Wright, J.V. *Dr. Wright's Guide to Healing with Nutrition* (Emmaus, PA: Rodale Press, 1984), p.76; Heinerman, J. *Dr. Heinerman's Encyclopedia of Nature's Vitamins and Minerals* (Paramus, NJ: Prentice Hall, 1998); Cheraskin, Emanuel, M.D., D.M.D. *Vitamin C: Who Needs It?* (Birmingham, AL: Arlington Press, 1993).

[15] Standing Committee on the Scientific Evaluation of Dietary Reference Intakes, Food and Nutrition Board, Institute of Medicine. *Dietary Reference Intakes for Calcium, Phosphorus, Magnesium, Vitamin D, and Fluoride* (Washington, D.C.: National Academies Press, 1999), Chapter 7.

[16] Vieth, R., P.C. Chan, and G.D. MacFarlane. "Efficacy and Safety of Vitamin D3 Intake Exceeding the Lowest Observed Adverse Effect Level." *Am J Clin Nutr* 73:2(2001), 288–294.

[17] Trivedi, D.P., R. Doll, and K.T. Khaw. "Effect of Four Monthly Oral Vitamin D3 (Cholecalciferol) Supplementation on Fractures and Mortality in Men and Women Living in the Community: Randomised Double-blind Controlled Trial." *BMJ* 326:7387(2003), 469.

[18] Maras, J.E., O.I. Bermudez, N. Qiao, et al. "Intake of Alpha-tocopherol Is Limited

among U.S. Adults." *J Am Diet Assoc* 104:4(2004), 567–575.

[19] Hutton, Eric. "The Fight over Vitamin E." *Maclean's Magazine* (June 15, 1953).

[20] Vivekananthan, D.P., M.S. Penn, S.K. Sapp, et al. "Use of Antioxidant Vitamins for the Prevention of Cardiovascular Disease: Meta-analysis of Randomised Trials." *The Lancet* 361(2003), 2017–2023.

[21] Vasdev, S., V. Gill, S. Parai, et al. "Dietary Vitamin E Supplementation Lowers Blood Pressure in Spontaneously Hypertensive Rats." *Mol Cell Biochem* 238:1–2(2002), 111–117; Vaziri, N.D., Z. Ni, F. Oveisi, et al. "Enhanced Nitric Oxide Inactivation and Protein Nitration by Reactive Oxygen Species in Renal Insufficiency." *Hypertension* 39:1(2002) 135–141; Galley, H.F., J. Thornton, P.D. Howdle, et al. "Combination Oral Antioxidant Supplementation Reduces Blood Pressure." *Clin Sci* (London) 92:4(1997), 361–365.

[22] Shute, E.V., Vogelsang, A.B., Skelton, F.B., Shute, W.E. *Surg Gyn Obst 86:1(1948).*

[23] Koo, J.R., Z. Ni, F. Oviesi, et al. "Antioxidant Therapy Potentiates Antihypertensive Action of Insulin in Diabetic Rats." *Clin Exp Hypertens* 24:5(2002), 333–344.

[24] Cheraskin, E. "Antioxidants in Health and Disease: The Big Picture." J Orthomol Med 10:2(1995), 89–96. Meydani, S.N., M.P. Bark-

lund, S. Liu, et al. "Effect of Vitamin E Supplementation on Immune Responsiveness of Healthy Elderly Subjects." *FASEB J* 3(1989), A1057.

[25] Malmberg, K.J., R. Lenkei, M. Petersson, et al. "A Short-term Dietary Supplementation of High Doses of Vitamin E Increases T Helper 1 Cytokine Production in Patients with Advanced Colorectal Cancer." *Clin Cancer Res* 8:6(2002), 1772–1778.

[26] Rosenberg, H., and A. N. Feldzamen. *The Book of Vitamin Therapy* (New York: Berkley Publishing, 1974).

[27] The Associated Press. "Vita-Mania: RDA for C, E Raised; Limits Set." (April 11, 2000). Available on the Internet: abcnews.go.com/sections/living/DailyNews/vitamin000411.html.

[28] Sano, M., C. Ernesto, R.G. Thomas, et al. "A Controlled Trial of Selegiline, Alpha-tocopherol, or Both as Treatment for Alzheimer's Disease. The Alzheimer's Disease Cooperative Study." *N Engl J Med* 336:17(1997), 1216–1222.

[29] Ogunmekan, A.O., and P.A. Hwang. "A Randomized, Double-blind, Placebo-controlled, Clinical Trial of D-alpha-tocopheryl Acetate (Vitamin E), as Add-on Therapy, for Epilepsy in Children." *Epilepsia* 30:1(1989), 84–89.

[30] www.stayinginshape.com/4union/libv/k09.shtml.

[31] For more detailed information on wheatgrass, consider reading the following books: Kulvinskas, Viktoras. *Survival into the 21st Century* (Wethersfield, CT: Omangod Press, 1975); Meyerowitz, S., M. Parman, and B. Robbins. *Sprouts The Miracle Food: The Complete Guide to Sprouting,* rev. ed. (Great Barrington, MA: Sproutman Publications, 1998); Wigmore, A. *The Sprouting Book* (New York: Avery Publishing, 1986); Wigmore, Ann. *Why Suffer?* (New York: Hemisphere Press, 1964); Wigmore, Ann. *Be Your Own Doctor* (Garden City Park, NY: Avery, 1983).

Discovering the Nature-Cure

[1] Natural Hygiene Society (of America). The Greatest Health Discovery (Natural Hygiene Press, 1972), p.55. Though out of print, your public library can get you a copy through interlibrary loan.

[2] Clara Barton Chapter No.1, founded 1881, is still located at 57 Elizabeth Street, Dansville, NY 14437 (dansville.lib.ny.us/clara.html).

[3] Oursler, F. "The Most Unforgettable Character I've Met." *Reader's Digest* (July 1951), 78–82. Posted at: www.riverflow.com/Macfadden/mucim.html.

[4] Ernst, R. *Weakness Is a Crime: The Life of Bernarr Macfadden* (Syracuse, NY: Syracuse University Press, 1991); Hunt, W.R. *Body Love: The Amazing Career of Bernarr Macfadden* (Bowling Green, OH: Popular Press, 1989).

[5] Gilbert, D. Dansville's "Castle on the Hill." Published by the Dansville Area Historical Society, 4 Church Street, Dansville, NY 14437. On the Internet: dansville.lib.ny.us/historyo.html.

[6] Bookman, R. "101 Hints, Tips and Bits of Wisdom from the President's Allergist: Timely Help for People with Allergies and Asthma." *Rodale's Allergy Relief* 3:7 (July 1988), 1–8. Posted at: healthandenergy.com/101_allergy_tips.htm. See also: Bookman, R. *The Dimensions of Clinical Allergy* (Springfield, IL: Charles C. Thomas, 1985).

[7] Bennett, J. Article is available on the Internet: www.bernarrMacfadden.com (the site also has an extensive bibliography of Bernarr Macfadden's books).

[8] Bennett, J. On the Internet: www.riverflow.com/Macfadden/atlas.html.

[9] Sinclair, U. *The Fasting Cure* (Whitefish, MT: Kessinger Publishing Company, 2003). First published in 1911.

[10] Walford, R.L. *Maximum Life Span* (New York: W.W. Norton, 1983). Reviewed at: www .doctoryourself.com/lifespan.html.

[11] Cott, A. *Fasting: The Ultimate Diet* (New York: Bantam, 1975); Cott, A. *Fasting As a Way of Life* (New York: Bantam, 1981).

[12] Burns, D., ed., *The Greatest Health Discovery: Natural Hygiene and Its Evolution, Past, Present and Future* (Chicago: Natural Hygiene Press, 1972), p.86.

[13] Portions of this chapter appeared as part of my "Taking the Cure" column in the *Journal of Orthomolecular Medicine,* 19:3(2004). Reprinted with permission.

PART II: Natural Healing Protocols for All-Too-Common Health Problems

Acne

[1] *Merck Manual of Diagnosis and Therapy* (Rahway, NJ: Merck, 2004), Section 1, Chapter 3.

AIDS

[1] Haney, D. "For lucky few, HIV simmers but never boils." *The Associated Press,* (February 13, 1994).

[2] Tang, A.M., N.M. Graham, A.J. Kirby, et al. "Dietary Micronutrient Intake and Risk of Progression to Acquired Immunodeficiency Syndrome (AIDS) in Human Immunodeficiency Virus Type 1 (HIV-1)-infected Homosexual Men." *Am J Epidemiol* 138:11(1993), 937–951.

[3] Fawzi, W.W., G.I. Msamanga, D. Spiegelman, et al. "A Randomized Trial of Multivitamin Supplements and HIV Disease Progression and Mortality." *N Engl J Med* 351:1(2004), 23–32.

[4] Cathcart, R.F. "Vitamin C in the Treatment of Acquired Immune Deficiency Syndrome (AIDS)." *Med Hypotheses* 14:4(1984), 423–433.

[5] Cathcart, R.F. "Vitamin C in the Treatment of Acquired Immune Deficiency Syndrome (AIDS)." *Med Hypotheses* 14:4(1984), 423–433; Cathcart, R.F. "Clinical Trial of Vitamin C." (Letter to the Editor.) *Medical Tribune* (June 25, 1975); Cathcart, R.F. "The Method of Determining Proper Doses of Vitamin C for the Treatment of Disease by Titrating to Bowel Tolerance." *J Orthomolecular Psychiatr* 10 (1981), 125–132; Cathcart, R.F. "Vitamin C: Titrating to Bowel Tolerance, Anascorbemia, and Acute Induced Scurvy." *Med Hypotheses* 7(1981), 1359–1376; Cathcart, R.F. "Vitamin C Function in AIDS. Current Opinion." *Medical Tribune* (July 13, 1983); Klenner, F.R. "Virus Pneumonia and Its Treatment with Vitamin C."

J South Med Surg 110(1948), 60–63; Klenner, F.R. "The Treatment of Poliomyelitis and Other Virus Diseases with Vitamin C." *J South Med Surg* 111 (1949), 210–214;. Klenner, F.R. "Massive Doses of Vitamin C and the Virus Diseases." *J South Med Surg* 113(1951), 101–107; Klenner, F.R. "Observations on the Dose and Administration of Ascorbic Acid When Employed Beyond the Range of a Vitamin in Human Pathology." *J App Nutr* 23(1971), 61–88; Murata, A. "Virucidal Activity of Vitamin C: Vitamin C for the Prevention and Treatment of Viral Diseases." *Proceedings of the First Intersectional Congress of Microbiological Societies, Science Council of Japan* 3(1975), 432–442; Cathcart, R.F. "Vitamin C Function in AIDS." *Bay Area Reporter* (Nov 17, 1983), 18; Cathcart, R.F. "Vitamin C Treatment Protocol for AIDS." *Bay Area Reporter* (Jan5, 1984), 14–15.

[6] Taylor, E.W. "Selenium and Viral Disease Facts and Hypotheses." *J Orthomolecular Med* 12(1997), 227–239.

[7] Foster, H.D. *What Really Causes AIDS?* (Victoria: Trafford Publishing, 2002). Also posted at: www.hdfoster.com and available for downloading.

Anxiety and Panic Attacks

[1] Smith, S., and C. Smith. *Personal Health Choices* (Boston: Jones and Bartlett, 1990), p.18.

[2] Holford, P., and S. Heaton. "Vitamin B6: Extract of Submission to the UK's Food Standards Agency." *J Orthomolecular Med* 18:3–4(2003), 161; Vos, E. "A Comment on Safe Upper Levels of Folic Acid, B6 and B12." *J Orthomolecular Med* 18:3–4(2003), 166.

[3] Hawkins, D., and L. Pauling. *Orthomolecular Psychiatry: Treatment of Schizophrenia* (New York: W.H. Freeman, 1973); Hoffer, A., and M. Walker. *Orthomolecular Nutrition* (New Canaan, CT: Keats, 1978).

[4] Whalen, R. "Caffeine Anaphylaxis: A Progressive Toxic Dementia." *J Orthomolecular Med* 18:1(2003), 25.

Arthritis

[1] Pottenger, F.M., Jr. *Pottenger's Cats* (Lemon Grove, CA: Price-Pottenger Nutrition Foundation, 1995).

[2] The benefits of a primarily raw food diet are discussed in: Kulvinskas, Viktoras. *Survival into the 21st Century* (Wethersfield, CT: Omangod Press, 1975); Wigmore, Ann. *Why Suffer?* (New York: Hemisphere Press,

1964); Wig-more, Ann. *Be Your Own Doctor* (Garden City Park, NY: Avery, 1983).

[3] Jonas, W.B., C.P. Rapoza, and W.F. Blair. "The Effect of Niacinamide in Osteoarthritis: A Pilot Study." *Inflamm Res* 45:7(1996), 330–334. Also, see the original study: Kaufman, W. *The Common Form of Joint Dysfunction: Its Incidence and Treatment* (Brattleboro, VT: E.L. Hildreth, 1949).

[4] Rivers, J.M. "Ascorbic Acid in Metabolism of Connective Tissue." *New York State Journal of Medicine* 65(1965), 1235–1238.

[5] Dr. Kaufman's detailed clinical experience treating arthritis with megadoses of niacinamide has been posted in its entirety at: www.doctoryourself.com. Special thanks are due to Mrs. Charlotte Kaufman for her kind permission in making this important work freely available to the public.

[6] Kaufman, William. "Niacinainide, A Most Neglected Vitamin." (1978 Tom Spies Memorial Lecture.) *J Intl Academy Preventive Med* 8(1983), 5–25.

[7] Kaufman, William. "The Use of Vitamins to Reverse Certain Concomitants of Aging." *J Amer Geriat Society* 3(1955), 927–936.

[8] *Ellis, John M. Free of Pain* (Dallas: Southwest Publishing, 1983).

[9] Pauling, Linus. *How To Live Longer and Feel Better* (New York: Avon, 1996).

Behavior and Learning Disorders

[1] Ray, O.S., and C. Ksir. *Drugs, Society and Human Behavior,* 5th ed. (St. Louis: Mosby, 1990), 121.

[2] *The Massachusetts News.* Holliston, MA (November 1, 1999).

[3] Reprinted with the kind permission of Charlotte Kaufman from: Kaufman, William. M.D., Ph.D. *The Common Form of Joint Dysfunction,* 73–74.

[4] For more information, I highly recommend Hoffer, Abram, M.D., Ph.D. *Dr. Hoffer's ABC of Natural Nutrition for Children* (Kingston, Ontario: Quarry Press, 1999).

Bipolar Disorder
(Manic-Depressive Disorder)

[1] Cheraskin, E. "Antioxidants in Health and Disease." *J Orthomolecular Med* 10:2(1995), 89–96.

[2] Hoffer, A. Megavitamin therapy for psychosis. (2000) www.doctoryourself.com/hoffer _psychosis.html.

[3] For further reading and additional scientific studies: Whalen, R. Welcome to the Dance: Caffeine Allergy, A Masked Cerebral Allergy and Progressive Toxic Dementia (In press); Werbach, M. Nutritional Influences on Illness (New

Canaan, CT: Keats, 1988), 85–91; Werbach, M., M.D., with Jeffrey Moss, D.D.S. Textbook of Nutritional Medicine (Tarzana, CA: Third Line Press, 1999), pp.174–179.

Caffeine Addiction

[1] Jacobson, M.F. "Liquid Candy: How Soft Drinks Are Harming Americans' Health." In: Center for Science in the Public Interest. *Nutrition Action.* www.cspinet.org/sodapop/liquid_candy.htm.

[2] Carper, Jean. "Your Food Pharmacy." (June 15, 1994).

[3] Wilcox, A., C. Weinberg, and D. Baird. "Caffeinated Beverages and Decreased Fertility." *The Lancet* 1988 Dec24–31;2(8626–8627):1453–1456.

[4] Cheraskin, E., W.M. Ringsdorf Jr., A.T. Setyaadmadja, et al. "Effect of Caffeine versus Placebo Supplementation on Blood-glucose Concentration." *The Lancet* 1:7503(1967), 1299–1300. Cheraskin, E., W.M. Ringsdorf Jr. "Blood-glucose Levels after Caffeine." *The Lancet* 2:7569(1968), 689.

[5] Cameron, E., and G. Baird. "Ascorbic Acid and Dependence on Opiates in Patients with Advanced and Disseminated Cancer." *J Intl Res Comm* 1 (1973), 38; Levin, E.D., F. Behm, E. Carnahan, et al. "Clinical Trials Using Ascorbic Acid Aerosol to Aid Smoking Cessa-

tion." *Drug Alcohol Dependence* 33:3(1993), 211–223.

Cancer

[1] Padayatty, S.J., H. Sun, Y. Wang, et al. "Vitamin C Pharmacokinetics: Implications for Oral and Intravenous Use." *Ann Intern Med* 140:7(2004), 533–537; Riordan, H.D., R.B. Hunninghake, N.H. Riordan, et al. "Intravenous Ascorbic Acid: Protocol for Its Application and Use." *P R Health Sci J* 22:3(2003), 287–290; Gonzalez, M. J., J.R. Miranda-Massari, E.M. Mora, et al. "Orthomolecular Oncology: A Mechanistic View of Intravenous Ascorbate's Chemotherapeutic Activity." *P R Health Sci J* 21:1(2002), 39–41; Jackson, J.A., H.D. Riordan, N.L. Bramhall, et al. "Case From the Center: Sixteen-year History with High Dose Intravenous Vitamin C Treatment for Various Types of Cancer and Other Diseases." *J Orthomolecular Med* 17:2(2002), 117.

[2] This is described in great detail in the book *Hyaluronidase and Cancer,* by Ewan Cameron, M.D. (Oxford: Pergamon Press, 1966).

[3] Hoffer, A. *Vitamin C and Cancer* (Kingston, ON, Canada: Quarry Press, 2000).

[4] Cameron, E., and L. Pauling. *Cancer and Vitamin C,* rev. ed. (Philadelphia: Camino Books, 1993).

[5] Cathcart, Robert F. "The Method of Determining Proper Doses of Vitamin C for the Treatment of Disease by Titrating to Bowel Tolerance." *J Orthomolecular Psychiatr* 10(1981), 125–132; Cathcart, Robert F. "Titration to Bowel Tolerance, Anascorbemia, and Acute Induced Scurvy." *Med Hypotheses* 7(1981), 1359–1376.

[6] Riordan, H.D., J.A. Jackson, M. Schultz. "Case Study: High-dose Intravenous Vitamin C in the Treatment of a Patient with Adenocarcinoma of the Kidney." *J Orthomolecular Med* 5(1990), 5–7; Jackson, J.A., H.D. Riordan, R.E. Hunninghake, et al. "High Dose Intravenous Vitamin C and Long Term Survival of a Patient with Cancer of Head of the Pancreas." *J Orthomolecular Med* 10:2(1995), 87–88; Riordan, N.H., H.D. Riordan, X. Meng, et al. "Intravenous Ascorbate as a Tumor Cytotoxic Chemotherapeutic Agent." *Med Hypotheses* 44(1995), 207–213; Riordan, N.H., J.A. Jackson, and H.D. Riordan. "Intravenous Vitamin C in a Terminal Cancer Patient." *J Orthomolecular Med* 11:2(1996), 80–82; Riordan, H.D., et al. "High-Dose Intravenous Vitamin C in the Treatment of a Patient with Renal Cell Carcinoma of the Kidney." *J Orthomolecular Med* 13:2(1998), 72; Gonzalez, M.J., E. Mora, N.H. Riordan, et al. "Rethinking Vitamin C and Cancer: An Update on Nutritional Oncology." *Cancer Prevention Intl* 3(1998),

215–224; Gonzalez, M.J., N.H. Riordan, and H.D. Riordan. "Antioxidants as Chemopreventive Agents for Breast Cancer." *BioMedicina* 1:4(April 1998); Riordan, N.H., H.D. Riordan, and J.J. Casciari. "Case from the Center: Clinical and Experimental Experiences with Intravenous Vitamin C." *J Orthomolecular Med* 15:4(2000), 201; Mikirova, N., J.A. Jackson, J.J. Casciari, et al. "Case From the Center: The Effect of Alternating Magnetic Field Exposure and Vitamin C on Cancer Cells." *J Orthomolecular Med* 16:3(2001), 177; Casciari, J.J., N.H. Riordan, T.L. Schmidt, et al. "Cytotoxicity of Ascorbate, Lipoic Acid, and Other Antioxidants in Hollow Fibre *in vitro* Tumours." *Brit J Cancer* 84:11(2001), 1544–1550; Gonzalez, M.J., E.M. Mora, J.R. Miranda-Massari, et al. "Inhibition of Human Breast Carcinoma Cell Proliferation by Ascorbate and Copper." *P R Health Sci J* 21:1 (March 2002), 21–23; Gonzalez, M.J., J.R. Miranda-Massari, E.M. Mora, et al. "Orthomolecular Oncology: A Mechanistic View of Intravenous Ascorbate's Chemotherapeutic Activity." *PR Health Sci J* 21:1(2002), 39–41; Rivers, J.M. "Safety of High-level Vitamin C Injection," in "Third Conference on Vitamin C," *Ann NY Acad Sci* 498(1987), 95–102.

[7] These studies are discussed in Dr. Hoffer's book *Vitamin C and Cancer* (Kingston, ON: Quarry Press, 1999) and in the Ewan

Cameron–Linus Pauling book *Cancer and Vitamin C* (Philadelphia: Camino Books, 1993).

[8] Riordan, N.H., H.D. Riordan, X. Meng, et al. "Intravenous Ascorbate as a Tumor Cytotoxic Chemotherapeutic Agent." *Med Hypotheses* 44(1995), 207–213.

[9] Padayatty, S.J., H. Sun, Y. Wang, et al. "Vitamin C Pharmacokinetics: Implications for Oral and Intravenous Use." *Ann Intern Med* 140:7(2004), 533–537.

[10] Dr. Riordan's team's instructions for physicians seeking to administer vitamin C by I.V. are presented in this paper: Riordan, H.D., R.B. Hunninghake, N.H. Riordan, et al. "Intravenous Ascorbic Acid: Protocol for Its Application and Use." *P R Health Sci J* 22:3(2003), 287–290.

[11] McCormick, W.J. "Have We Forgotten the Lesson of Scurvy?" *J Appl Nutr* 15:1–2(1962), 4–12;. McCormick, W.J. "Cancer: The Preconditioning Factor in Pathogenesis." *Arch Pediatr NY* 71(1954), 313; McCormick, W.J. "Cancer: A Collagen Disease, Secondary to a Nutritional Deficiency?" *Arch Pediatr* 76(1959), 166.

[12] Hoffer, Abram, M.D., Ph.D. "Orthomolecular Treatment of Cancer." www.doctoryourself.com/cancer_hoffer.html.

[13] Hoffer, Abram, M.D., Ph.D. "Clinical Procedures in Treating Terminally Ill Cancer

Patients with Vitamin C." www.doctoryourse lf.com/hoffer_cancer_2.html.

[14] Hoffer, A. *Orthomolecular Medicine for Physicians* (New Canaan, CT: Keats Publishing, 1989).

[15] Hoffer, Abram, M.D., Ph.D. "Orthomolecular Treatment of Cancer." www.doctoryourself.com/cancer_hoffer.html.

[16] Ibid.

[17] Ibid.

[18] Reprinted from *Clinical Procedures in Treating Terminally Ill Cancer Patients with Vitamin C* by Abram Hoffer, M.D., Ph.D., with the permission of the author. www.doctoryourself.com/hoffer_cancer_2.html.

[19] Gerson, Charlotte, and Morton Walker. *The Gerson Therapy* (New York: Kensington Publishing, 2001), p.31 and personal communication.

[20] www.doctoryourself.com/cancer.html.

[21] Straus, Howard. *Dr. Max Gerson: Healing the Hopeless* (Kingston, Ontario, Canada: Quarry Press, 2002); Gerson, Charlotte, and Morton Walker. *The Gerson Therapy* (New York: Kensington Publishing, 2001); Gerson, M. *A Cancer Therapy: Results of Fifty Cases and the Cure of Advanced Cancer,* 6th ed. (San Diego, CA: Gerson Institute, 1958).

Cardiovascular Disease

[1] Ornish, D. *Dr. Dean Ornish's Program for Reversing Heart Disease* (New York: Random House/Ivy Books, 1995).

[2] Rinse, J. *The Rinse Formula* (New Caanan, CT: Keats Publishing, 1988)]; Rinse, Jacobus. "Atherosclerosis: Prevention and Cure (Parts 1 and 2)." *Prevention* (November and December 1975); Rinse, Jacobus. (1978) "Cholesterol and Phospholipids in Relation to Atherosclerosis." *American Laboratory Magazine* (April 1978).

[3] McBeath, M., and L. Pauling. "A Case History: Lysine/Ascorbate-related Amelioration of Angina Pectoris." *J Orthomolecular Med* 8(1993), 77–78; Pauling, L. "Case Report: Lysine/Ascorbate-related Amelioration of Angina Pectoris." J Orthomolecular Med 6 (1991), 144–146; Rath, M., and L. Pauling. "Hypothesis: Lipoprotein(a) is a Surrogate for Ascorbate." *Proc Natl Acad Sci USA* 87(1990), 6204–6207; Rath, M., and L. Pauling. "Solution to the Puzzle of Human Cardiovascular Disease: Its Primary Cause Is Ascorbate Deficiency, Leading to the Deposition of Lipoprotein(a) and Fibrinogen/fibrin in the Vascular Wall." *J Orthomolecular Med* 6(1991), 125–134; Rath, M., and L. Pauling. "A Unified Theory of Human Cardiovascular Disease Leading the Way to the Abolition of

This Disease As a Cause for Human Mortality." *J Orthomolecular Med* 7(1992), 5–15. www.orthomed.org/links/papers/rathpau.htm.

[4] Garcia, J. "Hypertensives spell relief T-M." *Ashland Daily Tidings,* Ashland, Oregon. Aug13, 1997.

[5] "Reduced Health Care Utilization in Transcendental Meditation Practitioners." Paper presented at the Conference of the Society for Behavioral Medicine, Washington, D.C., March 22, 1987.

[6] Schneider, R.H., C.N. Alexander, and R.K. Wallace. "In Search of an Optimal Behavioral Treatment for Hypertension: A Review and Focus on Transcendental Meditation." In: Johnson, E.H., W.D. Gentry, and S. Julius, eds., *Personality, Elevated Blood Pressure, and Essential Hypertension* (Washington, D.C.: Hemisphere Publishing, 1992); Alexander, C.N., E.J. Langer, R.I. Newman, et al. "Transcendental Meditation, Mindfulness, and Longevity: An Experimental Study with the Elderly." *J Personality Social Psych* 57:6(1989), 950–964.

Additional References

Ornish, D., Denke, M. "Dietary treatment of hyperlipidemia." *J Cardiovasc Risk.* 1994 Dec;1(4):283–6.

Ornish, D. "Can lifestyle changes reverse coronary heart disease?" *World Rev Nutr Diet.* 1993;72:38–48. Review.

Ornish, D. "Can lifestyle changes reverse coronary atherosclerosis?" *Hosp Pract* (Off Ed). 1991 May 15;26(5):123–6, 129–32.

Ornish, D.R "eversing heart disease through diet, exercise, and stress management: an interview with Dean Ornish." Interview by Elaine R. Monsen. *J Am Diet Assoc.* 1991 Feb;91(2):162–5.

Ornish, D., Brown, S.E., Scherwitz, L.W., Billings, J.H., Armstrong, W.T., Ports, T.A., McLanahan, S.M., Kirkeeide, R.L., Brand, R.J., Gould, K.L. "Lifestyle changes and heart disease." *Lancet.* 1990 Sep 22;336(8717):741–2.

Ornish, D., Brown, S.E., Scherwitz, L.W., Billings, J.H., Armstrong, W.T., Ports, T.A., McLanahan, S. M., Kirkeeide, R.L., Brand, R.J., Gould, K.L. "Can lifestyle changes reverse coronary heart disease?" The Lifestyle Heart Trial. *Lancet.* 1990 Jul21;336(8708):129–33.

Ornish, D., Scherwitz, L.W., Doody, R.S., Kesten, D., McLanahan, S.M., Brown, S.E., DePuey, E., Sonnemaker, R., Haynes, C., Lester, J., McAllister, G.K., Hall, R.J., Burdine, J.A., Gotto, A. M., Jr. "Effects of stress management training and dietary changes in treating ischemic heart disease." *JAMA.* 1983 Jan7;249(l):54–9.

Stroke and Heart Attack

[1] McCormick, W.J. "Coronary Thrombosis: A New Concept of Mechanism and Etiology." *Clin Med* 4:7(1957), 839–845.

[2] Enstrom, J.E., et al. "Vitamin C Intake and Mortality among a Sample of the United States Population." *Epidemiol* 3:3(1992), 194–202.

[3] McCully, K.S., and R.B. Wilson. "Homocysteine Theory of Arteriosclerosis." *Atherosclerosis* 22:2(1975), 215–227.

[4] Rinehart, J.F., and L.D. Greenberg. "Arteriosclerotic Lesions in Pyridoxine Deficient Monkeys." *Am J Pathol* 25(1949), 481–496; Rinehart, J.F., and L.D. Greenberg. "Pathogenesis of Experimental Arteriosclerosis in Pyridoxine Deficiency with Notes on Similarities to Human Arteriosclerosis." *Arch Pathol* 51(1951),12–29; Rinehart, J.F., and L.D. Greenberg. "Vitamin B6 Deficiency in the Rhesus Monkey, with Particular Reference to the Occurrence of Atherosclerosis, Dental Caries and Hepatic Cirrhosis." *Am J Clin Nutr* 4(1956), 318–325.

[5] Shute, E.V. "Alpha Tocopherol in Cardiovascular Disease." *Oxford University Med Gaz* 9:96(1957).

[6] "Amelioration of oxidative stress by high-dose vitamin E enhances nitric oxide availability, (and) improves hypertension." Vaziri, N.D., Z.Ni, F. Oveisi, et al. "Enhanced Nitric Oxide Inactivation and Protein Nitration by Reactive Oxygen Species in Renal Insufficiency." *Hypertension* 39:1(2002), 135–141.

[7] For more information on vitamin E, see the following: Shute, E.V., et al. *The Heart and Vitamin E* (London, Canada: The Shute Foundation for Medical Research, 1963); Shute, E.V., and W.E. Shute. *Alpha Tocopherol in Cardiovascular Disease* (Toronto, Canada: Ryerson Press, 1954); Shute, Wilfrid E. *The Vitamin E Book* (New Canaan, CT: Keats Publishing, 1978); Shute, W.E., and H.J. Taub. *Vitamin E for Ailing and Healthy Hearts* (New York: Pyramid House, 1969).

Chronic Fatigue and Immune Dysfunction

[1] Cheraskin, E. "Vitamin C and Fatigue." *J Orthomolecular Med* 9:1(1994), 39–45.

[2] Chandra, R.K. "Nutrition and Immunity: Basic Considerations, Part 1." *Contemporary Nutr* 11:11(1986).

[3] Alexander, M., et al. "Oral Beta-carotene Can Increase the Number of OKT4

Cells in Human Blood." *Immunol Lett* 9 (1985), 221–224.

[4] Williams, S.R. *Nutrition and Diet Therapy,* 7th ed. (St. Louis: Mosby, 1989), 201.

[5] A considerable number of supporting references appear in: Werbach, M.R., M.D. *Nutritional Influences on Illness* (New Canaan, CT: Keats, 1988). Pages 243–251 and 418–423 can be applied to CFIDS.

[6] Klenner, F.R. "Virus Pneumonia and Its Treatment with Vitamin C." *South Med Surg* (February 1948), 36–46.

[7] Murray, F. "Vitamin C and AIDS: Another Direction?" *Today's Living* (September 1987), 5–25.

[8] Cathcart, R.F. "Vitamin C in the Treatment of Acquired Immune Deficiency Syndrome." *Med Hypotheses* 14(1984), 423–433; Cathcart, R.F. "Vitamin C in Massive Doses Does Work." *Today's Living* (December 1981), 10–11, 60–64.

[9] "MRCA Census for the Calendar Year 1975." General Mills, Inc., Minneapolis, MN, 1980.

[10] Anderson, R., and A. Kozlovsky. "Chromium Intake, Absorption, and Excretion of Subjects Consuming Self-Selected Diets." *Am J Clin Nutr* 41:6 (1985), 1177–1183.

[11] Anderson, R. "Chromium Metabolism and Its Role in Disease Processes in Man." *Clin Physiol Biochem* 4(1986), 31–41.

[12] Burton, J.L., B.A. Mallard, and D.N. Mowat. "Effects of Supplemental Chromium on Immune Responses of Periparturient and Early Lactation Dairy Cows." *J Anim Sci* 71:6(1993), 1532–1539; Moonsie-Shageer, S., and D.N. Mowat. "Effect of Level of Supplemental Chromium on Performance, Serum Constituents, and Immune Status of Stressed Feeder Calves." *J Anim Sci* 71:1(1993), 232–238. Also see: "Chromium Improves Immune Responsiveness." *Manitoba Co-Operator* (December 2, 1993).

[13] Bogden, J.D., et al. "Zinc and Immuno-competence in the Elderly: Baseline Data on Zinc Nutriture in Unsupplemented Subjects." *Am J Clin Nutr* 46(1987), 101.

[14] Prasad, A.S. "The Role of Zinc in Human Health." *Contemporary Nutr* 16(1991), 5.

[15] Elby, G.A., D.R. Davis, and W.W. Halcomb. "Reduction in Duration of Common Colds by Zinc Gluconate Lozenges in a Double-blind Study." *Antimicrob Agents Chemother* 25:1(1984) 20–24; "Cold duration was an additional 4.3 days in zinc-treated patients compared with 9.2 days for placebo-treated patients. Cough, nasal drainage, and congestion were the symptoms most affected, and only mild side effects were noted." Godfrey, J.C., B.

Conant-Sloane, D. S. Smith, et al. "Zinc Gluconate and the Common Cold: A Controlled Clinical Study." *J Int Med Res* 20:3(1992), 234–246; "The duration of symptoms was 2.3 days in the zinc group and 9.0 days in the control group, a statistically significant difference." Hirt, M., S. Nobel, and E. Barron. "Zinc Nasal Gel for the Treatment of Common Cold Symptoms: A Double-blind, Placebo-controlled Trial." *Ear Nose Throat J* 79:10(2000), 778–780, 782.

[16] "Supplemental zinc was administered to 15 subjects over 70 years of age (220mg zinc sulfate twice daily for a month). The data suggest that the addition of zinc to the diet of old persons could be an effective and simple way to improve their immune function." Duchateau, J., G. Delepesse, R. Vrijens, et al. "Beneficial Effects of Oral Zinc Supplementation on the Immune Response of Old People." *Am J Med* 70:5(1981), 1001–1004.

Chronic Pain

[1] For more information on phenylalanine, see: Balagot, R.C., S. Ehrenpreis, J. Greenberg, et al. "D-Phenylalanine in Human Chronic Pain." In: Ehrenpreis, S., and F. Sicuteri, eds., *Degradation of Endogenous Opioids: Its Relevance in Human Pathology and Therapy* (New York: Raven Press, 1983); Balagot, R.C., S.

Ehrenpreis, K. Kubota, et al. In: Bonica, J.J., J.C. Liebeskind, and D.G. Albe-Fessard, eds., *Advances in Pain Research and Therapy,* Vol.5 (New York: Raven Press, 1983), pp.289–293; Beckman, H., et al. "DL Phenylalanine in Depressed Patients: An Open Study." *J Neural Transmission* 41(1977), 123–134; Budd, K. "Use of D-Phenylalanine, an Enkephalinase Inhibitor, in the Treatment of Intractable Pain." In: Bonica, J.J., J.C. Liebeskind, and D.G. Albe-Fessard, eds., *Advances in Pain Research and Therapy,* Vol.5 (New York: Raven Press, 1983), pp.305–308; Ehrenpreis, S., R.C. Balagot, J.E. Comaty, et al. "Naloxone Reversible Analgesia in Mice Produced by D-Phenylalanine and Hydrocinnamic Acid, Inhibitors of Carboxypeptidase A." In: Bonica, J.J., J.C. Liebeskind, and D.G. Albe-Fessard, eds., *Advances in Pain Research and Therapy,* Vol.3 (New York: Raven Press, 1978), pp.479–488; Ehrenpreis, S., R.C. Balagot, S. Myles, et al. "Further Studies on the Analgesic Activity of D-Phenylalanine in Mice and Humans." Proceedings of the International Narcotic Research Club Convention, 1979, 379–382; Heller, B. "Pharmacological and Clinical Effects of D-Phenylalanine in Depression and Parkinson's Disease." In: Mosnaim, A.D., and M.E. Wolf, eds., *Modern Pharmacology-Toxicology, Non-catecolic Phenylethylamines, Part 1* (New

York: Marcel Dekker, 1978), pp.397–417; Sabelli, H.C., and A.D. Mosnaim. "Phenylethylamine Hypothesis of Affective Behavior." *Am J Psychiatr* 131(1974), 695.

[2] Cameron, Ewan, and Linus Pauling. *Cancer and Vitamin C* (New York: Warner Books, 1981), xii.

Colitis, Ulcers, and Other Intestinal Problems

[1] Benjamin, H. *Everybody's Guide to Nature Cure* (North Hollywood, CA: Newcastle Publishing 1982).

[2] Williams, S.R. *Nutrition and Diet Therapy,* 7th ed. (St. Louis: Mosby, 1993), p.29.

[3] Cheney, G. "Vitamin U Therapy of Peptic Ulcer." *Calif Med* 77:4(October 1952), 248–252.

[4] Cheney, Garnett. "Antipeptic Ulcer Dietary Factor." *J Am Dietetics Assoc* 26 (September 1950), 9; Cheney, Garnett. "The Nature of the Antipeptic-ulcer Dietary Factor." *Stanford Med Bull* 8(1950), 144; Cheney, Garnett. "Prevention of Histamine-induced Peptic Ulcers by Diet." *Stanford Med Bull* 6 (1948), 334; Cheney, Garnett. "Rapid Healing of Peptic Ulcers in Patients Receiving Fresh Cabbage Juice." *Calif Med* 70:10(1949), 10–14.

[5] "Cruciferous vegetables such as broccoli and cauliflower seem to be especially protective against cancer. Most studies show that phytochemicals in crucifers up-regulate many detoxification enzyme systems in the animal that consumes them." Finley, J.W. "The Antioxidant Responsive Element (ARE) May Explain the Protective Effects of Cruciferous Vegetables on Cancer." *Nutr Rev* 61:7(2003), 250–254; "(C)ruciferous vegetables decrease the risk of both stomach and colorectal cancer." Hara, M., T. Hanaoka, M. Kobayashi, et al. "Cruciferous Vegetables, Mushrooms, and Gastrointestinal Cancer Risks in a Multicenter, Hospital-based Case-control Study in Japan." *Nutr Cancer* 46:2(2003), 138–147.

[6] Cantorna, M.T., C. Munsick, C. Bemiss, et al. "1,25-Dihydroxycholecalciferol Prevents and Ameliorates Symptoms of Experimental Murine Inflammatory Bowel Disease." *J Nutr* 130:11(2000), 2648–2652.

[7] Kloss, J. *Back to Eden* (Lotus Press, 1989), pp.82–83; 549–550.

Down Syndrome

[1] Harrell, R.F., R.H. Capp, D.R. Davis, et al. "Can Nutritional Supplements Help Mentally Retarded Children? An Exploratory Study." *Proc Natl Acad Sci USA* 78(1981), 574–578.

[2] Bennett, F.C., S. McClelland, E.A. Kriegsmann, et al. "Vitamin and Mineral Supplementation in Down's Syndrome." *Pediatrics* 72:5(1983), 707–713; Bidder, R.T., P. Gray, R.G. Newcombe, et al. "The Effects of Multivitamins and Minerals on Children with Down Syndrome." *Dev Med Child Neurol* 31:4(1989), 532–537; Menolascino, F.J., J.Y. Donaldson, T.F. Gallagher, et al. "Vitamin Supplements and Purported Learning Enhancement in Mentally Retarded Children." *J Nutr Sci Vitaminol* (*Tokyo*) 35:3(1989), 181–192; Smith, G.F., D. Spiker, C.P. Peterson, et al. "Failure of Vitamin/Mineral Supplementation in Down Syndrome." *The Lancet* 2(1983), 41; Weathers, C. "Effects of Nutritional Supplementation on IQ and Certain Other Variables Associated with Down Syndrome." *Am J Ment Defic* 88:2(1983), 214–217; Pruess, J.B., R.R. Fewell, and F.C. Bennett. "Vitamin Therapy and Children with Down Syndrome: A Review of Research." *Except Child* 55:4(1989) 336–341.

[3] Harrell, R.F., R.H. Capp, D.R. Davis, et al. "Can Nutritional Supplements Help Mentally Retarded Children? An Exploratory Study." *Proc Natl Acad Sci USA* 78(1981), 574–578.

[4] Harrell, Ruth Flinn. "Effect of Added Thiamine on Learning." *The Health Seeker* (New York: AMS Press, 1972), 18–19. www.geocities.com/HotSprings/2194/vitamin.html.

[5] Winter, A. "Differential Diagnosis of Memory Dysfunction: Finding the Cause When Your Patient Can't Remember." www.afpafitness.com/articles/Memory.htm.

[6] Garrison, R.H., and E. Somer. *The Nutrition Desk Reference* (New Canaan, CT: Keats, 1990), p.43.

[7] Ibid., 45.

[8] Ibid., 46, 48.

[9] Ibid., 49.

[10] Ibid., 51.

[11] Pincheira, J., M.H. Navarrete, C. de la Torre, et al. "Effect of Vitamin E on Chromosomal Aberrations in Lymphocytes From Patients with Down Syndrome." *Clin Genet* 55:3(1999), 192–197.

[12] Harrell, R.F., R.H. Capp, D.R. Davis, et al. "Can Nutritional Supplements Help Mentally Retarded Children? An Exploratory Study." *Proc Natl Acad Sci USA* 78(1981), 574–578.

[13] Craft, D. "Can Nutritional Supplements Help Mentally Retarded Children?" www.diannecraft.com/nut-sup1.html; Turkel, H. "Medical Amelioration of Down's Syndrome Incorporating the Orthomolecular Approach." *J Orthomolecular Psychiatr* 4(1975), 102–115. Turkel, H. *The Medical Treatment for Down's Syndrome* (Southfield, MI: Ubiotica, 1985).

Earaches and Ear Infections

[1] Cantekin, E.I., E.M. Mandel, C.D. Bluestone, et al. "Lack of Efficacy of a Decongestant-antihistamine Combination for Otitis Media with Effusion ("Secretory" Otitis Media) in Children. Results of a Double-blind, Randomized Trial." *N Engl J Med* 308:6(1983), 297–301.

Eczema (Atopic Dermatitis)

[1] www.aad.org/pamphlets/eczema.html.

[2] Kirjavainen, P.V., T. Arvola, S.J. Salminen, et al. "Aberrant Composition of Gut Microbiota of Allergic Infants: A Target of Bifidobacterial Therapy at Weaning?" *Gut* 51:1(2002), 51–55; Kalliomaki, M., S. Salminen, H. Arvilommi, et al. "Probiotics in Primary Prevention of Atopic Disease: A Randomised Placebo-controlled Trial." *The Lancet* 357:9262(2001), 1076–1079; Kalliomaki, M., S. Salminen, T. Poussa, et al. "Probiotics and Prevention of Atopic Disease: 4-year Follow-up of a Randomised Placebo-controlled Trial." *The Lancet* 361:9372(2003), 1869–1871; Rautava, S., M. Kalliomaki, and E. Isolauri. "Probiotics During Pregnancy and Breast-feeding Might Confer Immunomodulatory Protection against Atopic Disease in the Infant." *J Allergy Clin Immunol* 109:1(2002), 119–121.

542

[3] "Severe Atopic Dermatitis Responds to Ascorbic Acid." *Med World News* (April 24, 1989), 41.

[4] Reynolds, N.J., V. Franklin, J.C. Gray, et al. "Narrowband Ultraviolet B and Broadband Ultraviolet A Phototherapy in Adult Atopic Eczema: A Randomised Controlled Trial." *The Lancet* 357:9273(2001), 2012–2016.

Emphysema and Chronic Respiratory Diseases

[1] www.nhlbi.nih.gov/meetings/workshops/copd_wksp.htm.

[2] If you would like to help prevent another generation of tobacco addiction and disease, go to www.SmokefreeAir.org and send a "Smokefree EZ-Letter" to a key decision maker.

[3] Massaro, G.D., and D. Massaro. "Retinoic Acid Treatment Abrogates Elastase-induced Pulmonary Emphysema in Rats." *Nat Med* 3:6(1997), 675–677.

Fever

[1] Schmitt, B.D. *Your Child's Health* (New York: Bantam Books, 1991).

[2] Kluger, M.J. "Is Fever Beneficial?" *Yale J Biol Med* 59:2(1986), 89–95. "Moderate fevers decrease morbidity and increase survival rate."

[3] A simple guide to the handiest remedies is *The Prescriber* by John H. Clarke, M.D. (Essex, England: C.W. Daniel, 1972). I'm especially keen on Dr. Schuessler's Biochemistry by J.B. Chapman, M.D. (London: New Era, 1973) and *Who is Your Doctor and Why* by Alonzo Shad-man, M.D. (New Canaan, CT: Keats, 1958). All these books contain practical dosage information.

Gallstones

[1] Simon, J.A., and E.S. Hudes. "Serum Ascorbic Acid and Other Correlates of Gallbladder Disease among U.S. Adults." *Am J Public Health* 88:8(1998), 1208–1212.
[2] Simon, J.A. "Ascorbic Acid and Cholesterol Gallstones." *Med Hypotheses* 40:2(1993), 81–84.

Headaches

[1] To learn other pressure points, please refer to *The Natural Healer's Acupressure Handbook* by Michael Blate (New York: Holt, Rinehart and Winston, 1977).
[2] Gerson, C., and M. Walker. *The Gerson Therapy* (New York: Kensington Publishing, 2001). Gerson, M. *A Cancer Therapy: Results of Fifty Cases and the Cure of Advanced Cancer,* 6th ed. (San Diego, CA: Gerson Institute,

1958); Straus, H. *Dr. Max Gerson: Healing the Hopeless* (Kingston, Ontario, Canada: Quarry Press, 2002).

[3] Prousky, J.E., and E. Sykes. "Two Case Reports on the Treatment of Acute Migraine with Niacin: Its Hypothetical Mechanism of Action upon Calcitonin-Gene Related Peptide and Platelets." *J Orthomolecular Med* 18:2(2003), 108.

Herpes, Cold Sores, HPV (Human Papilloma Virus), Shingles (Herpes Zoster)

[1] Cathcart, R.F. "Vitamin C in the Treatment of Acquired Immune Deficiency Syndrome (AIDS)." *Med Hypotheses* 14:4(1984), 423–433.

[2] Cathcart, R.F. "Vitamin C, Titrating to Bowel Tolerance, Anascorbemia, and Acute Induced Scurvy." *Med Hypotheses* 7(1981), 1359–1376.

Boosting Your Immunity (SIDEBAR)

[1] From: Cheraskin, E., M.D., D.M.D. "The Health of the Naturopath: Vitamin Supplementation and Psychologic State." *J Orthomolecular Med* 13:4(1998), 223–224.

[2] Chandra, R.K. "Effect of Vitamin and Trace-element Supplementation on Immune Responses and Infection in Elderly Subjects." *The Lancet* 340:8828 (1992), 1124–1127; Pike, J., and R.K. Chandra. "Effect of Vitamin and Trace Element Supplementation on Immune Indices in Healthy Elderly." *Intl J Vitamin Nutr Res* 65:2(1995), 117–120.

[3] Meydani, S.N., M.P. Barklund, S. Liu, et al. "Effect of Vitamin E Supplementation on Immune Responsiveness of Healthy Elderly Subjects." *FASEB J* 3(1989), A1057; Meydani, S.N., M.P. Barklund, S. Liu, et al. "Vitamin E Supplementation Enhances Cell-Mediated Immunity in Healthy Elderly Subjects." *Am J Clin Nutr* 52:3(1990), 557–563.

[4] Incidentally, even people with the weakest of immune systems (AIDS patients) have benefitted from huge carotene dosages. Alexander, M., H. Newmark, and R.G. Miller. "Oral Beta Carotene Can Increase the Number of OKT4+Cells in Human Blood." *Immunol Lett* 9 (1985), 221–224.

Lupus

[1] Gerson, Charlotte, and Morton Walker. *The Gerson Therapy* (New York: Kensington Publishing, 2001).

[2] Levy, T. *Vitamin C, Infectious Diseases, and Toxins: Curing the Incurable* (Philadelphia: XLibris, 2002), p.404.

[3] From a talk given October 7, 2000, to the Lupus Foundation of Northern California at Stanford University Medical Center: "Hypothesis for the Cause and Treatment of Various Inflammatory Diseases."

Motor Neuron Diseases

[1] www.mndassociation.org.

[2] Klenner, F.R. "Treating Multiple Sclerosis Nutritionally." *Cancer Control J* 2:3 (undated reprint), 16–20; Klenner, F.R. "Response of Peripheral and Central Nerve Pathology to Mega-doses of the Vitamin B-complex and Other Metabolites." *J Appl Nutr* 25(1973), 16.

[3] Goldberg, P., M. Fleming, and E. Picard. "Multiple Sclerosis: Decreased Relapse Rate through Dietary Supplementation with Calcium, Magnesium and Vitamin D." *Med Hypotheses* 21(1986), 193–200.

[4] Embry, A.F. "Vitamin D Supplementation in the Fight against Multiple Sclerosis." *J Orthomolecular Med* 19:1(2004). 27–38; Saul, A.W. "Vitamin D: Deficiency, Diversity and Dosage." *J Orthomolecular Med* 18:3–4(2003), 194–204; Cantorna, M., C. Hayes, and H. DeLuca. "1,25Dihydroxyvitamin D3 Reversibly Blocks the Progression of Relapsing En-

cephalomyelitis, A Model of Multiple Sclerosis." *Proc Natl Acad Sci* 93(1996), 7861–7864; Hayes, C.E., M.T. Cantorna, and H.F. DeLuca. "Vitamin D and Multiple Sclerosis." *Proc Soc Exp Biol Med* 216:1(1997), 21–27; Hayes, C.E. "Vitamin D: A Natural Inhibitor of Multiple Sclerosis." *Proc Nutr Soc* 59:4(2000), 531–535.

[5] The treatment protocol is more fully described in: Smith, Lendon H. *Clinical Guide to the Use of Vitamin C: The Clinical Experiences of Frederick R. Klenner, M.D.* (Portland, OR: Life Sciences Press, 1988), pp.42–53.

Muscular Dystrophy

[1] www.ninds.nih.gov/health_and_medical/disorders/md.htm (accessed April 2004).

[2] *American Heritage Dictionary of the English Language,* 4th ed. (Boston: Houghton Mifflin, 2000), p.407.

[3] Folkers, K., J. Wolaniuk, R. Simonsen, et al. "Biochemical Rationale and the Cardiac Response of Patients with Muscle Disease to Therapy with Coenzyme Q10." *Proc Natl Acad Sci USA* 82:13(1985), 4513–4516.

[4] Folkers, K., and R. Simonsen. "Two Successful Double-blind Trials with Coenzyme Q10 (Vitamin Q10) on Muscular Dystrophies and Neurogenic Atrophies." *Biochim Biophys Acta* 1271:1 (1995), 281–286.

[5] Dr. Pauling's comments are reprinted with permission of the Linus Pauling Institute, Oregon State University. Pauling, Linus, Ph.D. *How to Live Longer and Feel Better* (New York: Avon Books, 1996).

[6] Backman, E., and K.G. Henriksson. "Effect of Sodium Selenite and Vitamin E Treatment in Myotonic Dystrophy." *J Intern Med* 228:6(1990), 577–581.

[7] Gamstorp, I., K.H. Gustavson, O. Hellstrom, et al. "A Trial of Selenium and Vitamin E in Boys with Muscular Dystrophy." *J Child Neurol* 1:3(1986), 211–214.

[8] Orndahl, G., U. Sellden, S. Hallin, et al. "Myotonic Dystrophy Treated with Selenium and Vitamin E." *Acta Med Scand* 219:4(1986), 407–414.

[9] Bicknell, F., and F. Prescott. *The Vitamins in Medicine,* 3rd ed. (Milwaukee, WI: Lee Foundation for Nutritional Research, 1953).

[10] Jackson, M.J., D.A. Jones, and R.H. Edwards. "Vitamin E and Muscle Diseases." *J Inherit Metab Dis* 8:Suppl1(1985), 84–87. (This review explains how vitamin E and the phospholipids in lecithin benefit the muscles.); Milhorat, A.T., and W.E. Bartels. "The Defect in Utilization of Tocopherol in Progessive Muscular Dystrophy." *Science* 101(1945), 93–94; Milhorat, A.T., et al. "Effect of Wheat Germ on Creatinuria in Dermatomyositis and Progressive Muscular

Dystrophy." *Proc Soc Exp Biol Med* 58(1945), 40–41.

[11] Werbach, M. *Nutritional Influences on Illness* (New Canaan, CT: Keats, 1988), 310–311; Orndahl, G., et al. "Selenium Therapy of Myotonic Dystrophy." *Acta Med Scand* 213(1983), 237; Hidiroglou, M., K. Jenkins, R.B. Carson, et al. "Selenium and Coenzyme Q10 Levels in the Tissues of Dystrophic and Healthy Calves." *Can J Physiol Pharmacol* 45:3(1967), 568–569.

[12] Ihara, Y., A. Mori, T. Hayabara, et al. "Free Radicals, Lipid Peroxides and Antioxidants in Blood of Patients with Myotonic Dystrophy." *J Neurol* 242:3(1995), 119–122.

Osteoporosis

[1] Recker, R.R., M.D. "Osteoporosis." *Contemporary Nutr* 8:5(1983).

[2] McCormick, C.C. "Passive Diffusion Does Not Play a Major Role in the Absorption of Dietary Calcium in Normal Adults." *J Nutr* 132:11(2002), 3428–3430.

[3] Dawson-Hughes, B., S.S. Harris, E.A. Krall, et al. "Effect of Calcium and Vitamin D Supplementation on Bone Density in Men and Women 65 years of Age or Older." *N Engl J Med* 337(1997), 670–676.

[4] Mitric, J.M. Maturity News Service (November 15, 1992).

[5] "BluePrint for Health Herb Index: Vitamin D." Blue Cross and Blue Shield of Minnesota, Inc. (2002). blueprint.bluecrossmn.com/topic/topic100587894.

[6] Glerup, H., K. Mikkelsen, L. Poulsen, et al. "Commonly Recommended Daily Intake of Vitamin D is Not Sufficient if Sunlight Exposure is Limited." *J Intern Med* 247(2000), 260–268.

[7] Vieth, R. "Vitamin D Supplementation, 25-hydroxyvitamin D Concentrations, and Safety." *Am J Clin Nutr* 69:5(1999), 842–856.

[8] Recker, R.R. "Osteoporosis." *Contemporary Nutr* 8:5(1983).

[9] Neilsen, F.H. "Ultratrace Minerals." *Contemporary Nutr* 15:7(1990).

[10] Barnett, L.B., M.D. "New Concepts in Bone Healing." *J Appl Nutr* 7(1954), 318–323.

[11] A review of the subject entitled "Fluoridation and Osteoporosis" was authored by John R. Lee, M.D., and published in the *National Fluoridation News* 32:1–2(1986–7); *Medical World News* ran articles on increased fractures due to fluoride on October 23, 1989 and November 13, 1989; "Fluoridation of Water." *Chem Eng News* 66 (August 1, 1988), 26–42; Additional confirmation of fluoride's contribution to fractures will be found in: Bayley, T.A., J.E. Harrison, T.M. Murray, et al. "Fluoride-induced Fractures: Relation to Osteogenic Effect." *J Bone Miner Res* 5:Suppl 1(1990), S217–S222.

"(F)luoride therapy may be implicated in the pathogenesis of hip fractures which may occur in treated patients despite a rapid, marked increase in bone mass." Danielson, C., J.L. Lyon, M. Egger, et al. "Hip Fractures and Fluoridation in Utah's Elderly Population." *JAMA* 268:6(1992), 746–748. "We found a small but significant increase in the risk of hip fracture in both men and women exposed to artificial fluoridation at 1ppm, suggesting that low levels of fluoride may increase the risk of hip fracture in the elderly." Hedlund, L.R., and J.C. Gallagher. "Increased Incidence of Hip Fracture in Osteoporotic Women Treated with Sodium Fluoride." *J Bone Miner Res* 4:2(1989), 223–225.

[12] Toxicology Program. Fact Sheet (January 22, 1990); and "Review of Fluoride Benefits and Risks," U.S. Public Health Service (February 1991).

Prostate Problems

[1] Fair, W.R., and W. Heston. "Prostate Inflammation Linked to Zinc Shortage." *Prevention* 113 (June 1977).

[2] Taylor, D.S. "Nutrients Can Remedy Prostate Problems." *Today's Living* (February 1990), 12–13.

[3] Ibid.

552

[4] Hoffer, Abram, M.D., Ph.D. "Orthomolecular Treatment of Cancer." www.doctoryourself.com/cancer_hoffer.html.

[5] *USA Weekend* (December 3–5, 1993), 14.

[6] "Prostate Cancer Cure Questioned." The Associated Press (January 27, 1994).

[7] Dr. Gerson's entire program is set forth in his tremendously valuable book: Gerson, Max. *A Cancer Therapy: Results of 50 Cases* (San Diego, CA: Gerson Institute, 1958). Visit the website: www.gerson.org.

[8] La Vecchia, C. "Tomatoes, Lycopene Intake, and Digestive Tract and Female Hormone-related Neoplasms." *Exp Biol Med* (Maywood) 227:10(2002), 860–863; La Vecchia, C. "Mediterranean Epidemiological Evidence on Tomatoes and the Prevention of Digestive-tract Cancers." *Proc Soc Exp Biol Med* 218:2(1998), 125–128; Franceschi, S., E. Bidoli, C. La Vecchia, et al. "Tomatoes and Risk of Digestive-tract Cancers." *Intl J Cancer* 59:2(1994), 181–184; Wu, K., J.W. Erdman Jr., S.J. Schwartz, et al. "Plasma and Dietary Carotenoids, and the Risk of Prostate Cancer: A Nested Case-control Study." *Cancer Epidemiol Biomarkers Prev* 13:2(2004), 260–269.

[9] Awad, A.B., K.C. Chan, A.C. Downie, et al. "Peanuts as a Source of Beta-sitosterol, A

Sterol with Anticancer Properties." *Nutr Cancer* 36:2(2000), 238–241.

[10] "Soybean Products May Lower Prostate Cancer." *Lancaster Intelligencer-Journal* (January 12, 1994); "Our study suggests that men with high consumption of soy milk are at reduced risk of prostate cancer." Jacobsen, B.K., S.F. Knutsen, and G.E. Fraser. "Does High Soy Milk Intake Reduce Prostate Cancer Incidence? The Adventist Health Study (United States)." *Cancer Causes Control* 9:6(1998), 553–557.

Psoriasis

[1] Hoffer, Abram, and Morton Walker. *Orthomolecular Nutrition* (New Canaan, CT: Keats Publishing, 1978), pp.156–157.

[2] Morimoto, S., K. Yoshikawa, T. Kozuka, et al. "An Open Study of Vitamin D3 Treatment in Psoriasis Vulgaris." *Br J Dermatol* 115:4(1986), 421–429.

Respiratory Infections

[1] Pauling, Linus. Vitamin C, The Common Cold and the Flu (Cutchogue, NY: Buccaneer Books, 1995), chapter 14.

[2] Evans, A.T., S. Husain, L. Durairaj, et al. "Azithromycin for Acute Bronchitis: A

Randomised, Double-blind, Controlled Trial."
The Lancet 359:9318(2002), 1648–1654.

[3] Klenner, F.R. "Virus Pneumonia and Its Treatment with Vitamin C." *South Med Surg* (February 1948); Klenner, F.R. "Massive Doses of Vitamin C and the Virus Diseases." *South Med Surg* 103:4(1951), 101–107; Klenner, F.R. "The Use of Vitamin C as an Antibiotic." *J Appl Nutr* 6 (1953), 274–78; Klenner, F.R. "The Role of Ascorbic Acid in Therapeutics." *Tri-State Med J* (November 1955); McCormick, W. J. "The Changing Incidence and Mortality of Infectious Disease in Relation to Changed Trends in Nutrition." *Med Record* (September 1947); McCormick, W.J. "Have We Forgotten the Lesson of Scurvy?" *J Appl Nutr* 15(1962), 4–12.

Sinus Congestion

[1] Bookman, Ralph, M.D., interviewed in Rodale's *Allergy Relief* 3:7(July 1988), 6.

Sugar Cravings

[1] Williams, R.J. *Nutrition and Alcoholism* (Norman, OK: University of Oklahoma Press, 1951); Williams, R.J. *Alcoholism: The Nutritional Approach* (Austin, TX: University of Texas Press, 1959); Williams, R.J. *Nutri-*

555

tion against Disease (New York: Pitman, 1971). Williams, R.J. Physicians' Handbook of Nutritional Science (Springfield, IL: Charles C. Thomas, 1975); Williams, R.J. The Prevention of Alcoholism through Nutrition (New York: Bantam, 1981).

Tobacco Addiction

[1] Levin, E.D., F. Behm, E. Carnahan, et al. "Clinical Trials Using Ascorbic Acid Aerosol to Aid Smoking Cessation." *Drug Alcohol Dependence* 33:3(1993), 211–223.

[2] Monahan, R.J. "Secondary Prevention of Drug Dependence through the Transcendental Meditation Program in Metropolitan Philadelphia." *Intl J Addictions* 12:6(1977), 729–754.

[3] Boericke, William. Homoeopathic Materia Medica, 9th ed. (Philadelphia: Boericke and Tafel, 1927); Clarke, John H. *The Prescriber,* 9th ed. (Essex, England: C.W. Daniel, 1972).

[4] Cherner, Joseph W. SmokeFree Educational Services, www.SmokefreeAir.org.

[5] Rimm, E.B. J., E. Manson, M.J. Stampfer, et al. "Cigarette Smoking and the Risk of Diabetes in Women." *Am J Public Health* 83:2(1993), 211–214.

Tooth Care

[1] Erickson, A.W. "Deaf Smith's Secret." *Field Notes Crop Reporting Service* (1945).

[2] *Chemical and Engineering News* (May 8, 1989).

[3] A lengthy and remarkably unbiased review of the detrimental effects of fluoride, "Fluoridation of Water," appeared in *Chemical and Engineering News* 66(August 1, 1988), 26–42.

[4] Skolnick, A. "New Doubts about Benefits of Sodium Fluoride." *JAMA* 263:13(1990), 1752–1753; See also: *Environment Week* (August 15, 1991). *Environment Week* reviewed studies "demonstrating adverse effects to bone caused by fluoride at levels to which the majority of the U.S. population on public water supplies are exposed."

QUICK REFERENCE GUIDE TO ADDITIONAL HEALTH CONDITIONS

Drug Addiction

[1] Monahan, R.J. "Secondary Prevention of Drug Dependence through the Transcendental Meditation Program in Metropolitan

Philadelphia." *Intl J Addictions* 12:6(1977), 729–754.

[2] Cameron, E., and G. Baird. "Ascorbic Acid and Dependence on Opiates in Patients with Advanced and Disseminated Cancer." *J Intl Res Comm* 1(1973), 38.

Epilepsy (in Children)

[1] Ogunmekan, A.O., and P.A. Hwang. "A Randomized, Double-blind, Placebo-controlled, Clinical Trial of D-alpha-tocopheryl Acetate (Vitamin E), as Add-on Therapy, for Epilepsy in Children." *Epilepsia* 30:1(1989), 84–89.

Glaucoma

[1] Head, K.A. "Natural Therapies for Ocular Disorders, Part Two: Cataracts and Glaucoma." *Altern Med Rev* 6:2(2001), 141–166; Shen, T.M. and M.C. Yu. "Clinical Evaluation of Glycerin-sodium Ascorbate Solution in Lowering Intraocular Pressure." *Chin Med J* (Engl) 1:1(1975), 64–68; Tams, G. "The Pressure-lowering Action of Glycerin Ascorbate-Na." *Klin Monatsbl Augenheilkd* 158:5(1971), 663–667; Moschini, G.B. "Modifications of Hematic Osmotic Pressure and Ocular Tonus after Intravenous Infusions of High Doses of Vitamin C (Sodium Ascorbate)." *Boll Ocul* 47:2(1968), 143–152; Bietti, G.B. "Possibilities of Vitamin

C Administration As an Intraocular Pressure Lowering Agent. Studies on Its Mode of Action." *Ber Zusammenkunft Dtsch Ophthalmol Ges* 68(1968), 190–206; Missiroli, A., R. Neuschuler, and J. Pecori Giraldi. "Therapeutic Possibilities of the Association of Oral Glycerol and Ascorbic Acid in the Treatment of Glaucoma." *Boll Ocul* 46:11(1967), 877–890; Suzuki, Y., Y. Kitazawa, and K. Kawanishi. "The Effect of Intravenous Ascorbic Acid on IOP in Man." *Nippon Ganka Gakkai Zasshi* 71:5(1967), 481–488; Virno, M., M.G. Bucci, J. Pecori-Giraldi, et al. "Findings on the Hypotensive Intraocular Effect of High Oral Doses of Ascorbic Acid. Preliminary Results in Glaucoma Therapy." *Boll Ocul* 46:4(1967), 259–274; Hilsdorf, C. "On the Decrease of Intraocular Pressure by Intravenous Drop Infusion of 20 Percent Sodium Ascorbinate." *Klin Monatsbl Augenheilkd* 150:3(1967), 352–358; Suzuki, Y., and Y. Kitazawa. "The Effects of Topical Administration of Ascorbic Acid on Aqueous Humor Dynamics of Glaucomatous Eyes." *Nippon Ganka Gakkai Zasshi* 71:1(1967), 57–60; Virno, M., M.G. Bucci, J. Pecori-Giraldi, et al. "Intravenous Glycerol-Vitamin C (Sodium Salt) as Osmotic Agents to Reduce Intraocular Pressure." *Am J Ophthalmol* 62:5(1966), 824–833.

Schlerodoma

[1] Humbert, P., J.L. Dupond, P. Agache, et al. "Treatment of Scleroderma with Oral 1,25-dihydroxyvitamin D3: Evaluation of Skin Involvement Using Non-invasive Techniques. Results of an Open Prospective Trial." *Acta Derm Venereol* 73:6(1993), 449–451.

About the Author

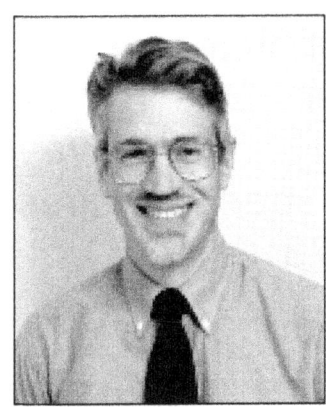

Image I

Andrew W. Saul, Ph.D., has taught clinical nutrition at the New York Chiropractic College and health science and biology at the State University of New York. He has been in practice as a natural therapeutics consultant for nearly thirty years. Dr. Saul publishes the *Doctor Yourself Newsletter* and is the author of *Doctor Yourself: Natural Healing That Works.* He is also a contributing editor for the *Journal of Orthomolecular Medicine.* His website (www.do ctoryourself.com) is an important orthomolecular nutrition resource on the Internet.

Back Cover Material

FIRE YOUR DOCTOR!

If you want something done right, you have to do it your self. This especially includes your health care.

Natural healing is not about avoiding doctors; it is about not needing to go to doctors. The idea is to be well. Each of us is ultimately responsible for our own wellness, and we should consider all options in our search for better health. That is the focus of this book: how we can get better using practical, effective, and safe natural therapies.

The biggest deception ever perpetrated upon the American people is the myth that improving your health with vitamins and natural living is somehow difficult or dangerous. Better health is not difficult, and it is conventional drug treatments for disease that are dangerous. The effective use of food supplements and natural diet saves money, pain, and lives.

The good news is that therapeutic nutrition is cheap, simple, effective, and safe. It comes down to this: living healthfully is prevention and cure for most chronic killer diseases. That is indeed simple; it is also true and it works. *Fire Your Doctor!* provides information on:

- Nutritional therapy for over 80 health conditions.
- How to change your diet and lifestyle to improve your health.
- Practical tips on juicing and growing your own vegetables.
- Ways to educate yourself on natural alternatives to drugs.
- The latest scientifically validated supplement recommendations.

Mostly, *Fire Your Doctor!* is about asserting yourself. For nearly thirty years, Dr. Saul has worked with people who have been transformed from fear-filled patients to self-reliant, naturally healthy people. It can be done, and you can do it.

About the Author: Andrew W. Saul, Ph.D., has taught clinical nutrition at the New York Chiropractic College and health science and biology at the State University of New York. He has been in practice as a natural therapeutics consultant for nearly thirty years. Dr. Saul publishes the *Doctor Yourself* Newsletter and is the author of *Doctor Yourself: Natural Healing That Works*. He is also a contributing editor for the *Journal of Orthomolecular Medicine*. His website (www.doctoryourself.com) is an important orthomolecular nutrition resource on the Internet.

A

Acne, *253, 256*
Acupressure, *369*
ADHD, *277, 280*
AIDS, *257, 260, 323*
Airola, Paavo, *21*
Alcohol, *65, 89, 136, 409*
Allergies, *267*
Alternative and Natural Therapies for Cancer Prevention and Control, *43*
American Association of Poison Control Centers' Toxic Exposure Surveillance System, *188*
American Cancer Society, *173*
American Heart Association, *307*
American Journal of Clinical Nutrition, *406*
American Lung Association, *356*
American Medical Association, *316*

American Red Cross, *235*
Amyotrophic lateral sclerosis, *395*
Angell, Marcia, *28*
Antioxidants, *85, 192, 201, 295, 356, 381*
Anxiety attacks, *264, 267, 270*
    foods to avoid for, *270*
    homeopathic remedies for, *270*
Arthritis, *272, 275*
Ascorbate: The Science of Vitamin C, *43*
Ascorbic acid,
    See Vitamin C,
Atherosclerosis, *307, 310, 313*
Atlas, Charles, *242*
Atopic dermatitis,
    See Eczema,
Attention deficit hyperactivity disorder,
    See ADHD,
Australian National University, *21, 224, 264*
Ayurvedic medicine, *428*

M

migraines, *369, 372*
Macfadden, Bernarr, *235, 238, 242, 248*
Maclean's Magazine, *201*
Macular degeneration, *391*
Mad cow disease, *120*
Mag phos, *369*
Magnesium, *182, 206, 298, 323, 409, 451*
Malaise, *85*
Manganese, *182, 211*
Manic-depressive disorder, *282*
Massage, *428*
McCormick, William J., *21, 313, 426*
Mears, Ainslie, *264*
Meat, *67, 92, 94, 97, 99, 112, 114, 117, 120, 124, 127, 133, 136, 384, 445*
   reasons to stop eating, *112, 114, 117, 120, 124, 127*
   reducing intake, *127*
Meditation, *76, 313*
Mendelsohn, Robert, *21, 28, 359*
Merck Manual, *36, 39, 79, 188, 253*
Migraines, *369, 372*

Milk products,
   See Dairy products,
Minerals, *182, 206, 211-212*
   chelated, *212*
Miso, *127*
Molasses, *217, 339, 448*
Molière, Jean-Baptiste Poquelin de, *12*
Moniliasis, *453*
Mosher, John I., *18*
Motivation, *8*
Motor Neuron Disease Association, *395*
Motor neuron diseases, *395*
Mowat, Farley, *97*
Muscles, sore, *431*
Muscular dystrophy, *398, 401, 404*

N

National Academy of Sciences, Institute of Medicine, *206*
National Institutes of Health, *398*
National Library of Medicine, *404*
Native diets, *120, 124, 448*
Natural food,
   See Food, natural,

Books For ALL Kinds of Readers

At ReadHowYouWant we understand that one size does not fit all types of readers. Our innovative, patent pending technology allows us to design new formats to make reading easier and more enjoyable for you. This helps improve your speed of reading and your comprehension. Our EasyRead printed books have been optimized to improve word recognition, ease eye tracking by adjusting word and line spacing as well as minimizing hyphenation. Our EasyRead SuperLarge editions have been developed to make reading easier and more accessible for vision-impaired readers. We offer Braille and DAISY formats of our books and all popular E-Book formats.

We are continually introducing new formats based upon research and reader preferences. Visit our web-site to see all of our formats and learn how you can Personalize our books for yourself or as gifts. Sign up to Become A RHYW Registered Reader.

www.readhowyouwant.com

Lightning Source UK Ltd.
Milton Keynes UK
UKOW05f1806020915
257970UK00004B/214/P